AF342702

An Atlas of Investigation and Diagnosis

PRIMARY HYPERLIPIDEMIAS

To all the students we had the pleasure of working with during our careers.

An Atlas of Investigation and Diagnosis

PRIMARY HYPERLIPIDEMIAS

Jean Davignon OC, GOQ, MD, MSc, FRCP(C), FACP, FACN, FAHA, FRSC
Director, Hyperlipidemia and Atherosclerosis Research Group
Clinical Research Institute of Montreal (IRCM)
Montreal, Quebec
CANADA

Robert Dufour MD, MSc
Director, Lipid Clinic
Hyperlipidemia and Atherosclerosis Research Group
Clinical Research Institute of Montreal (IRCM)
Montreal, Quebec
CANADA

CLINICAL PUBLISHING

OXFORD

Clinical Publishing
an imprint of Atlas Medical Publishing Ltd
Oxford Centre for Innovation
Mill Street, Oxford OX2 0JX, UK

Tel: +44 1865 811116
Fax: +44 1865 251550
Email: info@clinicalpublishing.co.uk
Web: www.clinicalpublishing.co.uk

Distributed in USA and Canada by:
Clinical Publishing
30 Amberwood Parkway
Ashland, OH 44805, USA

tel: 800-247-6553 (toll free within USA and Canada)
fax: 419-281-6883
email: order@bookmasters.com

Distributed in UK and Rest of World by:
Marston Book Services Ltd
PO Box 269
Abingdon
Oxon OX14 4YN, UK

tel: +44 1235 465500
fax: +44 1235 465555
email: trade.orders@marston.co.uk

A catalogue record of this book is available from the British Library

ISBN-13 978 1 904392 44 6

ISBN-10 1 904392 44 X

The publisher makes no representation, express or implied, that the dosages in this book are correct. Readers must therefore always check the product information and clinical procedures with the most up-to-date published product information and data sheets provided by the manufacturers and the most recent codes of conduct and safety regulations. The authors and the publisher do not accept any liability for any errors in the text or for the misuse or misapplication of material in this work.

Project manager: Gavin Smith, GPS Publishing Solutions, Herts, UK
Typeset by Phoenix Photosetting, Chatham, Kent, UK
Printed by T G Hostench SA, Barcelona, Spain

Contents

Preface

Why are primary hyperlipidemias so important, and why do they warrant the writing of this atlas? The main reason for being concerned about these conditions is that they are harbingers of dire consequences for the cardiovascular system. Lipoprotcins such as low-density lipoproteins (LDL), oxidized LDL and remnant lipoproteins (β-very-low-density lipoproteins [β-VLDL], and intermediate-density lipoproteins [IDL]) are potently atherogenic. Dyslipoproteinemia remains asymptomatic for a long time, and when its presence is recognized, it is too late as the damage has been done. By the time the early clinical manifestations appear, arterial narrowing is already of the order of 50% or more. However, its presence needs to be recognized to proceed with diagnosis, treatment and prevention of the life-threatening and catastrophic consequences, such as angina pectoris, myocardial infarction, transient ischemic attack, stroke, intermittent claudication, gangrene of a limb and renovascular hypertension. Cardiovascular disease remains the primary cause of morbidity and mortality in developed countries. Thus it follows that physicians must actively look for clues to allow detection. This is a major objective of this atlas.

Furthermore, normal levels of LDL may be associated with an increased susceptibility to atherosclerosis. High proportions of oxidized, glycated or small, dense LDL, very low levels of HDL, an abundance of circulating lipoprotein(a), or dysfunctional high-density lipoproteins (HDL) for instance may be atherogenic. The diagnosis of such disturbances is often difficult and requires at least minimal knowledge of lipoprotein metabolism and of the pathophysiology of conditions leading to such abnormalities. The discussions on dyslipoproteinemias in this text are accompanied by explanatory diagrams of the metabolic abnormalities where possible.

Genetic abnormalities leading to hyper- or dyslipoproteinemias are considered systematically. Confusion may arise when the same phenotype is shared by different genetic defects. These are conditions in which the family history is an essential clue, but acquired causes of dyslipoproteinemia must also be ruled out in any patient presenting with abnormal lipid or lipoprotein levels. This is important because the treatment is directed at the cause and not at the dyslipoproteinemia itself, as is the case for many hereditary lipid disorders in which there is no treatment available for the causal defect. An accurate diagnosis should always be the first step in establishing a rational treatment strategy.

For the patient, manifestations of lipid transport disorders may be a source of concern unrelated to cardiovascular disease as awareness of the link is limited among the general public. Patients may consult a dermatologist for aesthetic reasons (unsightly xanthelasma, eruptive xanthomas), a rheumatologist (painful Achilles' tendon xanthomas), an ophthalmologist (arcus corneae, corneal opacities) or even an orthopaedic surgeon (prepatellar, plantar, Achilles' xanthomas) without thinking that these may be clinical signs of dyslipidemia. In these situations the tell-tale signs are apparent, but there again, several conditions may be associated with the same or similar clinical/biochemical manifestation and knowledge of these sources of confusion is mandatory. Typical examples are syringomas being mistaken for xanthelasmas, lesions of primary biliary cirrhosis being confused with those of dysbetalipoproteinemia (type III), tendon xanthomas of homozygous familial hypercholesterolemia and those of cerebro-tendinous xanthomatosis, or hypercholesterolemia of unrecognized hypothyroidism being treated with a statin, etc. This atlas reviews such pitfalls and differential diagnosis is considered throughout.

In writing this atlas the authors have aimed to provide an up-to-date, informative and practical book with helpful images to guide physicians through the complexity of lipid transport disorders. The volume is aimed at non-specialists in the field, and also provides enough key information, details and diagnostic finesse for the fledgling lipidologist, whether or not he or she is preparing for specialty examinations. The book not only covers common diseases referred to a lipid clinic, such as familial hypercholesterolemia, familial combined hyperlipidemia and familial dysbetalipoproteinemia, but also describes disease entities that are infrequently seen, such as inherited hypercholesterolemia due to a *PCSK9* gene defect, cholesterol 7α-hydroxylase deficiency, autosomal recessive hypercholesterolemia, sea-blue histiocytosis syndrome, familial phytosterolemia, Wolman's disease, hepatic lipase deficiency, cholesteryl ester transfer protein deficiency, multiple symmetric lipomatosis, and Alagille's syndrome. The astute physician should be able to unravel difficult cases, find the tell-tale diagnostic clue, understand the pathophysiology of disease and save on time required to scan the literature. This atlas has several features to help with the above, including addresses of useful websites, further reading, explanation of discrepancies in nomenclature in the literature, metabolic diagrams, key laboratory techniques, information on gene and/or protein structure and on the important mutations causing hyperlipidemias. The authors were inspired to undertake this atlas by the great books written in the past that have achieved similar goals with success, such as *French's Index of Differential Diagnosis*, the *Ciba Collection of Medical Illustrations* by Frank Netter and *Braverman's Skin Signs of Systemic Diseases*. They hope the reader will find that this first edition responds well to an unmet need and will help them in facing the current explosion of information that physicians need to be aware of in their daily practice. The atlas does not focus on treatment but on patient evaluation, mechanism of disease and diagnosis.

Authors' note on the lipoprotein metabolism illustrations

The diagrams representing lipoprotein metabolism throughout this atlas were inspired by similar drawings by Scott M Grundy, University of Texas in Dallas, and H Bryan Brewer Jr, National Heart Lung and Blood Institute at the National Institutes of Health, with their permission. It is obvious that apolipoproteins look more like ribbons on a sphere than little circles, but we believe the complex message is more easily understood using simplified schematic diagrams. A recurrent basic diagram is modified throughout the atlas to adapt to the topic under discussion.

Acknowledgements

We extend our most sincere gratitude to Lise Bernier PhD, Research Associate, for her sound advice and invaluable help with the molecular biology aspects of this atlas.

The hard work of Lise St-Germain in bibliographic research and help with the illustrations is also deeply appreciated.

We gratefully acknowledge the many colleagues from the lipid research community who generously provided their help and advice in the preparation of this atlas and contributed several key figures. We are particularly indebted for this to Gerd Assmann, Philip J. Barter, H. Bryan Brewer Jr, Lise Bernier, Katherine Cianflone, Michael H. Davidson, Claude Gagné, Robert A. Hegele, Henry F. Hoff, Murrray W. Huff, G. Kees Hovingh, John P. Kastelein, Jan Albert Kuivenhoven, Émile Lévy, David Mymin, Giorgio Noseda, Ernst J. Schaefer, Gerd Schmitz, Nabil Seidah, Ann K. Soutar, Anton F. H. Stalenhoef, and Arnold Von Eckardstein.

Finally, we would like to thank our graduate students Geneviève Dubuc and Hanny Wassef, our technicians Lucie Boulet, Hélène Jacques and Michel Tremblay, our secretarial assistants Laurent Castellucci and Carole Tremblay and our nursing staff for their support and for the time they generously contributed to this work.

Abbreviations

ABCA1	ATP-binding cassette family G type 1		HDL	high-density lipoprotein(s)
ACAT	acyl-CoA:cholesterol acyl transferase		HDL-C	high-density lipoprotein-cholesterol
ADH	autosomal dominant hypercholesterolemia		HERS	Heart and Estrogen/progestin Replacement Study
AGS	Alagille's syndrome		HL	hepatic lipase
apoB	apolipoprotein B		HRT	hormone replacement therapy
apoCII	apolipoprotein CII		IDL	intermediate-density lipoprotein(s)
ARH	autosomal recessive hypercholesterolemia		IEF	isoelectric focusing
ASP	acylation stimulating protein		Ig	immunoglobulin
ATP	adenosine triphosphate		IL	interleukin
BRIC	benign recurrent intrahepatic cholestasis		IMT	intima-media thickness
BSEP	bile salt export pump		K	kringle
CAC	coronary artery calcium		LAL	lysosomal acid lipase
CAD	coronary artery disease		LCAT	lecithin:cholesterol acyl transferase
CE	cholesteryl ester		LDL	low-density lipoprotein(s)
CESD	cholesteryl ester storage disease		LDL-C	low-density lipoprotein-cholesterol
CETP	cholesteryl ester transfer protein		LDLR	LDL receptor
CGS	continuous gene syndrome		Lp(a)	lipoprotein(a)
CHD	coronary heart disease		LPL	lipoprotein lipase
CLASP	clathrin-associated sorting protein		LpX	lipoprotein X
CM	centi-Morgan		LRP	LDL receptor-related protein
CRO	C-reactive protein		LXR	liver X receptor
CVD	cardiovascular disease		MCT	medium-chain triglycerides
CYP7A1	cytochrome P450 7A1 or cholesterol 7α-hydroxylase		MEDPED	make an early diagnosis, prevent an early death
EBCT	electron beam computed tomography		MHTG	(familial) mixed hypertriglyceridemia
ELISA	enzyme-linked immunosorbent assay		MTP	microsomal triglyceride transfer protein
FATS	Familial Atherosclerosis Treatment Study		MSL	multiple symmetric lipomatosis
FCH	familial combined hyperlipidemia		NARC	neural apoptosis regulated convertase
FCHL	familial combined hyperlipidemia		NHLBI	National Heart, Lung and Blood Institute
FDB	familial defective apolipoprotein B-100		NIH	National Institutes of Health
FDH	familial dyslipidemic hypertension		NPC1L1	Niemann–Pick C-1 like-1 protein
FEHTG	familial endogenous hypertriglyceridemia		OCRL	oculocerebrorenal syndrome of Lowe
FFA	free fatty acids		OMIM	Online Mendelian Inheritance in Man
FH	familial hypercholesterolemia		PAI-1	plasminogen activator inhibitor-1
	familial hyperchylomicronemia		PCSK9	proprotein convertase subtilisin/kexin type 9
FHALP	familial hyperalphalipoproteinemia		PFIC	progressive familial intrahepatic cholestasis
FHTG	familial hypertriglyceridemia		PPAR	peroxisome proliferation activated receptor
FLDB	familial ligand-defective apoB-100		PRIME	Prospective Epidemiological Study of Myocardial Infarction
FXIIa	activated factor XII			
FXR	farnesoid X receptor			
HALP	hyperalphalipoproteinemia		PTB	phosphotyrosine binding

PT-III	pseudo type III hyperlipoproteinemia
PUFA	polyunsaturated fatty acid
RCT	reverse cholesterol transport
sdLDL	small dense LDL
SMC	smooth muscle cell
SNP	single nucleotide polymorphism
SR-A	scavenger receptor type A
SR-B1	scavenger receptor class B type 1
SREBP	sterol regulatory element binding protein
SR-PSOX	scavenger receptor for phosphatidyl-serine and oxidized LDL
TAT	thrombin–antithrombin complex
TG	triglyceride(s)
Tg	transgenic
t-PA	tissue plasminogen activator
TRL	triglyceride-rich lipoprotein(s)
VLDL	very-low-density lipoprotein(s)
VLDLR	VLDL receptor
vWF	von Willebrand factor

Chapter 1

Hereditary Hypercholesterolemias

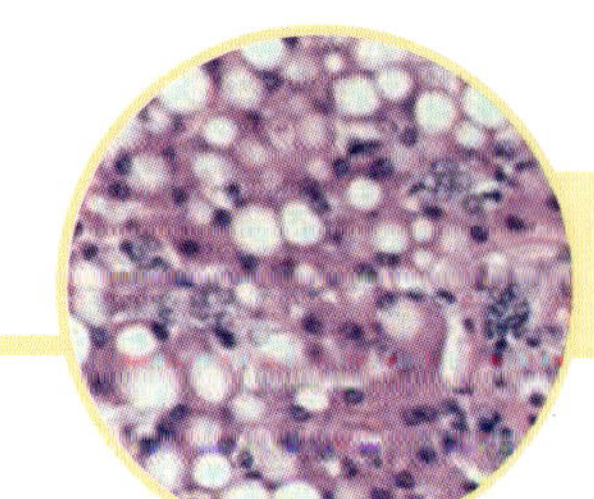

Introduction

The 'familial hypercholesterolemia phenotype' has clinical and laboratory features usually ascribed to the heterozygous form of familial hypercholesterolemia (FH) (*Table 1.1*) secondary to a mutation of the low-density lipoprotein (LDL) receptor gene (*LDLR*). Over time, this phenotype has been observed, albeit more rarely and often incompletely, in conditions with different etiologies, some inherited in a dominant fashion (i.e. homozygotes do not have a more severe phenotype than the heterozygote) and others as a recessive trait. They essentially mimic heterozygous FH, which is a co-dominantly inherited disease (i.e. homozygotes have a more severe phenotype than heterozygotes). These disorders are monogenic and include familial defective apolipoprotein B-100 (FDB) (*APOB* gene), autosomal dominant hypercholesterolemia (*PCSK9*), cholesterol 7α-hydroxylase deficiency (*CYP7A1*), familial sitosterolemia (*ABCG5* or *ABCG8*) and autosomal recessive hypercholesterolemia (ARH) (*ARH*). From this degree of heterogeneity, it is anticipated that other gene defects will also account for this phenotype. Autosomal dominant hypercholesterolemia (ADH) has been referred to as comprising 'FH1', the classical FH, 'FH2' (FDB) and 'FH3', attributed to a *PCSK9* defect. As discussed below, there are variations of the typical FH phenotype that might not fully justify this classification, such as dominance versus co-dominance, variable expression and less severe manifestations.

Dominant monogenic forms

Familial hypercholesterolemia

The classical nosological entity called familial hypercholesterolemia had been part of the medical literature for a

Table 1.1 Characteristics of familial hypercholesterolemia (FH)*

1. Severe hypercholesterolemia
2. Low-density lipoprotein (LDL)-cholesterol >95th percentile
3. Family history of premature coronary artery disease, other atherosclerotic vascular disease and typical manifestations of FH
4. Tendon xanthomas and other forms of lipid deposits (such as arcus corneae, xanthelasma, tuberous and plantar xanthomas)
5. Premature manifestations of atherosclerosis
6. Autosomal co-dominant inheritance with high penetrance
7. An LDL receptor defect with delayed LDL clearance

*These characterize the 'FH phenotype' and it is helpful if the family history also reveals the presence of tendon xanthomas or the presence of a homozygote.

long time before its mechanism was fully unraveled by the seminal work of the 1985 Nobel laureates, Joseph L Goldstein and Michael S Brown. For a monogenic disorder, it is relatively common, its frequency varying from 1 in 500 in most parts of the world to as much as 1 in 80 in regions where a founder effect exists due to factors such as endogamy, consanguinity, geographic isolation and limited genetic admixture. Such regions include, among others, Lebanon, Finland, South Africa (Afrikaners), Canada (French-Canadians) (**1.1**) and Israel (FH-Sephardic and FH-Lithuania). Its importance stems also from the devastating severe and premature cardiovascular consequences for the affected members (50%) of a family, stressing the need for early diagnosis. As there is treatment that will prevent or markedly delay the complications of this condition, early intervention may result in a normal life. In other words, it is a treatable killer and worldwide efforts have therefore been made to identify individuals and families at risk. MEDPED, '**m**ake an **e**arly **d**iagnosis, **p**revent an **e**arly **d**eath' is one such initiative (www.cholesterol.med.utah.edu/medped/). In certain communities, it may be a major health problem, disabling or killing many young adults.

The etiology of FH is well established. The metabolic defect (**1.2**), which leads to a large increase in plasma levels of LDL-cholesterol (LDL-C) (two to three times that of normal subjects), is attributed to mutations of the LDL receptor gene that result in a decreased number or total absence of LDL receptors or, alternatively, in expression of dysfunctional receptors. This ubiquitous receptor allows uptake and degradation in the liver of LDL, the major lipoprotein carrier of circulating cholesterol (mostly cholesteryl esters), allowing excretion of the latter into the bile (as free cholesterol). It is essential for bringing cholesterol, a major constituent of membranes, to cells. The

defect causes a considerable delay of LDL clearance from plasma. Normal subjects catabolize about 45% of their LDL pool per day, whereas the fractional catabolic rate is 25–30% for heterozygotes and 15% for homozygotes. There is also a delayed clearance of intermediate-density lipoproteins (IDL), which represent 'remnant' lipoproteins and an increased conversion of IDL into LDL. Recent studies by Tremblay and co-workers have shown that there is also a 50% increased production rate of very-low-density lipoprotein (VLDL) apolipoprotein B (apoB) – 100 in heterozygotes and 109% in homozygotes. This finding sheds light on an old debate. The LDL particles are large and buoyant in this condition because there is excess cholesterol associated with apoB, the main apolipoprotein associated with these cholesterol-rich particles. There are over 800 mutations of the LDL receptor gene (*LDLR*), which is located on the short arm of chromosome 19 (19p13.1–13.3) (**1.2**). They have been indexed continually in the UK since October 1996 on a dedicated website (www.ucl.ac.uk/fh/) and in France since April 1998 (www.umd.necker.fr/). A classification of the various defects of the *LDLR* gene has also been established (Hobbs *et al.*

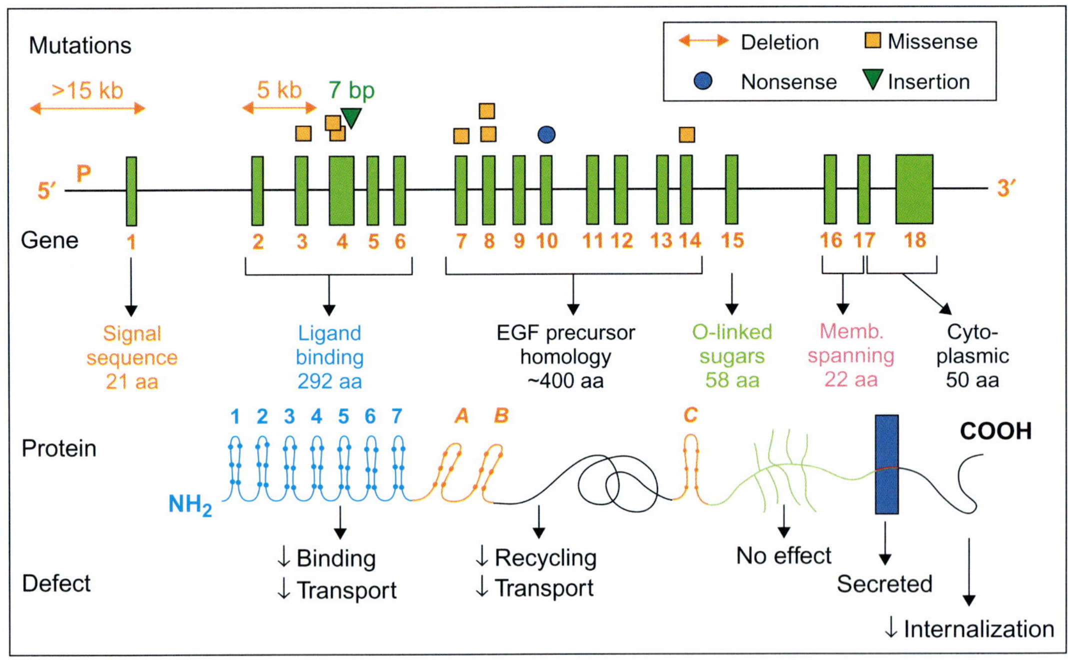

1.1 French-Canadian mutations of the LDL receptor gene. This figure provides information on the type of mutations (those most frequent in the Province of Quebec), the structure of the gene, what the exons (green vertical bars) code for, the structure of the protein (domains and number of amino acids), and what abnormalities might be expected when one such domain is affected by the mutation. The dots on the protein sequence represent cysteines. The mutations represented are reported in the following papers: Hobbs HH *et al.* (1987). *N Engl J Med*, **217**: 734; Leitersdorf E *et al.* (1990). *J Clin Invest*, **85**: 1014; Ma Y *et al.* (1989). *Clin Genet*, **36**: 219; Simard J *et al.* (1994). *Hum Mol Genet*, **3**: 1689; Assouline L *et al.* (1995). *Pediatrics*, **96**: 239; Couture P *et al.* (1998). *Hum Mutat*, **1**: S226.

1990). The abnormality may involve synthesis in the endo plasmic reticulum, transport of newly synthesized recep tors to the Golgi complex, transport to the cell surface, clustering in the surface-coated pits or binding affinity for LDL, depending on the portion of the receptor gene that is affected (**1.1**). For practical purposes, it is useful to know if the receptor activity is impaired (*receptor defective*) or not functional at all (*receptor negative*). Severity and resistance to treatment are greater in the latter. This is especially important for homozygotes and can be determined by identifying the mutation or testing LDL receptor activity in cultured skin fibroblasts or blood mononuclear cells.

The diagnosis of heterozygous FH (*Table 1.1*) is based essentially on:

- the family history (premature atherosclerosis and early deaths especially in males, tendon xanthomas, presence of a homozygote)
- premature atherosclerosis (a myocardial infarction may occur as early as in the third or fourth decade)
- the clinical manifestations of hypercholesterolemia (especially tendon xanthomas – Achilles or extensor tendons of the fingers – but also periosteal, prepatellar, plantar, tricipital and tuberous xanthomas as well as

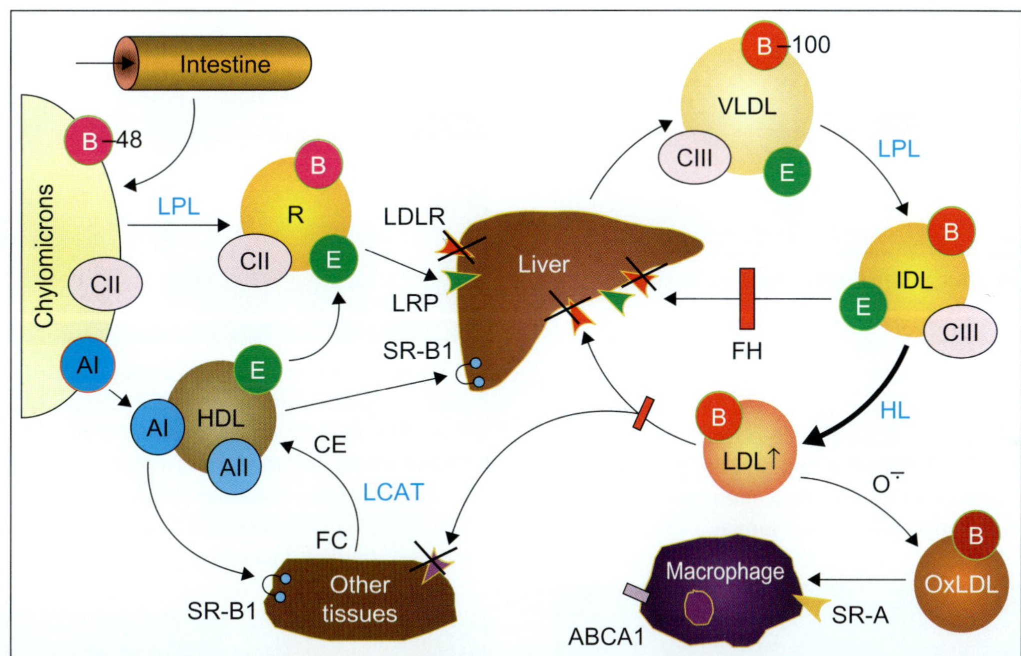

1.2 Metabolic defects in familial hypercholesterolemia (FH). Abnormalities of the low-density lipoprotein (LDL) receptor (LDLR, small red arrowheads marked with a cross) prevent the normal clearance of cholesteryl esters (orange in the circles) transported by LDL, which increase in plasma. Characteristically, these LDL particles transport as the main protein apolipoprotein B-100 (apoB-100) on their surface (red circles) that interact with the LDL receptor for uptake by the liver allowing eventual excretion of cholesterol into the bile. ApoB-100 is carried by very-low-density lipoproteins (VLDL) secreted by the liver, and their degradation products, including intermediate-density lipoproteins (IDL). This degradation takes place gradually by delipidation and loss of surface proteins such as apoCIII and apoE. Lipoprotein lipase (LPL) allows transformation of VLDL into LDL and hepatic lipase (HL), that of IDL into LDL.

In FH, IDL are still taken up by the remnant receptor, LDL receptor-related protein (LRP), but this pathway is limited (red bar) by the LDLR defect. On the other hand, more IDL are transformed into LDL (large black arrow). Some LDL particles, because of the prolonged residence time, may become oxidized (OxLDL), taken up by macrophages via various scavenger receptors (SR-A) and contribute to the formation of foam cells present in xanthomas and atheroma. ApoB-48, a smaller apoB formed by splicing of the *APOB* gene mRNA present on chylomicrons is not taken up by the LDL receptors but by another dedicated receptor. Breakdown delipidated products of chylomicrons become remnants (R) as they gain apoE which can interact with LRP for uptake by the liver. There is evidence from stable isotope studies that the high LDL levels in FH may also be due to some increase in VLDL apoB production rate relative to normal subjects. When one refers to apoB without the -100 or the -48, it is usually taken to be apoB-100 or, alternatively, all forms of apoB. SR-B1 refers to the scavenger receptor class B type 1 (also called Cla-1). It is a receptor that allows transfer of cholesteryl esters (CE) from high-density lipoproteins (HDL) to different tissues as well as transfer of cholesterol from tissues to HDL. Lecithin:cholesterol acyl transferase (LCAT) is an enzyme that esterifies free cholesterol to CE during HDL remodelling from discoid to spherical and mature HDL.

corneal arcus) (**1.3–1.7**) and atherosclerosis (arterial bruits, angina, intermittent claudication, Leriche syndrome, transient ischemic attacks, etc.)

- high levels of plasma LDL-C (>95th percentile) (**1.8**)
- identification of an LDL receptor defect.

Detection of affected individuals is more difficult in childhood. The family history, combined with a blood sample for LDL-C is most useful in children. In women, manifestations are delayed by about 10–15 years compared with men (**1.9**). Evolution of tendon xanthomas may be assessed and followed using standardized X-ray techniques (**1.10**), ultrasonography or magnetic resonance imaging. The xanthoma size correlates with the duration and severity of the disease

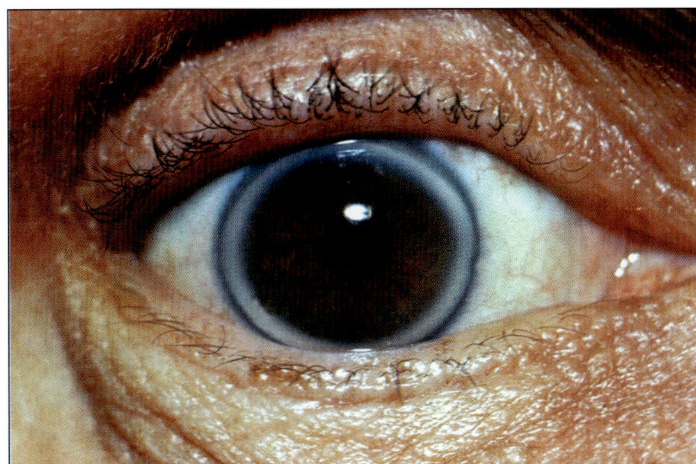

1.3 Corneal ring in a patient with heterozygous familial hypercholesterolemia. A corneal arcus usually starts as a small, barely visible whitish crescent in the upper and/or lower part of the cornea. Careful attention needs to be paid, using good lighting, in order to notice them. They may grow to the point, as seen here, where they form a quite obvious corneal ring. Note the clear space between the ring and the periphery of the cornea. Corneal arcus and rings may be seen in individuals of African origin in the absence of hyperlipidemia.

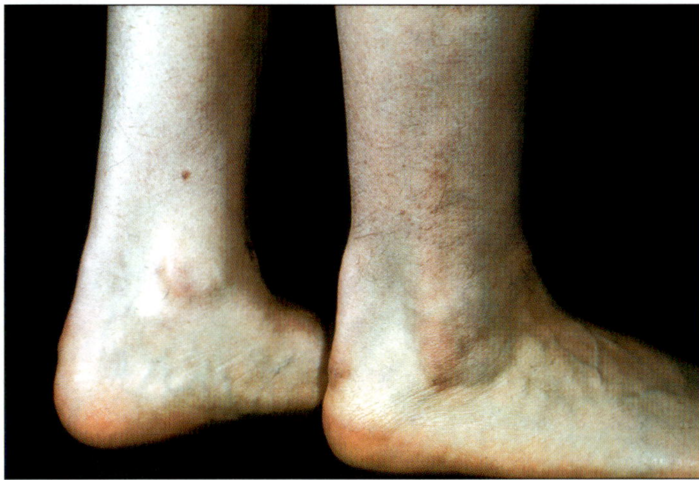

1.5 Lateral view of Achilles tendon xanthomas in familial hypercholesterolemia. This lateral view of tendon xanthomas shows the growth of these lesions anteroposteriorly as well as laterally. These xanthomas are often missed if smaller in size and the physician does not palpate carefully. Pinching this area while sliding the fingers downward will reveal olive-shaped lesions or diffuse thickening of the tendon.

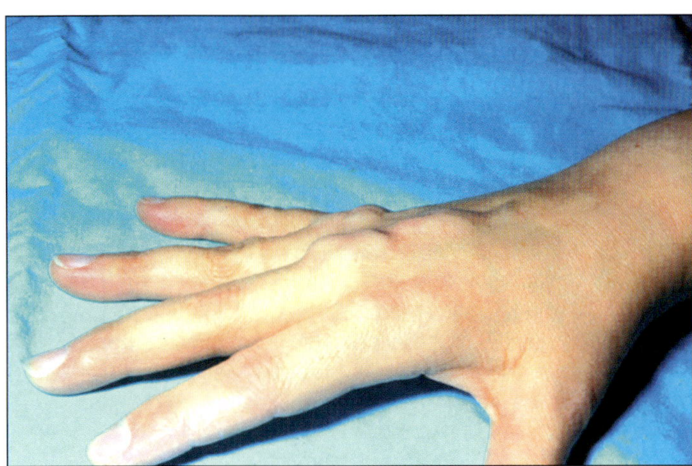

1.4 Extensor tendon xanthomas in familial hypercholesterolemia (FH). The presence of these xanthomas often allows a diagnosis of FH at first sight. They tend to regress readily with major reductions in LDL-C, e.g. with statin therapy. Even when discrete, they are rarely missed. Palpating the extensor tendons when FH is suspected may reveal incipient lesions.

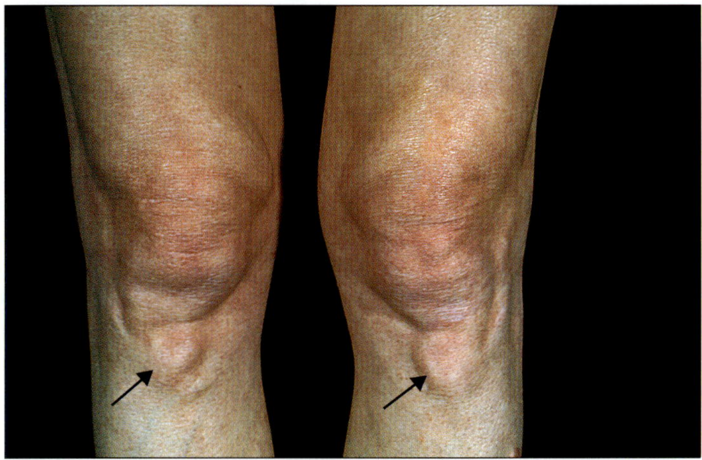

1.6 Periosteal xanthomas of the anterior tuberosity of the tibia. These lesions are not always noticed by the patients themselves as they progress very slowly, occasionally to huge proportions. They may become inflamed and painful or tuberous xanthomas may develop in the same area. Xanthomas often develop at sites of repeated trauma.

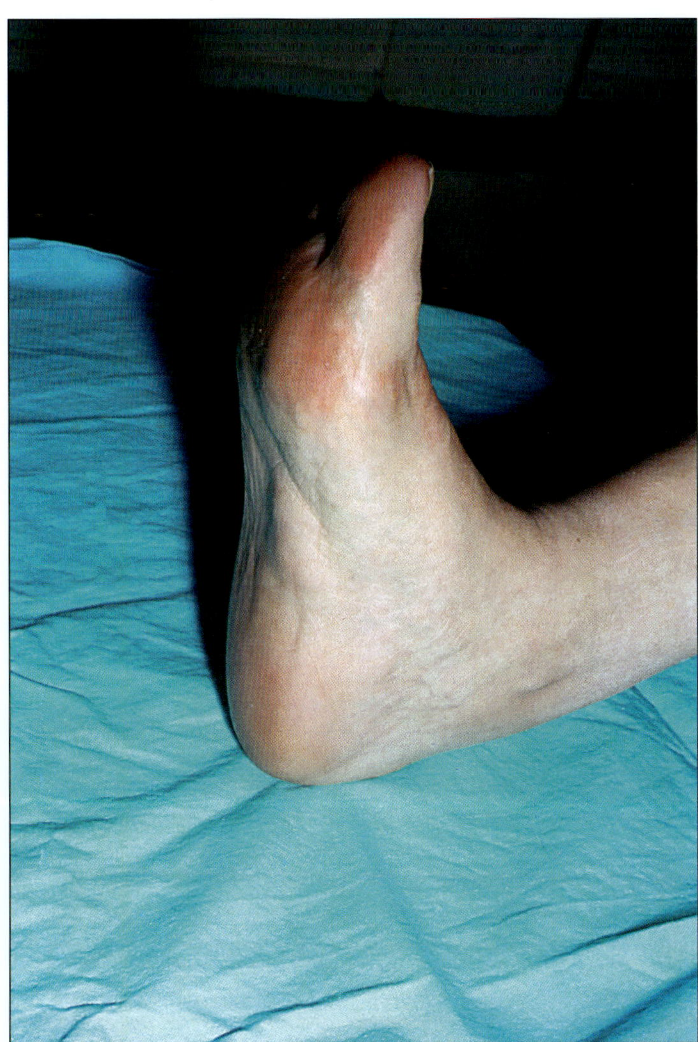

1.7 Plantar xanthoma in a woman with heterozygous familial hypercholesterolemia. Plantar xanthomas, like Achilles tendon xanthomas, become fibrotic and hard with time and regress poorly. They can become very debilitating and impair shoe fitting and walking.

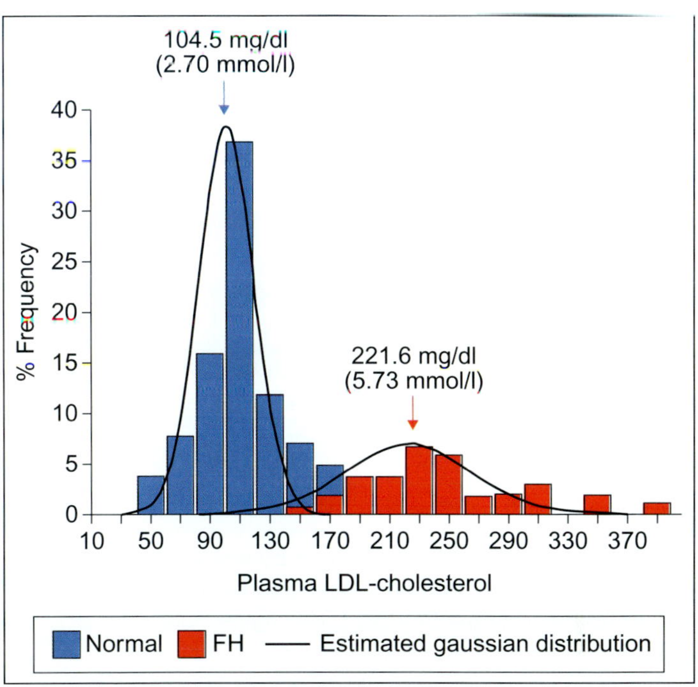

1.8 Bimodal frequency distribution of LDL-C in a large kindred with hypercholesterolemia. This diagram demonstrates the bimodal frequency distribution of low-density lipoprotein (LDL)-cholesterol in a single pedigree segregating for familial hypercholesterolemia (FH) (120 members). The red bars represent the patients in whom a clinical diagnosis of FH was made. The blue bars represent the non-affected members. Note the wide range of LDL-C in the affected subjects and the overlap with the normal population. The mutation of the *LDLR* segregating in this family was the French-Canadian-1 mutation (deletion >15 kb in the promoter region encompassing exon 1 and preventing expression of the LDL receptor). Reproduced with permission from Davignon J *et al.* (1991). In: Steiner G, Shafrir E (eds). *Primary Hyperlipidemia.* McGraw Hill, New York, p. 201.

(**1.11**). Achilles tendon xanthomas are prone to sporadic inflammation, causing painful acute tendinitis (**1.12**).

Because LDL-C level is the best biochemical marker of FH, the most threatening and most directly linked to the causal defect, it remains the centre of attention. FH was classified in the Fredrickson era among subjects presenting a 'type IIa' lipoprotein phenotype (isolated hypercholesterolemia), and 'type IIa' became wrongly synonymous with FH. Indeed, the hypercholesterolemia may occasionally be associated with hypertriglyceridemia (becoming Fredrickson's 'type IIb'). This associated hypertriglyceridemia may be due to a second gene defect, another medical condition or environmental factors, or may be part of the defect in a particular family (triglyceride-rich remnant lipoproteins are cleared to some extent by the LDL receptor). The diagnosis may be established in most cases without resorting to determination of the genetic defect(s) using molecular biology techniques. This task, when required, is easier in communities where a founder effect exists, because only a few mutations may explain a majority of cases (**1.1**). When a doubt exists, some specialized lipid clinics may be able to help with identification of the gene defect.

The differential diagnosis must include other causes of xanthoma tendinosum since they constitute quite a reliable diagnostic criterion; these include lesions that can be mistaken for xanthoma tendinosum (*Table 1.2*). Few hereditary dyslipidemias apart from heterozygous FH and

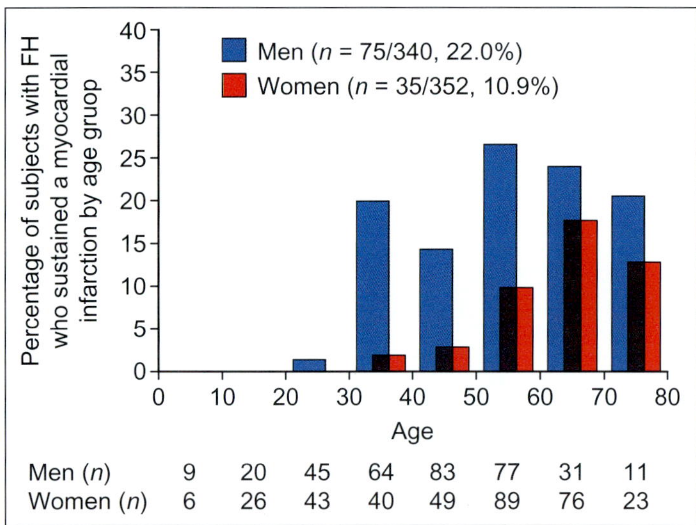

1.9 Myocardial infarction incidence by age group in men and women with heterozygous familial hypercholesterolemia (n = 692). This figure illustrates how myocardial infarction may occur early in life, even in the relatively protected Japanese population. It also shows the delay of 10–15 years (relative to men) before women develop myocardial infarctions. Reproduced with permission from Mabuchi H *et al.* (1989). Development of coronary heart disease in familial hypercholesterolemia. *Circulation*, **79**: 225–232.

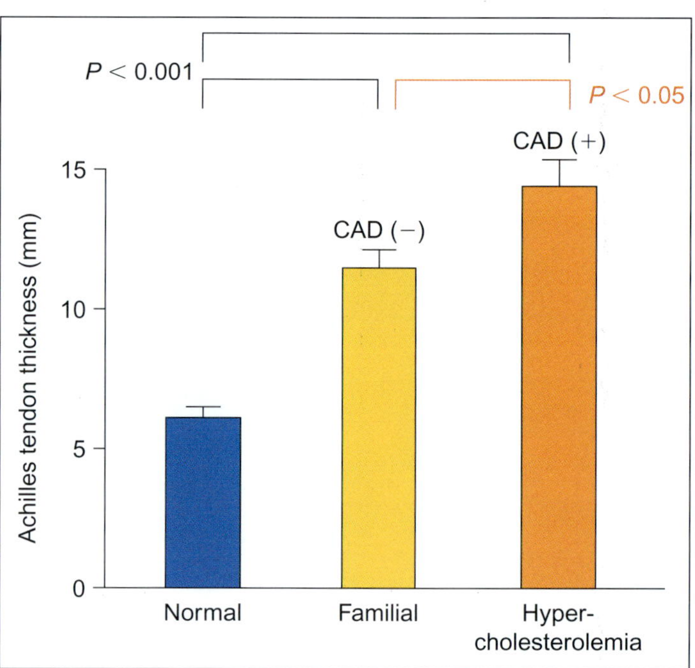

1.11 Tendon xanthoma thickness in FH patients without or with coronary artery disease. This figure shows that the size of Achilles tendon xanthomas is larger in subjects with coronary artery disease (CAD). The severity of the clinical manifestations is a function of the magnitude of the hypercholesterolemia, its duration and the presence of other cardiovascular risk factors. Redrawn from Mabuchi H *et al.* (1978). Achilles tendon thickness and ischemic heart disease in familial hypercholesterolemia. *Metabolism*, **27**: 1672–1678.

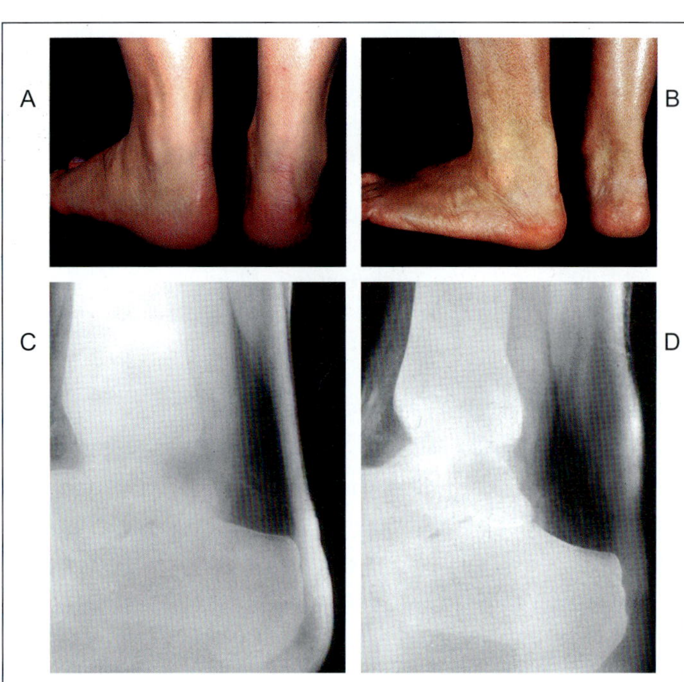

1.10 Normal and xanthomatous Achilles tendons and their radiological assessment. Panels A and C: Achilles tendons of a normal woman. Panels B and D: Nodular thickening of left Achilles tendon in a woman of the same age, heterozygotic for familial hypercholesterolemia. A soft tissue standardized radiological technique was used. The thickening of the Achilles tendon in the anteroposterior dimension is obvious with this radiological technique.

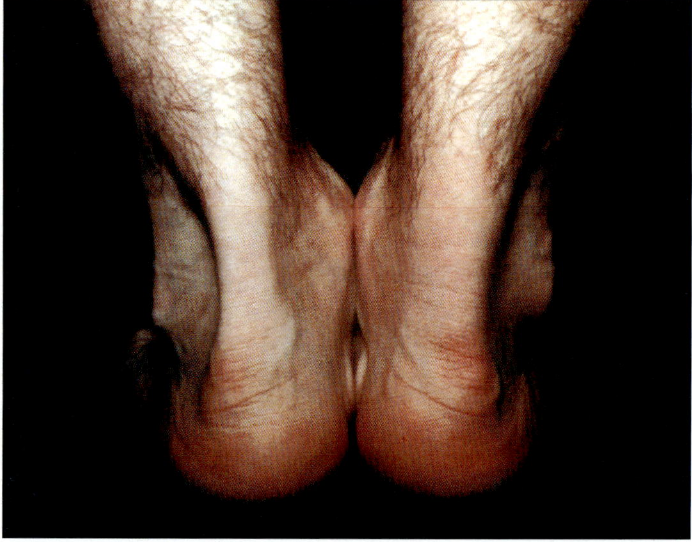

1.12 Tendinitis of xanthomatous right Achilles tendon in a heterozygous familial hypercholesterolemia (FH) patient. Both tendons are xanthomatous, but the right one is enlarged, inflamed and painful. This is not infrequent in patients with FH. In the authors' experience, it may occur in young men or women particularly responsive to treatment, after a large and rapid decrease in plasma low-density lipoprotein-cholesterol.

autosomal dominant hypercholesterolemia (FH3) have such high levels of cholesterol except the other monogenic forms discussed below and familial dysbetalipoproteinemia (type III), but in this condition, LDL-C measured directly is not elevated. Severe familial combined hyperlipidemia with isolated hypercholesterolemia (lipoprotein phenotype IIa) may rarely have LDL-C levels similar to those found in the lower distribution of FH, but tendon xanthomas have not been reported. Atherosclerotic vascular disease in the family tends to occur later in life than in FH and the variation in lipoprotein phenotype in first-degree relatives is typical. Among the secondary forms of hypercholesterolemia the most likely to be confused with FH are primary biliary cirrhosis, nephrotic syndrome and hypothyroidism, all potentially associated with very high levels of LDL-C.

Treatment almost always necessitates the addition of a statin (an HMG-CoA reductase inhibitor) to a cholesterol-lowering diet. Often, large doses of statin are needed and combination therapy with a resin (a bile acid absorption inhibitor) or with ezetimibe (a cholesterol absorption inhibitor) may be necessary. Various forms of LDL apheresis have been used in some very severe heterozygous FH refractory to drug therapy.

The homozygous (inheritance of two identical defective genes) or double heterozygous (two different gene defects at the same locus) forms are extremely rare (approximately 1 in 300 000 to 1 in 1 000 000). The clinical picture is so dramatic that the diagnosis is rarely missed (**1.13–1.17**). Xanthomas are diverse (tuberous, planar, tendinous, xanthelasma), extensive, ubiquitous (friction sites, elbows, knees, popliteal space, palms, plantar aponeurosis, gluteal crease) and may be present at birth. LDL-C levels may be four to six times the upper limit of normal and the type of mutation may also influence the plasma levels (**1.18**). Coronary death can occur as early as two years of age and the affected patients, whether male of female, rarely live beyond the third decade. One typical complication, in addition to myocardial ischemia and infarction, is aortic stenosis (**1.19**), which is sometimes seen in heterozygotes with severe disease. Differential diagnosis must include ARH and a condition reported in the past as pseudo-homozygous hypercholesterolemia (**1.20**). However, some of these cases may have had an *ARH* defect, especially when they responded well to dietary or statin treatment. Statins have a modest effect that is enhanced by combination with ezetimibe and LDL apheresis. Probucol, a major antioxidant, now withdrawn from the market but still available in Japan, has been reported to reduce the size of tendon xanthomas in homozygous FH. 'Last resort' treatments have been used, including porto-caval shunts, gene therapy and liver transplantation, with all but the latter having little success.

Table 1.2 Differential diagnosis of tendon xanthomas

- Familial hypercholesterolemia (FH1)
- Familial defective apoB-100 (FH2)
- Autosomal dominant FH3
- Autosomal recessive hypercholesterolemia (ARH)
- Dysbetalipoproteinemia type III
- Cerebrotendinous xanthomatosis (CTX)
- Familial phytosterolemia
- Alagille's syndrome
- Primary biliary cirrhosis
- Xanthomas associated with antiretroviral therapy
- ApoAI–ApoCIII deficiency
- ApoAI deficiency with analphalipoproteinemia*
- Gouty tophi
- Rheumatoid nodules
- Post-traumatic tendon lesions (asymmetrical)

*Reported by Ng *et al.* (1994). *J Clin Invest*, **93**: 223.

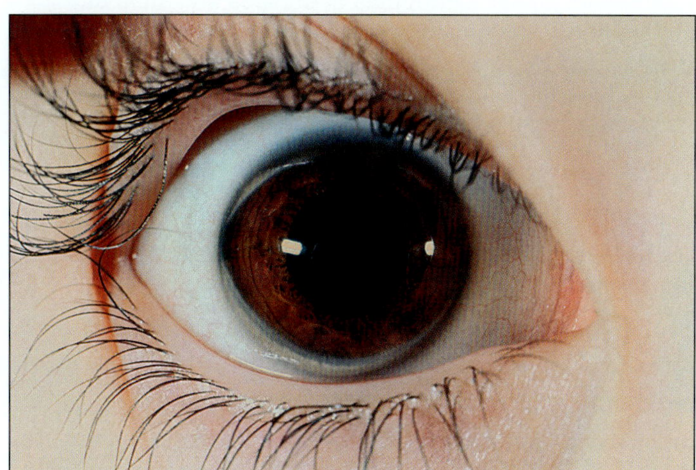

1.13 Corneal arcus in a 5-year-old with homozygous familial hypercholesterolemia (FH). Upper and lower corneal crescents in 5-year-old with homozygous FH. The lower arcus is unusual in not being separated from the sclera by a clear space as observed in the upper one and with the full corneal ring illustrated in **1.3**.

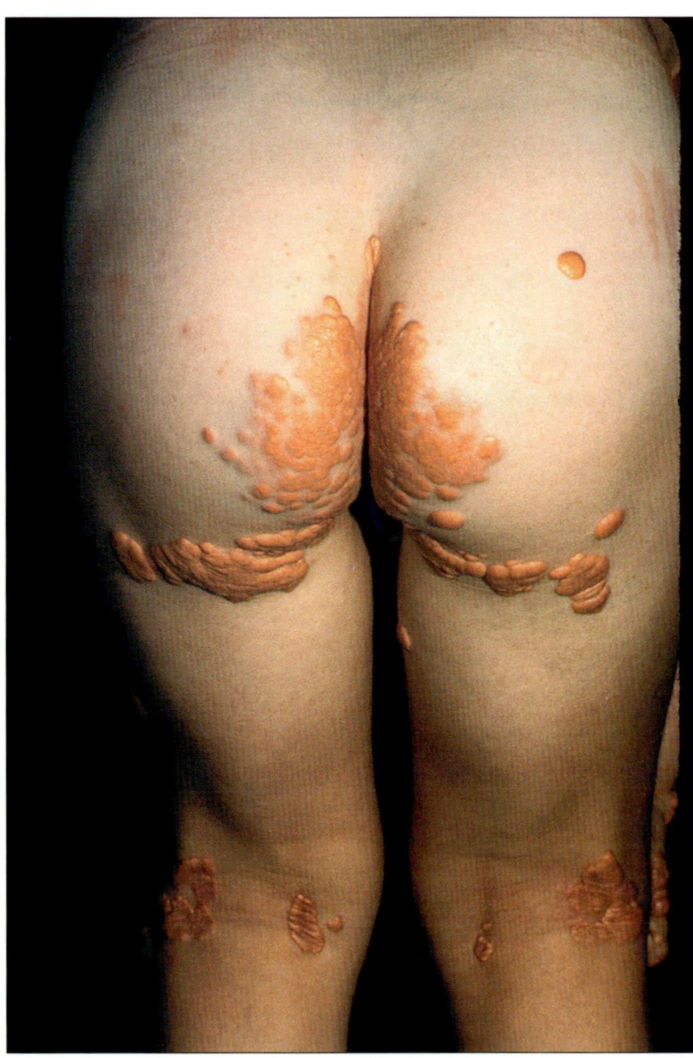

1.14 Raised planar xanthomas in creases and sites of friction in homozygous familial hypercholesterolemia (FH). These raised planar xanthomas in a 5-year-old homozygous FH boy have the typical orange colour and develop at sites of friction between the buttocks and in the popliteal space.

It is worth remembering that in FH, and especially in the homozygous form, the first concern of the doctor should be the accelerated atherosclerosis that accompanies this condition. The autopsy specimen presented in **1.21** showing severe aorto-femoral atheroma and aneurysmal weakening of the wall reminds us of the consequences of failing to intervene early and aggressively in these cases. A sense of urgency should always be uppermost in the mind of the doctor.

Familial defective apolipoprotein B-100

FDB was identified and its etiology determined in 1985–1986 by Grundy and colleagues at the University of Texas in Dallas and Mahley and co-workers at the Gladstone Research Foundation Laboratories in San Francisco. It is an autosomal dominant monogenic disorder due to point mutations in the *APOB* gene (**1.22**). This very large gene (43 kb, 29 exons) was mapped to the distal short arm of chromosome 2 (2p23–p24) in 1985–1986 by investigators from several laboratories (including Knotts, Chan, Law, Deeb and their co-workers). These mutations impair the affinity of apoB, the ligand, to its receptor, the LDL receptor (**1.23**), hence the synonym of 'familial ligand-defective apoB-100' (FLDB). Five mutations in exon 26 of *APOB* may cause this condition, $Arg_{3500} \rightarrow Gln$ (the first common mutation identified), $Arg_{3500} \rightarrow Trp$, $Arg_{3531} \rightarrow Cys$, and $Arg_{3480} \rightarrow Trp$ (Sweden) and $Thr_{3492} \rightarrow Ile$ (Poland). A sixth recently reported mutation $His_{3543} \rightarrow Tyr$ is four times more frequent than the R3500Q variant (for amino acid nomenclature see www.chem.qmul. ac.uk/iupac/AminoAcid/AA1n2.html#AA1). It appears to be associated with a variable but moderate degree of LDL-C elevation and a reduced apoB-100 fractional catabolic rate. An $Asn_{5316} \rightarrow Lys$ mutation of *APOB* has little impact on the lipoprotein profile but changes apoB conformation. FDB is inherited as an autosomal dominant trait with incomplete penetrance or variable phenotypic expression.

The prevalence of FDB varies widely from country to country. In Caucasians from the USA and Europe, it averages 1 in 500 to 1 in 700. It is high in Switzerland (1 in 209 to 1 in 230) and Poland (1 in 250) and rare in Mediterranean countries. It has not been found at all in the Turkish or Finnish populations, or among hypercholesterolemic Japanese or Israelis. From prevalence and haplotype studies, Miserez and Muller at the Basel University Clinics speculated that the common mutation originated from Celtic ancestors in a region between Lake Geneva, the Jura mountains and the Rhine (in the northwestern part of Switzerland the prevalence of this mutation is 1 in 114), perhaps as early as the Mesolithic period (6000–10 000 years ago) (**1.24**). This hypothesis is consistent with a previous study from Myant and colleagues who used a combined molecular and population genetic approach to estimate the age of the mutation to be 6000–7000 years.

The impaired ligand–receptor interaction (20–30% of normal binding to fibroblasts) results in delayed clearance of defective LDL particles with a residence time of LDL-apoB 3.6 times longer than that of normolipidemic controls (8.2 vs. 2.3 days). This is associated with decreased production of LDL and enhanced removal of the apoE-containing VLDL, as demonstrated by Schaefer and co-workers in 1997 in a subject homozygous for the common mutation R3500Q

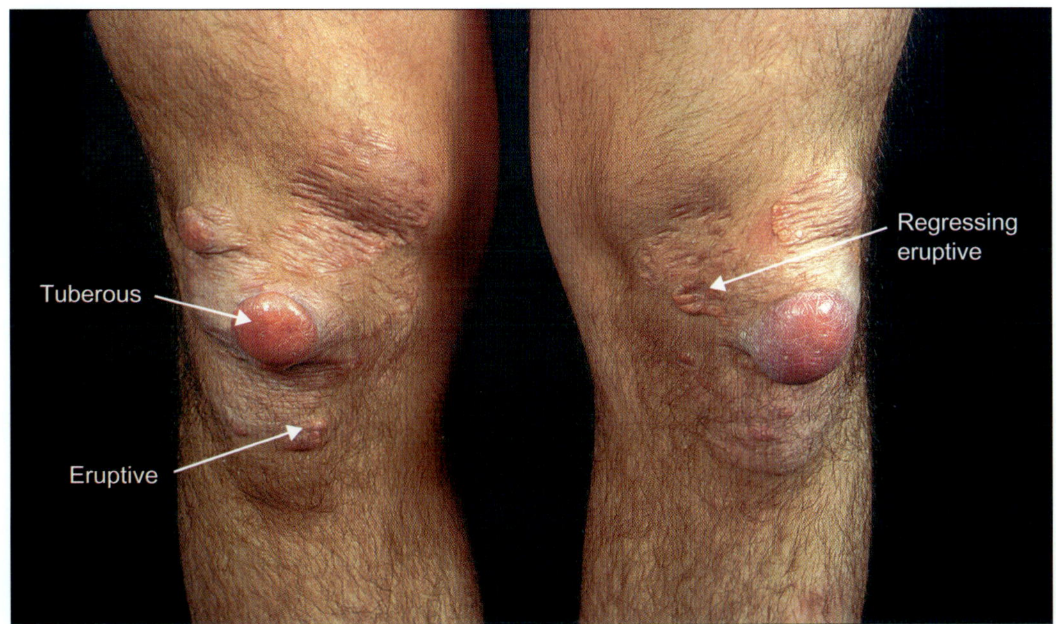

1.15 Tubero-eruptive xanthomas of the knees in a 17-year-old patient with homozygous familial hypercholesterolemia. Planar and tubero-eruptive xanthomas may co-exist in homozygous familial hypercholesterolemia patients. In this case some of the planar and eruptive xanthomas have regressed with treatment.

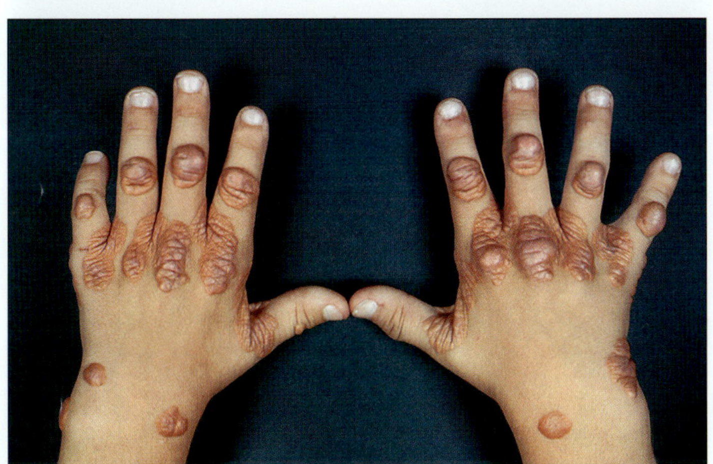

1.16 Tuberous and raised planar xanthomas of the hands in homozygous familial hypercholesterolemia. This picture was taken before puberty in a boy homozygous for the $Cys_{646} \rightarrow Tyr$ (C646Y) mutation in exon 14 of the low-density lipoprotein receptor.

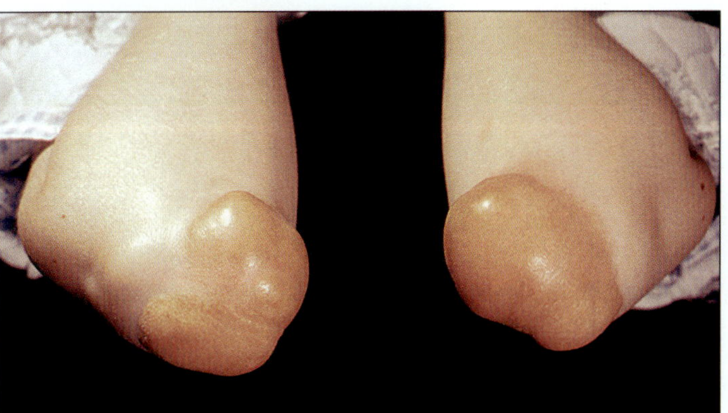

1.17 Large tuberous xanthomas in a 17-year-old girl homozygous for a null allele of the low-density lipoprotein (LDL) receptor gene. The lesions were large enough in this girl to prevent her wearing narrow sleeves, a major source of annoyance for her. She had the French-Canadian-1 mutation (>15 kb deletion of the promoter and exon-1 of the LDL receptor).

(**1.25**). The residence time of VLDL-apoB is also increased, but that of VLDL-apoE is reduced since apoE becomes the favoured ligand to clear particles via the LDL receptor and LDL receptor-related protein (LRP). In addition, LDL isolated from these subjects has increased susceptibility to oxidation. The molecular mechanism whereby the apoB-100 mutations cause the phenotype was unravelled by Borén and co-workers in 2001. Arginine at residue 3500 is essential for normal receptor binding. The carboxyl terminus of apoB-100 is necessary for mutations affecting this arginine at residue 3500 to disrupt LDL receptor binding. Borén

and colleagues drafted a model illustrating that Arg3500 interacts with Trp4369 and facilitates the conformation of apoB-100 required for normal receptor binding of LDL; the carboxyl terminal of apoB-100 interacts with the backbone of apoB-100, which in turn wraps around the LDL particle (**1.26**).

The clinical features of FDB range from no evidence of disease to a typical heterozygous FH phenotype including a positive family history of atherosclerotic vascular disease, early manifestations of atherosclerosis (fifth decade), and LDL-C concentrations ranging from 2.7 mmol/l to

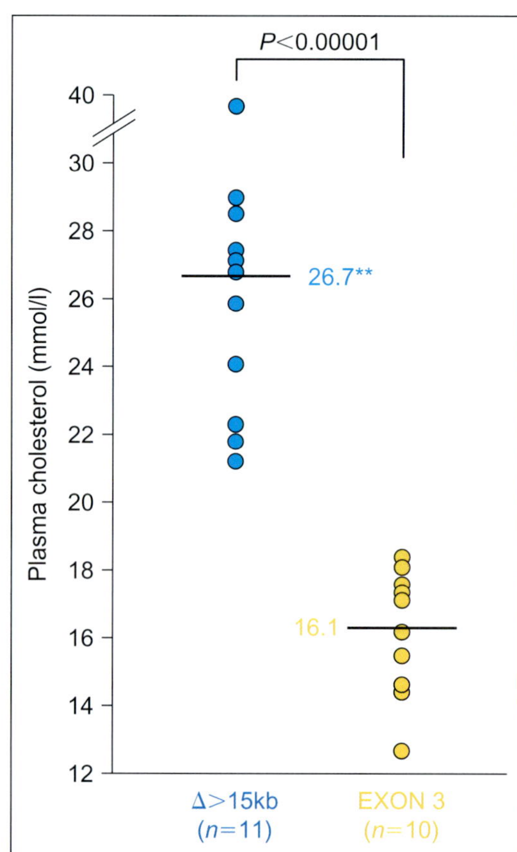

1.18 Plasma cholesterol in homozygous familial hypercholesterolemia (FH) patients with two different types of low-density lipoprotein (LDL) receptor mutation. This figure demonstrates the very high concentrations of total cholesterol in homozygous FH patients and that the type of mutation may influence these levels and their consequences. The large French-Canadian >15Kb deletion involving the promoter and exon 1 of the LDL receptor which results in a null allele (i.e. no LDL receptor produced) is associated with higher levels of cholesterol (mean of 26.7 mmol/l, 1032 mg/dl), and an earlier age of onset of CAD (12.7 years) compared with the exon 3 mutation. The latter (Trp$_{66}$→Gly, W66G) is a less severe French-Canadian mutation of the gene resulting in a 'defective' LDL receptor. The mean plasma cholesterol is lower at 16.1 mmol/l (622 mg/dl), and the age of onset of CAD is later (26.3 years). The difference is large enough that there is no overlap between the two for plasma cholesterol. Redrawn from Moorjani S *et al.* (1993). Mutations of low-density-lipoprotein-receptor gene, variation in plasma cholesterol, and expression of coronary heart disease in homozygous familial hypercholesterolemia. *Lancet,* **341**: 1303–1306.

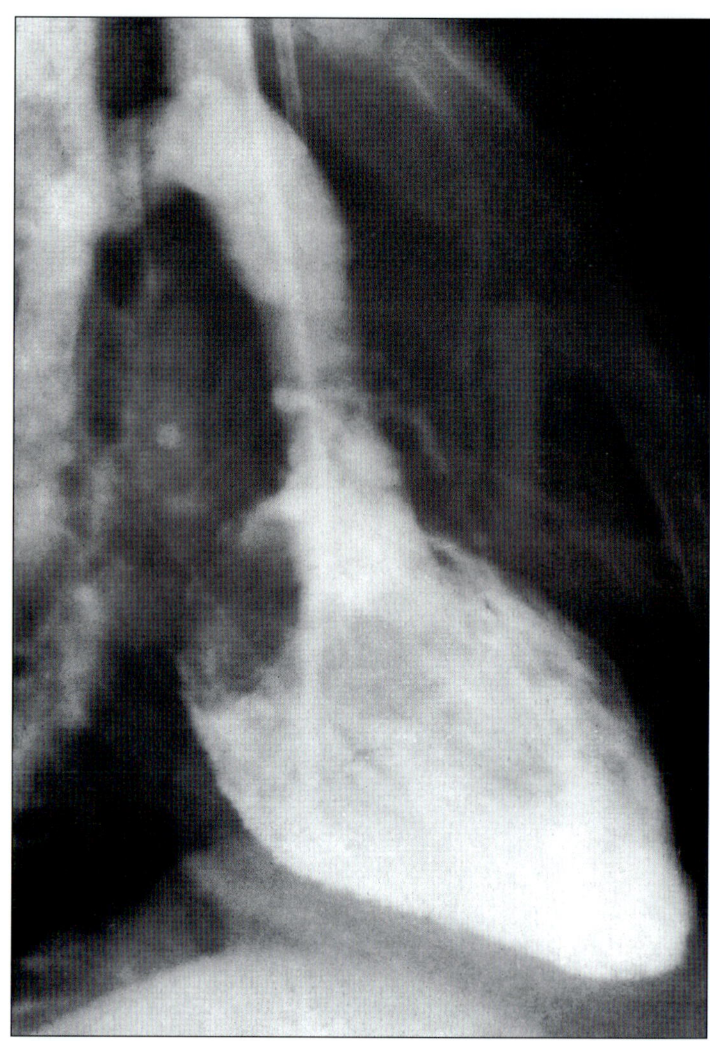

1.19 Diffuse aortic stenosis in a 21-year-old women with homozygous familial hypercholesterolemia. The aortic stenosis involves a long segment of the aorta and extends down into the sinus of Valsalva.

10.3 mmol/l (100 mg/dl to 400 mg/dl). The clinical picture therefore varies as a function of the severity of the hypercholesterolemia and the presence of accompanying genetic and/or environmental determinants of cardiovascular risk. We studied a kindred in which the severity of the pheno-type was a function of *APOE* polymorphism. Presence of the apoE ε4 allele was associated with high levels of cholesterol and the presence of atherosclerosis and tendon xanthomas, whereas the ε2 allele was associated with normal levels and no clinical manifestation (Davignon *et al.* 1992). Other cases have been reported in association with lecithin:cholesterol acyl transferase (LCAT) deficiency and *LDLR* defects. There are indications that the *FDB* gene may operate as a susceptibility gene with certain mutations (Arg$_{3531}$→Cys). Several reports have established the milder nature of FDB relative to FH in general. To attribute the FH phenotype to FDB, one must ideally eliminate co-existence of an LDL receptor gene defect by excluding common *LDLR* mutations in regions in which a founder

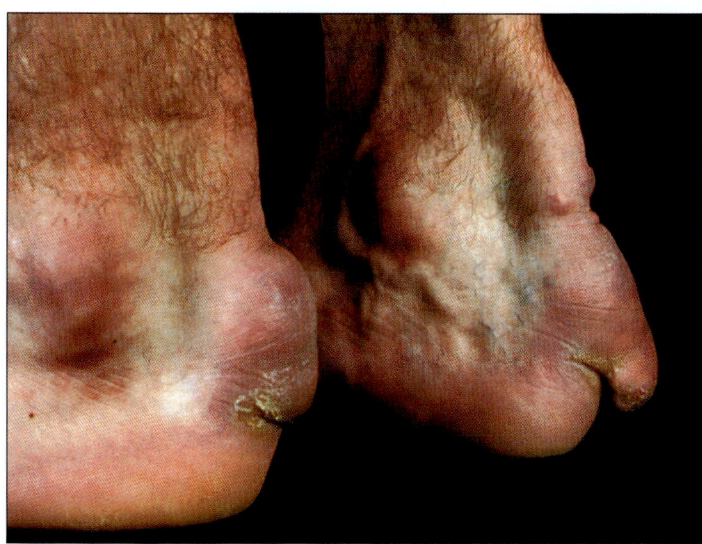

1.20 Severe tendinous and tuberous xanthomatosis of the Achilles tendons in pseudo-homozygous familial hypercholesterolemia. Only one parent of this man in his forties had hypercholesterolemia. He was seen many years ago and was lost to follow-up, so a molecular diagnosis could not be established.

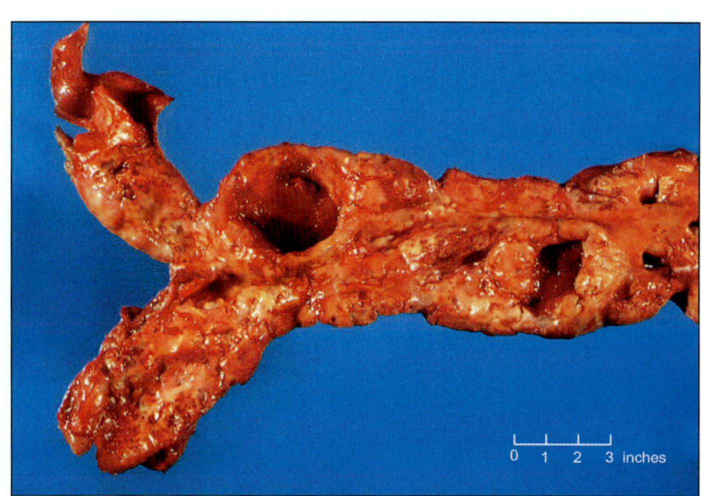

1.21 Severe aorto-femoral atherosclerosis in familial hypercholesterolemia.

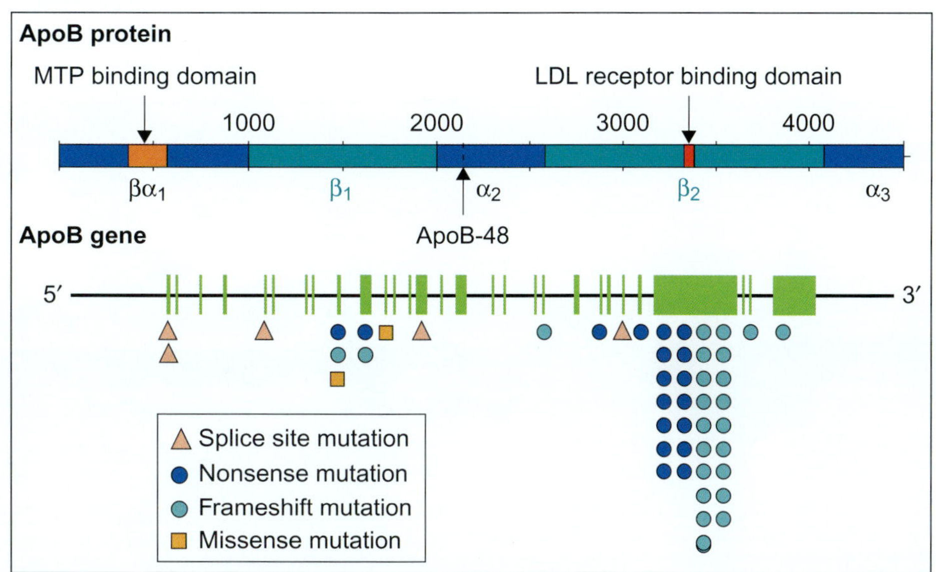

1.22 Apolipoprotein B (ApoB) protein and gene structure and mutations. ApoB is one of the most important proteins involved in lipoprotein metabolism. It is a huge amphipathic glycoprotein of 4536 amino acids (550 kD mature protein) made by the liver (apoB-100; 100 being an arbitrary number given to full length apoB, allowing nomenclature of the isoforms on a centile scale) and apoB-48 (2156 amino acids; 265 kD) made by the intestine. ApoB-100 comprises a series of amphipathic α-helices (α_1, α_2, α_3 for reversible lipid binding) and β-sheet (β, β_1, β_2) domains (β_1 and β_2 irreversibly associated with the lipid core of the lipoprotein).

Other functionally relevant domains (arrows) include the microsomal triglyceride transfer protein (MTP) binding domain of importance in very-low-density lipoprotein (VLDL) assembly, the LDL receptor binding domain for receptor-mediated endocytosis of lipoprotein particles and the apoB-48 splice site allowing chylomicron formation. Mutations of the *APOB* gene (43 kb, 29 exons) may cause familial defective apoB-100 (mutations in exon 26, *see text*) or hypobetalipoproteinemia associated with truncated forms of apoB. ApoB-48 (representing 48% of apoB-100) is produced by an enzyme, apobec-1 present only in the intestine, through a post-transcriptional mRNA editing process. Redrawn from Whitfield AJ *et al.* (2004). Lipid disorders and mutations in the APOB gene. *Clin Chem*, **50**: 1725–1732. For more details regarding the metabolic scheme see **1.2**.

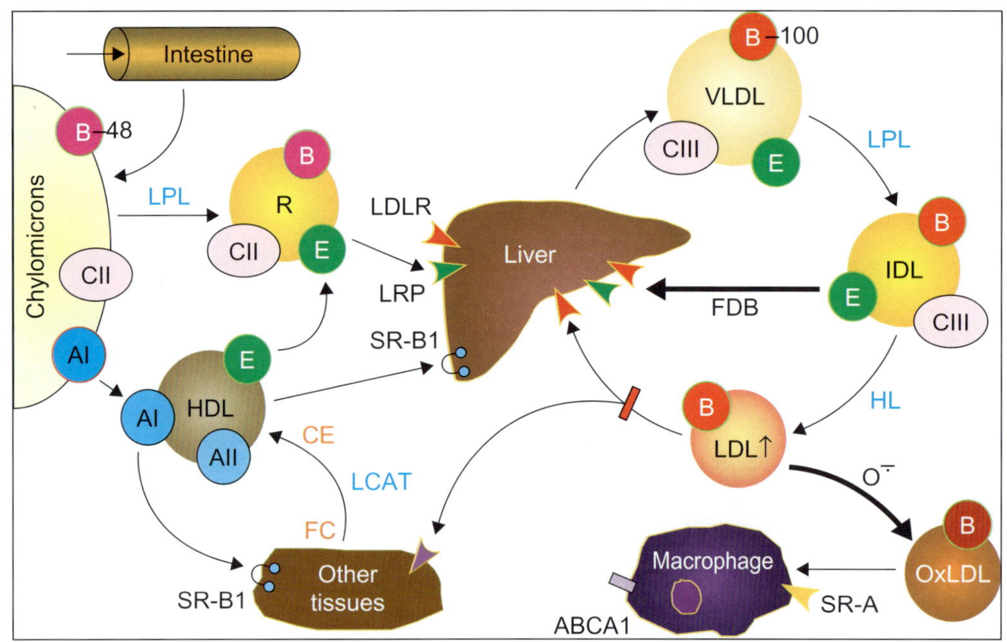

1.23 Metabolic defect in familial defective apolipoprotein B-100. In familial defective apolipoprotein B-100 (FDB), the primary defect is a point mutation in the *APOB* gene and production of a metabolically defective apoB-100 protein (represented by a B in a dark-red circle) with reduced affinity for the low-density lipoprotein (LDL) receptor and elevation of LDL-C. This is associated with a reduced production of LDL (thin arrows). In contrast, the residence time of very-low-density lipoprotein (VLDL) apoE (E on a green circle) is reduced because apoE becomes the favoured ligand to clear particles via the LDL receptor and the LDL receptor-related protein (LRP) (green arrowheads and direct arrow from IDL to the liver). Furthermore, the abnormal LDL are more susceptible to oxidation, increasing their atherogenic potential (thicker arrow, lower right). For more details regarding the metabolic scheme and abbreviations, see **1.2**

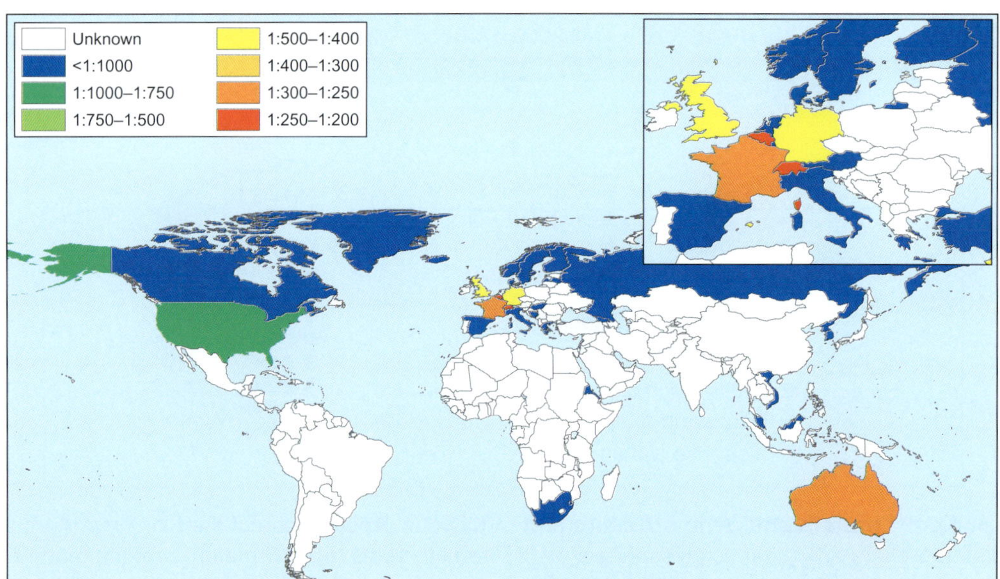

1.24 Estimated world prevalence of familial defective apolipoprotein B-100 (FDB). The prevalence of FDB, estimated to be 1 in 500 to 1 in 700 in Caucasians, varies widely from country to country. This figure demonstrates the very high prevalence in the countries of central Europe. From haplotype analysis of the mutations and population genetic studies, Miserez and Muller speculated that the common mutation originated from Celtic ancestors in a region between Lake Geneva, the Jura mountains and the Rhine, perhaps as early as the Mesolithic period (6000 to 10 000 years ago). Switzerland, Belgium and France stand out in Europe on this map and Australia in the rest of the world. In the northwestern part of Switzerland, the prevalence of this mutation is 1 in 114. These results are, in most cases, extrapolations from samples of hypercholesterolemic subjects attending their respective lipid clinics. The R3500Q mutation has been detected almost exclusively in Caucasian individuals. Redrawn from Miserez AR, Muller PY (2000). Familial defective apolipoprotein B-100: a mutation emerged in the Mesolithic ancestors of Celtic peoples? *Atherosclerosis*, **148**: 433–436.

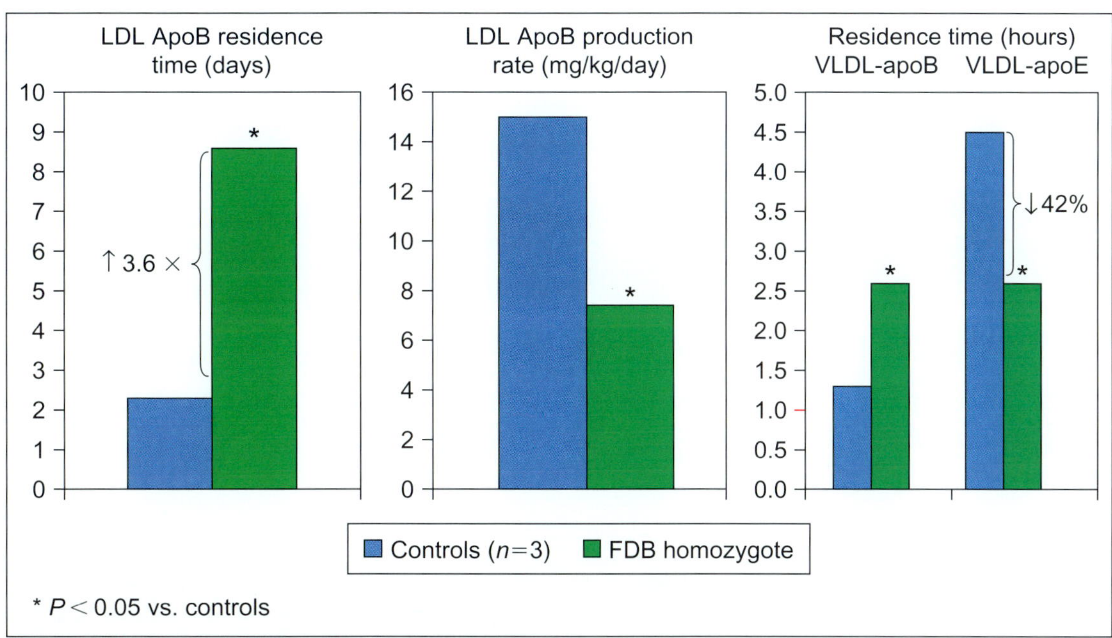

1.25 Lipoprotein kinetics in familial defective apoB-100 (FDB). The results of a stable-isotope-labelling lipoprotein kinetic study using a tritiated leucine-primed constant infusion carried out by Schaefer JR *et al.* are depicted in this figure. Three normal men were compared with a patient homozygous for FDB. Plasma low-density lipoprotein-cholesterol (LDL-C) (203 mg/dl) and apoB (254 mg/dl) concentrations of this patient were twice that of the normal subjects (92 mg/dl and 81 mg/dl), whereas his plasma apoE levels were low (20 mg/dl vs. 26 mg/dl). FDB is a dominant disease, accounting for the moderate levels of LDL-C in this homozygous patient, which contrasts with what is observed in FH patients in whom the homozygotes have much higher levels than the heterozygotes (a co-dominant disease). The LDL-apoB residence time is increased three-fold, the LDL-apoB production rate is halved, the VLDL-apoB residence time doubled and the VLDL-apoE residence time is reduced by 42% in the homozygous patient when compared with the normal controls ($P < 0.05$). Redrawn from data reported in Schaefer JR *et al.* (1997). Homozygous familial defective apolipoprotein B-100. Enhanced removal of apolipoprotein E-containing VLDL and decreased production of LDL. *Arterioscler Thromb Vasc Biol*, **17**: 348–353.

effect is present and/or demonstrate normal LDL receptor number or activity in cultured fibroblasts. This has been carried out in several studies.

The differential diagnosis depends on the severity of the hypercholesterolemia. When it is modest or moderate, familial combined hyperlipidemia with isolated hypercholesterolemia and polygenic hypercholesterolemia should be considered first, after exclusion of secondary causes or an unhealthy lifestyle. If the hypercholesterolemia is severe, the differential diagnosis is that of the FH phenotype. The family history and age at first manifestation assist in the diagnosis because clinical manifestations occur later in life than in FH. Treatment of FDB is identical to that of FH.

Autosomal dominant hypercholesterolemia (FH3)

The FH phenotype may occur in the absence of an *LDLR* or an *APOB* abnormality. It was the study of kindreds ascertained from a proband without such defects that led to the discovery of FH3. Varret, in the laboratory of Boileau, Junien and colleagues in Paris in 1999, mapped a third locus for the FH phenotype on the short arm of chromosome 1 (1p32–34.1),which they called *FH3*. The original demonstration was the result of a concerted international collaboration and involved the study of French, Spanish and Sardinian families. Other kindreds were identified in Utah, USA. More recently, in a collaboration with Seidah and co-workers in Montreal, Abifadel and colleagues in Boileau's Paris laboratory found that *FH3* was a proprotein convertase gene: the proprotein convertase subtilisin/kexin type 9 gene (*PCSK9*) which encodes the PCSK9 protein, also called the neural apoptosis regulated convertase-1 (NARC-1). Convertases are a family of enzymes responsible for the processing of multiple precursor proteins including growth factors, neuropeptides, receptors, membrane-bound transcription factors and enzymes. *PCSK9* mRNA is expressed in the liver, small intestine and brain. It is involved in neurogenesis, nephrogenesis and hepatogenesis and belongs to the proteinase subfamily of subtilases. Two mutations of this

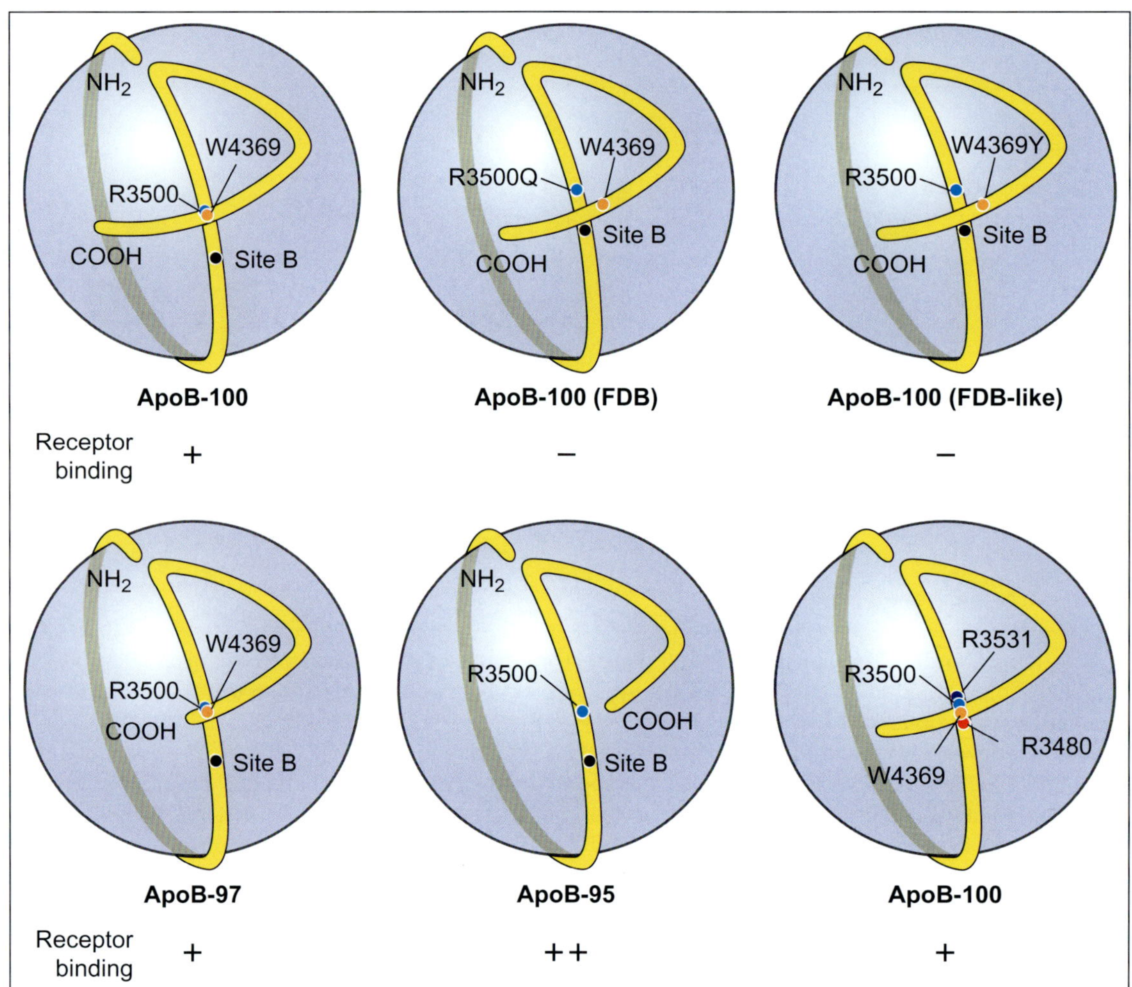

1.26 Model of low-density lipoprotein (LDL) receptor binding of Borén *et al.* In this drawing, the spheres represent the cholesteryl ester-rich LDL particle and the band is the apoB wrapped around it. Normal binding of apoB to its receptor involves an interaction between arginine 3500 and tryptophan 4369 (R3500-W4369) in the carboxyl tail of apoB-100 (overlap on top left drawing). This interaction drives the correct folding of the C-terminal end of apoB for interaction with the LDLR. In the metabolic diagrams throughout this atlas, this point is represented by a B in a red circle, depicting only the major ligand–receptor interaction site. The classic familial defective apoB-100 (FDB) mutation (R3500Q) displacing the carboxyl end of apoB away towards 'site B' causes improper folding and disruption of the ligand–receptor interaction (top middle). The same thing happens if the Trp at position 4369 is mutated (W4369Y, top right, FDB-like mutation). Mutated W4369Y LDL and R3500Q LDL isolated from transgenic mice have identical defective LDL binding as in FDB and a higher affinity for the monoclonal antibody MB47, which has an epitope flanking residue 3500.

Removing 3% of the carboxyl (apoB-97) allows the interaction and results in normal binding (lower left). The lack of the carboxyl tail (in apoB-95) induces a gain in function with enhanced receptor binding (lower middle). Therefore, the carboxyl terminal functions as a negative modulator of receptor binding and the same research group has shown that it inhibits binding of VLDL to the LDLR. Trp 4369 interacts not only with Arg 3500, but also with Arg 3480 and Arg 3531, explaining the occurrence of FDB in mutations affecting these sites. Site B (i.e. residues 3359–3369) is the receptor-binding site; as can be seen, it is slightly further from the major mutation sites. Redrawn with permission from Borén J *et al.* (2001). The molecular mechanism for the genetic disorder familial defective apolipoprotein B100. *J Biol Chem*, **276**: 9214–9218.

gene were reported to segregate with the FH phenotype in French families. They include Ser$_{127}$→ Arg (S127R) and Phe$_{216}$→Leu (F216L). A new mutation of *PCSK9* was identified in the Utah families, Asp$_{374}$→Tyr (D374Y) as well as in Norway and England. We have also observed a new mutation, Arg$_{237}$→Trp (R237W) in a 73-year-old French-Canadian patient attending the authors' lipid clinic. In addition, two polymorphisms of *PCSK9* are associated with elevated levels of LDL-C in Japan and another one in Caucasians. Later, other mutations were found to be associated with low plasma cholesterol levels (loss-of-function mutations). The major mutations are summarized in **1.27**.

The clinical picture of the affected individuals may be indistinguishable from that of FH although it may vary in severity within and across kindreds. There is also evidence that the affected subjects may be more responsive to treatment with statins. Our patient with the R237W mutation is alive at the age of 80 and presented with the FH phenotype including tendon xanthomas, xanthelasma, arcus corneae, LDL-C of 5.96 mmol/l (230 mg/dl) with normal triglycerides and HDL-cholesterol (HDL-C). He responded very well to 10 mg/day of simvastatin with a 41% fall in LDL-C (**1.28**). A *PCSK9* defect was sought because of the absence of any of the common *LDLR* mutations or the common FDB mutation (R3500Q). The mechanism whereby mutations of *PCSK9* are linked to the phenotype is not fully established. *PCSK9*

mRNA is downregulated by cholesterol in hepatocytes and by dietary cholesterol in mice. It is upregulated in the liver of sterol regulatory element binding protein-2 (SREBP-2) transgenic mice. *PCSK9* is markedly upregulated by statins and by cholesterol depletion in human hepatocytes as shown in the authors' laboratory. The *Pcsk9* transgenic mouse develops a phenotype similar to that of an Ldlr knockout, whereas mice lacking *Pcsk9* show hypocholesterolemia but statins are still active. There appears to be a close relationship of PCSK9 activity with the LDL receptor activity, perhaps a modulatory role. The current view is that PCSK9 promotes LDL receptor degradation (**1.29**). PCSK9 is secreted in plasma. In parabiotic mice the donor PCSK9 may degrade the LDLR of the recipient (Lagace *et al.* 2006). PCSK9 is sulphated and circulating PCSK9 is itself degraded by furin, another convertase (PC3) (Benjannet *et al.* 2006). *PCSK9* is

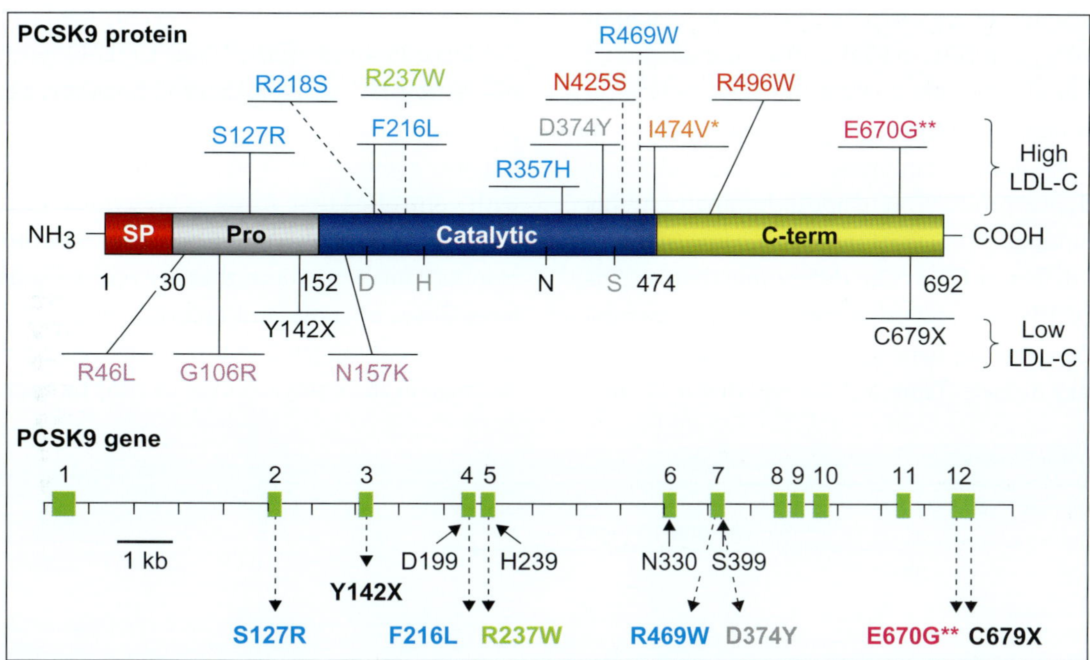

1.27 The PCSK9 (NARC-1) protein and gene mutations influencing plasma LDL-C. The PCSK9 protein (top) is a 692-amino acid pre-pro-peptide comprising a signal peptide (SP), a pro-segment (Pro), a catalytic domain (Catalytic) and a C-terminal domain. The catalytic pocket containing the nucleophiles aspartic acid (D), histidine (H), asparagine (N) and serine (S) takes an active conformation after cleavage of the pro-segment. The position and the amino acid substitutions of the mutations that are associated with high LDL-C levels are shown at the top of the protein, those that are associated with a reduced plasma LDL-C are shown at the bottom. Not shown among the latter is R237W that has been reported to be associated with hypercholesterolemia in Canada and with hypocholesterolemia in Norway. The colour code indicates the origin of the mutation, France (blue), USA and Norway (grey), Norway (pink), Italy (red) and Canada (green). The mutation in orange (Japan) with an asterisk is a common variant associated with high low-density lipoprotein-cholesterol (LDL-C) in the general population. The E670G coding SNP in mauve with two asterisks reported in Caucasians also influences the LDL-C levels (increased with the rare GG genotype). The mutations associated with low LDL-C reported in Dallas are shown in black; the others in pink are from Norway. The *PCSK9* gene (bottom) located on chromosome 1 contains 12 exons (squares). The locations of the mutations on the gene are given using the same colour code. The position of the codons coding for the nucleophiles of the catalytic pocket are also given.

regulated as a typical cholesterologenic gene. These findings undoubtedly establish a link between cholesterol homeostasis and *PCSK9*. The measurement of PCSK9 activity is based on its own autocatalytic zymogen processing for the time being because the natural substrate for PCSK9 is unknown. Two of the mutations reported, S127R and D374Y, partially and totally abrogated this processing, respectively.

FH3 is a rare condition and the prevalence of *PCSK9*-related hypercholesterolemia is not yet determined in the population at large. The metabolic abnormalities have been studied by Ouguerram and colleagues in two hypercholesterolemic subjects who were carriers of the S127R mutation. They were compared with controls or FH carriers of an *LDLR* mutation. The kinetics of VLDL, IDL and LDL apoB-100 were assessed using a stable isotope technique. The *PCSK9* mutation increased LDL-C due to a three-fold direct overproduction of VLDL and IDL and a five-fold overproduction of LDL. The fractional catabolic rate of LDL was only slightly reduced (30%). There was a decreased conversion of VLDL to IDL (10%) and IDL to LDL (30%) and a reduced catabolic rate of apoB. The cholesterol to triglyceride ratio was increased, which could account for a reduced rate of lipolysis of VLDL by lipoprotein lipase (LPL). Therefore, in contrast with FH, overproduction of apoB dominates in this disease. This preliminary work warrants further investigation of the metabolic defect in FH3. The differential diagnosis is essentially that of FH but responsiveness to statin therapy and a relatively less severe phenotype may help to focus on this new hereditary disease. Time will tell whether a *PCSK9*

mutation alone is sufficient to cause the phenotype or whether other genetic or environmental factors are needed for expression of the full clinical picture. On the other hand, because the loss-of-function mutations are associated with low LDL-C levels and protection against coronary artery disease (CAD), *PCSK9* has become a promising target for drug development.

Deficiency of cholesterol 7α-hydroxylase (CYP7A1)

This disease was discovered by Pullinger and co-workers in 2002 at the University of California in San Francisco. The proband was a 55-year-old man with fasting hypercholesterolemia (10.8 mmol/l or 419 mg/dl) and hypertriglyceridemia (10.4 mmol/l or 919 mg/dl) and history of gallstones (cholecystectomy at age 42), CAD (age 48) and aorto-femoral arteriosclerosis. Mean LDL-C was higher in homozygotes than in heterozygotes, which was in turn higher than in non-affected relatives (**1.30**). Only a few members of the large kindred studied had LDL-C levels close to those of classic FH. Total cholesterol, however, exceeded the 95th percentile. HDL-C was normal. Total fecal bile acid excretion was reduced 94% in one homozygote when compared with controls. These features are typical of the disease when added to the presence of remnant lipoproteins and poor responsiveness to statin therapy requiring a combination of large doses of statin and nicotinic acid for control. No xanthomas were reported, but there was no mention of physical findings in the study, so they cannot be excluded.

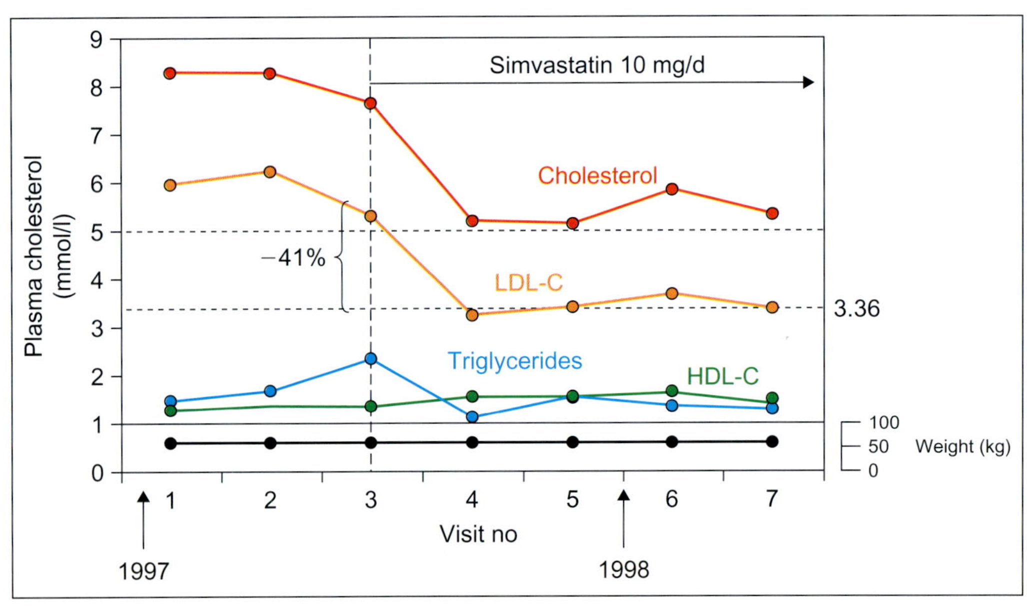

1.28 Sensitivity to treatment with a statin in FH3 (PCSK9 R237W). Sensitivity to treatment with a statin in a 73-year-old man with the Arg237→Trp mutation of *PCSK9* is part of the phenotype of FH3. This patient has clinical manifestations of familial hypercholesterolemia including tendon xanthomas, arcus corneae and xanthelasma. There is a history of myocardial infarction in the patient's family and in one sibling with the R237W mutation.

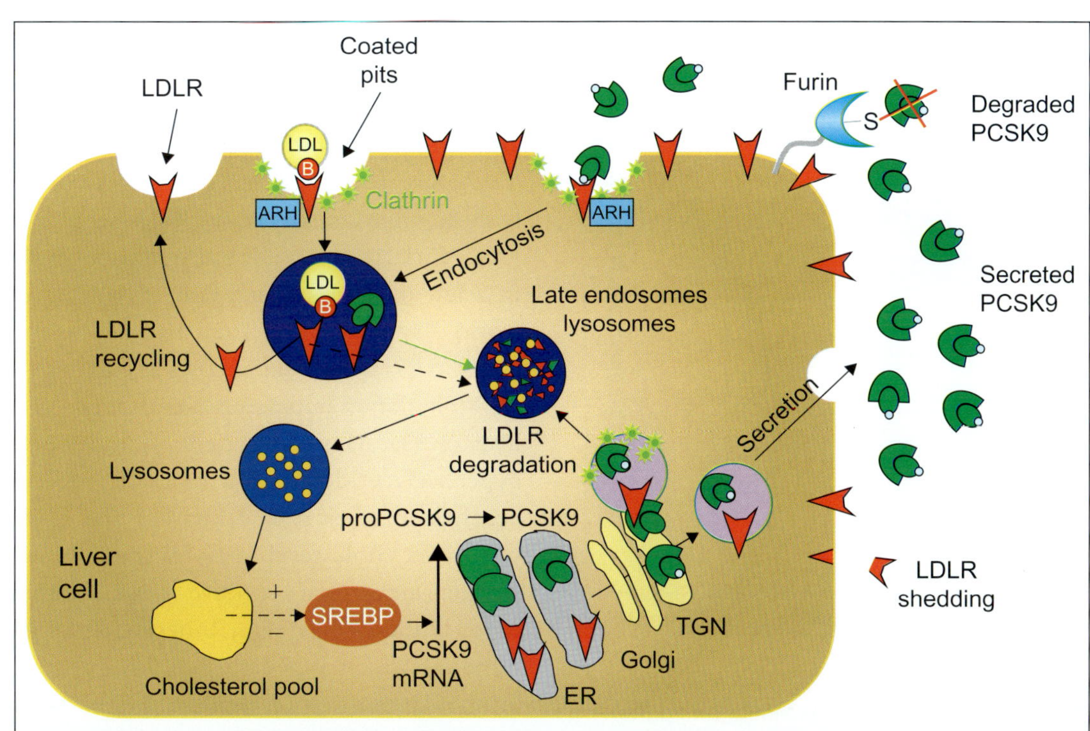

1.29 PCSK9 and low-density lipoprotein receptor (LDLR) protein metabolism. After binding of the LDL particle to its receptor via apolipoprotein B (apoB) (top left), the complex is internalized by endocytosis in clathrin-coated pits. Internalization requires ARH (autosomal recessive hypercholesterolemia) protein. It is believed that PCSK9 (in green) may contribute to LDLR degradation (coated pit on the right and green arrow) in the late endosome compartment. Inside the endocytotic vesicle, the LDL-apoB–LDLR complex is broken down. The freed LDLR can either be recycled to the cell surface or sent to the lysosomes for degradation. Cholesterol is unesterified and FC liberated into the cell where it contributes to the cholesterol pool. When cholesterol is low, SREBP is activated and stimulates the synthesis of both the LDLR and proPCSK9. In the endoplasmic reticulum (ER) proPCSK9 is cleaved into PCSK9 and remains tightly bound to PCSK9. The LDLR and PCSK9 move to the Golgi and the trans-Golgi network (TGN) where PCSK9 is post-transcriptionally sulphated within its prosegment at Tyr_{38} (white dot). At some point during this transit, the LDLR is directed either to the cell membrane (for surface expression or cleavage and shedding) or to a lysosomal compartment where it will be degraded. By a still unknown mechanism, this process is PCSK9 dependent. PCSK9 itself is secreted outside the cell. It may be degraded at the cell surface by furin (blue crescent) or another proprotein convertase (PC5/6A). When PCSK9 is overexpressed, fewer LDLRs appear at the surface and *vice versa* – when PCSK9 has a loss-of-function mutation, more receptors appear at the cell surface. Figure designed in collaboration with Nabil G Seidah and colleagues.

The defective enzyme, cholesterol 7α-hydroxylase, is a member of the cytochrome P450 mixed-function oxidase superfamily, hence the synonym CYP7A1 (**cy**tochrome **P**450 **7A1**) deficiency. It is a rate-regulating enzyme that induces 7-hydroxylation of cholesterol to initiate bile acid synthesis (**1.31**). Failure of this enzyme markedly reduces bile acids in the bile and feces, the major route of cholesterol excretion, and increases the pool of cholesterol in the liver, thereby inhibiting LDL receptor activity and raising plasma cholesterol. It also reduces the solubility of cholesterol in the bile, thus favouring gallstone formation. The gene encoding this enzyme in humans was mapped to chromosome 8 (8q11–q12) by Cohen in 1992. The mutation responsible for the original cases was a frameshift mutation in *CYP7A1* causing a Leu→Arg substitution at codon 413 (L413R) followed by a premature stop codon. This results in transcription of a truncated protein missing the last 91 C-terminal residues, which include a hem-binding domain essential for activity. A Taq1 restriction site is created that allows identification of the mutation. The mode of inheritance is co-dominant as in classic FH because of the intermediate phenotype in heterozygotes. More kindreds must be identified and more studies are needed to establish the full clinical picture, metabolic consequences, frequency and pathophysiology of this disease.

The diagnosis of this disease among dominant forms of hypercholesterolemia may be established on the basis of a plasma cholesterol level lower than expected for a classic FH,

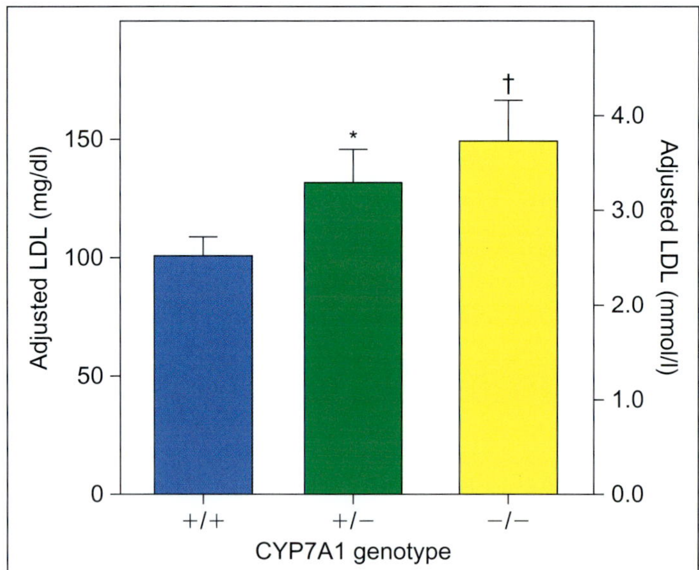

1.30 Effect of CYP7A1 genotypes on low-density lipoprotein (LDL)-cholesterol. Values (mean ± SEM) were adjusted for age and sex. There were three homozygotes (–/–), six heterozygotes (+/–) and 26 unaffected relatives (+/+) in this family where the *CYP7A1* defect segregated. The gene dosage effect is evident. Statistical analysis was by ANOVA; *P = 0.007 and †P = 0.002 vs. unaffected relatives. Redrawn with permission from Pullinger CR *et al.* (2002). Human cholesterol 7alpha-hydroxylase (CYP7A1) deficiency has a hypercholesterolemic phenotype. *J Clin Invest*, **110**: 109–117.

presence of gallstones in the patient or members of his or her family (relatively early gallstone disease in non-obese males is infrequent), hypertriglyceridemia (two of three homozygotes had hypertriglyceridemia) with the presence of remnant lipoproteins and resistance to lipid-lowering treatment. Reduced bile acid fecal excretion and demonstration of the mutation would clinch the diagnosis but imply referral to a specialist centre. Diagnostic accuracy will improve as more cases are reported and new diagnostic tools are developed.

Recessive forms

Autosomal recessive hypercholesterolemia (ARH)

In 1973, reviewing their experience with 52 cases of homozygous FH, Khachadurian and Uthman reported a Lebanese family in which all four children of normolipidemic parents had this phenotype, probably the first report of a recessive form of FH. In 1995 Zuliani and co-workers recognized the existence of a similar recessive disorder, this time in an

Italian family living in Sardinia. They reported two siblings in their twenties presenting marked hypercholesterolemia and clinical features of homozygous FH such as tuberous and tendinous xanthomas, which were first noted at age 10. They had severe aortic and coronary stenosis associated with angina. Unexpectedly, both parents were normolipidemic. Similar cases have also subsequently been identified in a few other Sardinian families and in other parts of the world (Japan, Turkey, Iran, Syria, England, India, Mexico and USA). Some patients in a Japanese family presented multiple large cutaneous xanthomas (**1.32**) and a fatty liver (**1.33**). Mexican patients were reported to be severely hypertriglyceridemic and markedly obese. Consanguinity, absence of vertical transmission and bimodal distribution of plasma cholesterol levels in the kindred were consistent with an autosomal recessive mode of inheritance. The disease (Online Mendelian Inheritance in Man, OMIM No. 603813) was mapped to the *ARH* gene in 2001 by Eden in the laboratory of Soutar and co-workers at Imperial College, London. Approximately 50 patients from different ethnic origins have been reported in the literature so far. *In vitro* studies with fibroblasts revealed that the LDL receptor of the affected subjects appeared intact as it bound and degraded LDL normally. Unexpectedly, however, it has been observed later that binding and degradation is defective in cultured lymphocytes and monocyte-derived macrophages. Familial defective ApoB-100, sitosterolemia and cholesteryl ester storage disease were also excluded. The new disease was identified as ARH (autosomal recessive hypercholesterolemia). Plasma total cholesterol concentration in ARH ranges from 12 mmol/l to 20 mmol/l (465–775 mg/dl) and plasma LDL-C from 10 mmol/l to 15 mmol/l (385–580 mg/dl). If left untreated, symptomatic cardiovascular disease may develop, beginning in the third decade. Fortunately, and contrary to homozygous FH, ARH is responsive to lipid-lowering therapy with bile acid sequestrants, ezetimibe and/or HMG-CoA reductase inhibitors capable of decreasing total cholesterol by 60–70%.

In recent years the molecular mechanism of ARH has been elucidated: mutations in the gene coding for a novel putative adaptor protein called ARH are responsible for the disease (**1.34**). To date, 12 mutations have been identified in the *ARH* gene located on the short arm of chromosome 1 (1p35–36). All but one of these introduces a premature stop codon that precludes the synthesis of detectable ARH protein necessary for the internalization of LDL after normal binding to the LDL receptor. The exception is the most

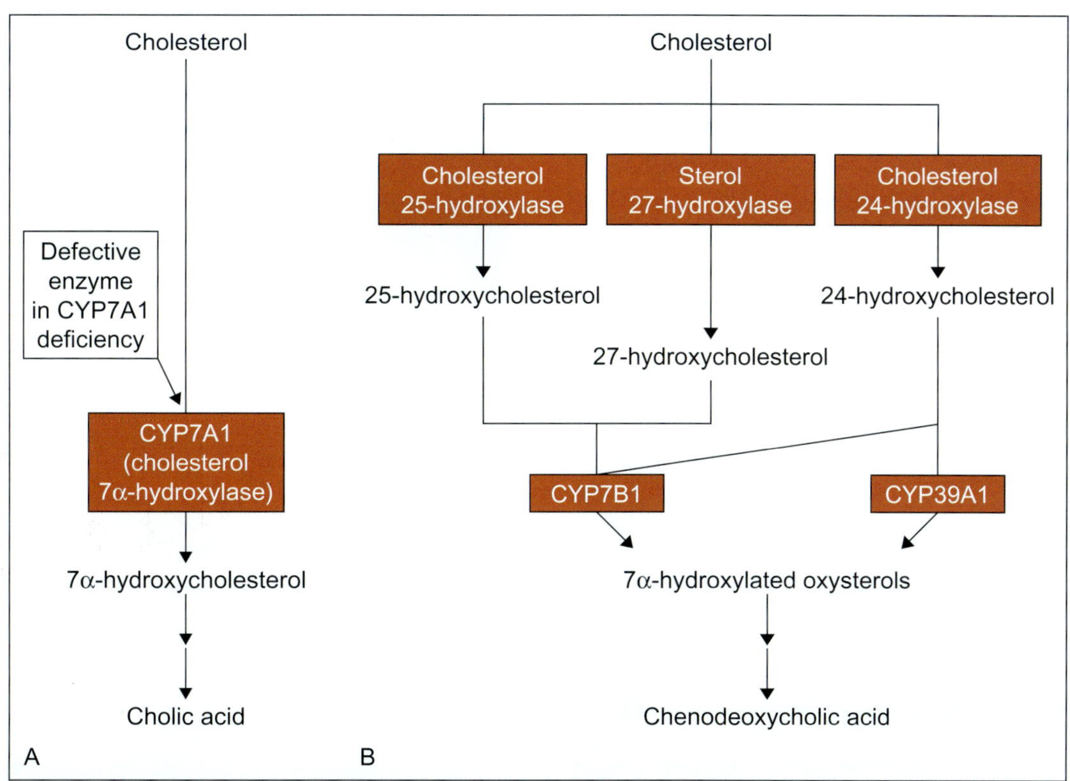

1.31 Metabolic defect in cholesterol 7α-hydroxylase deficiency. The classic pathway for bile acid synthesis shown in (A) begins with CYP7A1, which converts cholesterol into 7α-hydroxycholesterol. This pathway mainly produces cholic acid in humans. CYP7A1 deficiency markedly reduces bile acids in the bile and feces, the major route of cholesterol excretion, and increases the pool of cholesterol in the liver thereby inhibiting low-density lipoprotein (LDL) receptor activity and raising plasma cholesterol. The alternative pathways for bile acid synthesis are shown in (B). Cholesterol is first converted into oxysterols by one of three different enzymes: sterol 27-hydroxylase (CYP27), expressed in multiple tissues including the liver; cholesterol 25-hydroxylase, present at low levels in multiple tissues including the heart, lungs, and kidneys; and cholesterol 24-hydroxylase (CYP46), expressed predominantly in the brain. Oxysterols are transported through the bloodstream to the liver, where they are 7α-hydroxylated by oxysterol 7α-hydroxylase (CYP7B1) in the case of 25- and 27-hydroxycholesterol and by CYP39A1 in the case of 24-hydroxycholesterol. Alternative pathways preferentially produce chenodeoxycholic acid in humans. Redrawn with permission from Beigneux A *et al.* (2002). Human CYP7A1 deficiency: progress and enigmas. *J Clin Invest*, **110**: 129–131.

recently identified mutation, found in a Mexican family, which results in an in-frame deletion in the phosphotyrosine-binding (PTB) domain that is believed to interact directly with the LDL receptor. Interestingly, the reduced uptake of LDL is present in human lymphocytes, and monocyte-derived macrophages but not in fibroblasts. Ineffective hepatic LDL receptor activity has been postulated from experiments in *ARH* null mice showing abnormal accumulation of the LDL receptor on the cell surface of hepatocytes. Recent evidence indicates that ARH acts as a clathrin-associated sorting protein (CLASP) coupling the LDL receptor with clathrin machinery in the coated pits to promote endocytosis (see **1.29**). Therefore, in patients with ARH, LDL uptake in the liver is reduced to the same extent as it is in patients with homozygous FH, thus promoting the development of the same clinical phenotype. The differential diagnosis is the same as that of homozygous FH. Recognition of the mode of inheritance (**1.35**) and responsiveness to treatment should help the physician to make the correct diagnosis.

Lysosomal acid lipase deficiency: Wolman's disease and cholesteryl ester storage disease

Lysosomal acid lipase (cholesteryl ester hydrolase) deficiency is a recessive inborn error of metabolism that is classified among lysosomal diseases or lipidoses (OMIM No. 278000). It is characterized by massive accumulation of cholesteryl esters and triglycerides in most tissues of the body, especially in the liver. The severe pediatric form, Wolman's disease, occurs in infancy and is nearly always fatal in the first year of life causing hepatic or adrenal failure. It was initially termed

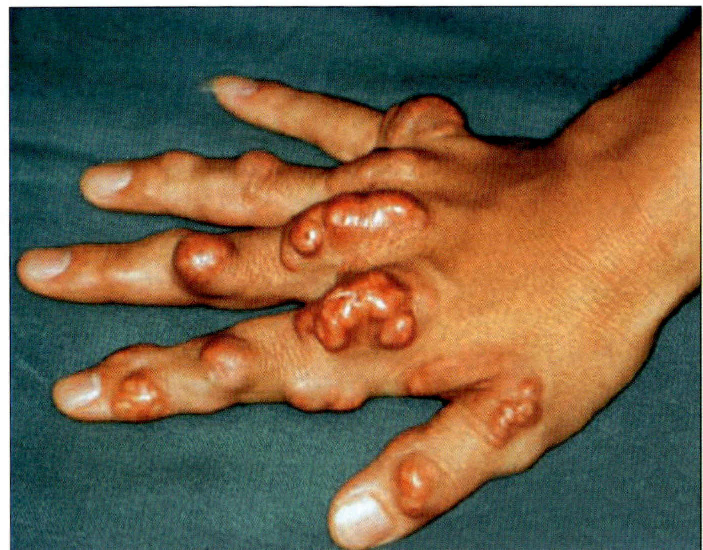

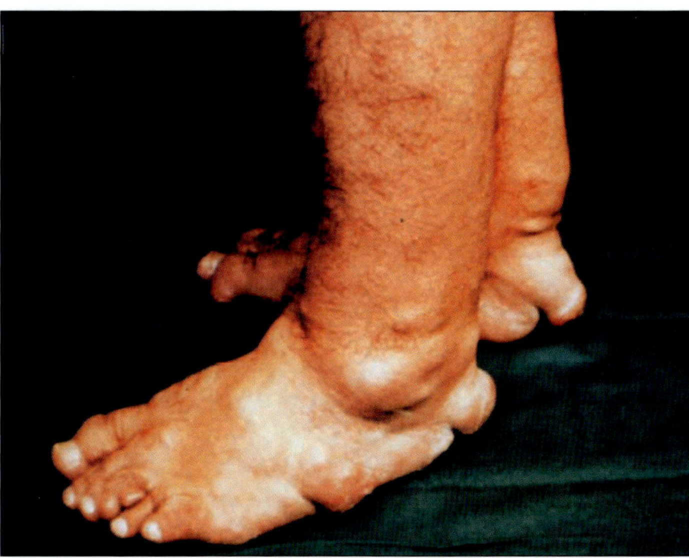

1.32 Severe tuberous xanthomatosis of hands and feet in autosomal recessive hypercholesterolemia (ARH). Note the resemblance with lesions of homozygous familial hypercholesterolemia (FH). Helpful clues to the diagnosis are the absence of hypercholesterolemia in the parents and the good response of plasma cholesterol to drug therapy in contrast to what is observed in homozygous FH. Reproduced with permission from Harada-Shiba M *et al.* (2003). Clinical features and genetic analysis of autosomal recessive hypercholesterolemia. *J Clin Endocrinol Metab*, **88**: 2541–2547.

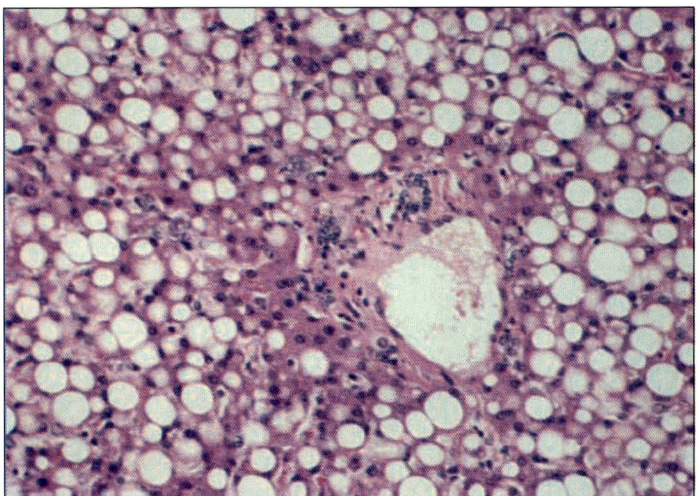

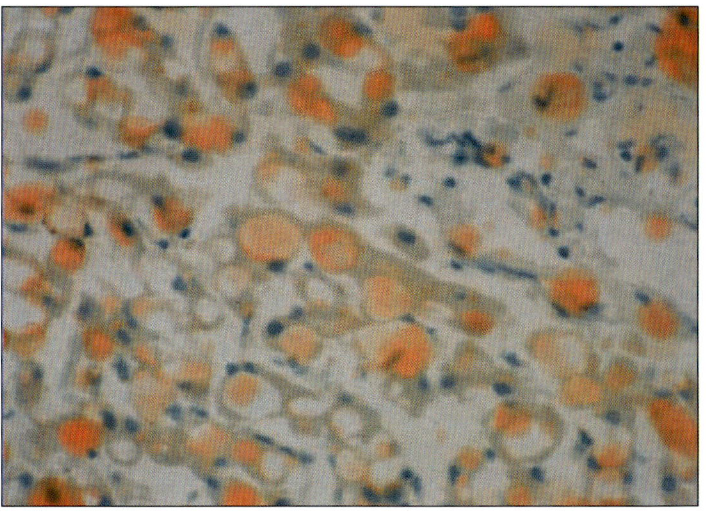

1.33 Liver steatosis in autosomal recessive hypercholesterolemia (ARH) reported in Japan. Microscopic sections of the liver demonstrate lipid accumulation in hepatocytes as clear vacuoles on the left (hematoxylin-eosin staining) and as pink vacuoles on the right at a higher magnification (Sudan III staining). Note that this feature has not been reported in other cases of ARH but it may not have been looked for in all cases. Reproduced with permission from Harada-Shiba M *et al.* (2003). Clinical features and genetic analysis of autosomal recessive hypercholesterolemia. *J Clin Endocrinol Metab*, **88**: 2541–2547.

a 'primary familial xanthomatosis with adrenal calcification'. It is estimated to occur with a frequency of less than 1 in 100 000 live births. It is manifested by hepatosplenomegaly, anemia, steatorrhoea, adrenal calcifications and failure to thrive. The punctate adrenal calcifications detected by X-rays are pathognomonic (**1.36**). Plasma lipid levels are usually at the low end of the normal range but a few cases with high triglycerides and/or low HDL-C have been reported. The only other disease that it may be confused with is glycogen storage disease type I, which may be excluded by the failure of an intravenous glucagon or galactose tolerance test to increase glucose and lactate. The diagnosis of this

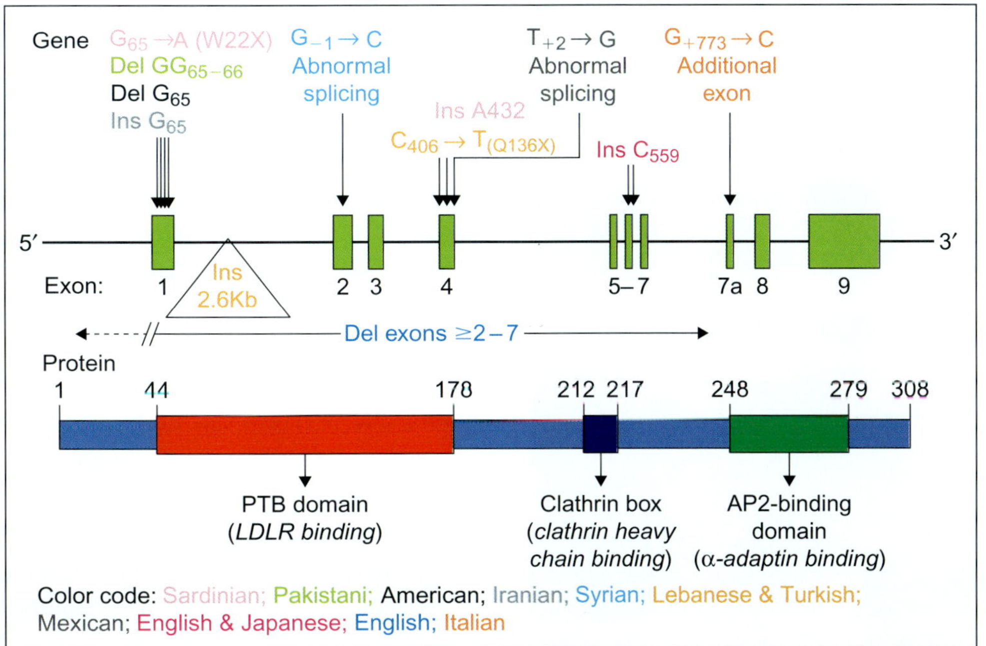

1.34 Mutations of the *ARH* gene causing autosomal recessive hypercholesterolemia. All known mutations (except exon 4, +2 T → G) result in premature termination and a null phenotype, i.e. no detectable protein. Colour code indicates the origin of the mutation: Sardinian (pink), Pakistani (light green), American (black), Iranian (grey), Syrian (light blue), Lebanese and Turkish (light orange), Mexican (dark grey), English and Japanese (red), English (dark blue), and Italian (dark orange). The major functional domains of the protein are shown in the lower part of the diagram. ins, insertion; del, deletion; AP-2, adaptor protein-2. Figure devised in collaboration with Anne K Soutar (Soutar AK, Naoumova RP (2004). Autosomal recessive hypercholesterolemia. *Semin Vasc Med*, **4**: 241–248).

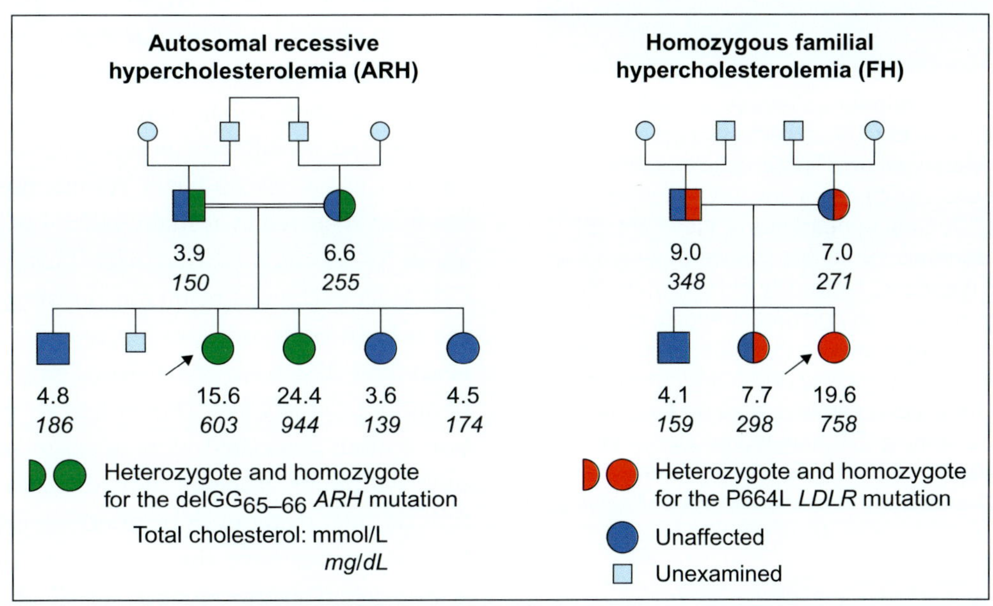

1.35 Typical autosomal recessive hypercholesterolemia (ARH) and homozygous familial hypercholesterolemia (FH) kindreds. The ARH kindred is that of an Asian-Indian family with two affected siblings. The recessive transmission is well illustrated by the normocholesterolemic parents, the presence of consanguinity, and the double dose of the abnormal gene needed for expression of the phenotype. The homozygous FH pedigree from an English family in contrast displays a typical co-dominant mode of inheritance with the heterozygotes having an intermediate phenotype between the homozygote and the unaffected. Arrows indicate the probands. Values of total cholesterol are given in mmol/l and mg/dl (italics). The double line indicates consanguinity. Redrawn with permission from Soutar AK, Naoumova RP (2004). Autosomal recessive hypercholesterolemia. *Semin Vasc Med*, **4**: 241–248.

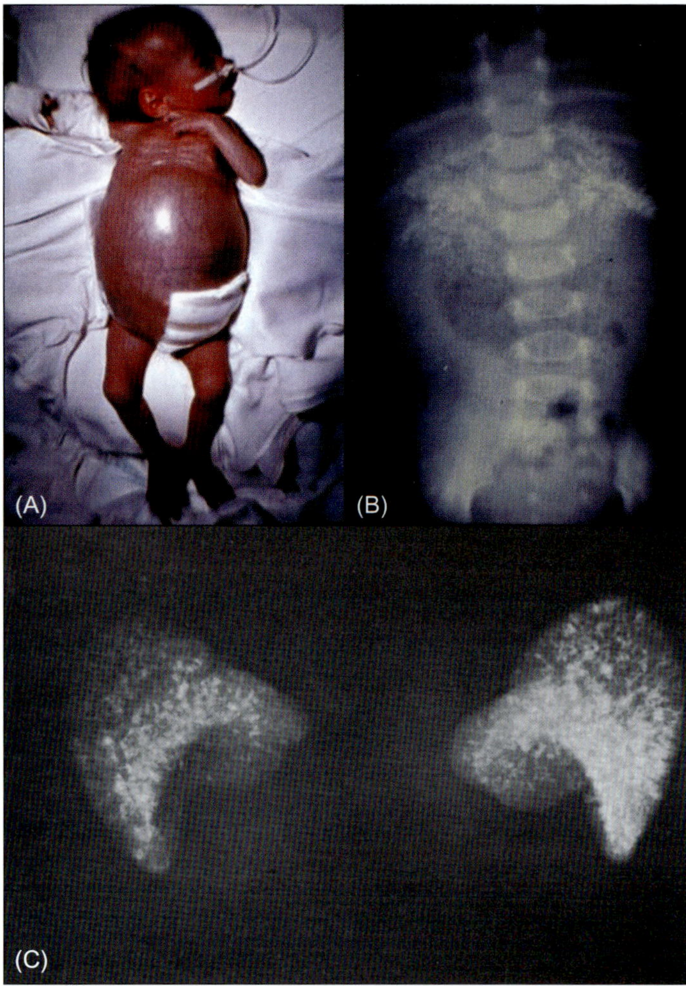

1.36 Calcified adrenals in Wolman's disease. In Wolman's disease, the severe pediatric form of cholesteryl ester storage disease secondary to lysosomal acid lipase deficiency, the adrenals are enlarged and calcified in a unique fashion as demonstrated here. (A) General appearance of the infant. (B) X-ray focusing on the adrenals. (Both pictures were generously contributed by Prof. G. Assmann, University of Muenster). (C) The extensive punctate deposits in enlarged adrenals are pathognomonic of Wolman's disease. In the adult form, which is associated with hypercholesterolemia, there are reports of calcified adrenals that have been demonstrated by X-ray or computed tomography scanning. CT scan reproduced with permission from Crocker AC *et al.* (1965). Wolman's disease: three new patients with a recently described lipidosis. *Pediatrics*, **35**: 627–640.

condition is based on the clinical picture and confirmed by measurement of lysosomal acid lipase (LAL) in peripheral blood leucocytes. There is no known effective treatment (see below).

The adult form, cholesteryl ester storage disease (CESD), in contrast, follows a milder clinical course and is associated with hypercholesterolemia. LDL-C may range from 4.5 mmol/l to 8.5 mmol/l (175–330 mg/dl). Triglycerides may be normal or modestly elevated. HDL-C is usually low, ranging between 0.2 mmol/l and 0.6 mmol/l (6–24 mg/dl). An inverse ratio of HDL_2 to HDL_3 of 10:1 rather than of 1:10 has been reported. CESD is discussed in this chapter because it may be a real, albeit very rare, source of confusion in the diagnosis of familial hypercholesterolemia: only about 100 cases of LAL deficiency have been described in published reports.

LAL's major function is to hydrolyse cholesteryl esters and triglycerides in various lipoproteins as they are removed from the plasma by receptor-mediated endocytosis in different tissues to be processed in the lysosome (**1.37**). LAL is ubiquitous and found in all nucleated cells. This 378 amino acid enzyme is coded by the *LIPA* gene on chromosome 10q23.2–23.3 (10 exons, spanning 36 kb). Mutations in this gene are responsible for both clinical forms of the disease. The severity of the phenotype is a function of the residual enzyme activity, which leads to various degree of accumulation of its substrates in all organs, particularly liver, spleen, adrenals, intestine, hemopoietic system, lymph nodes, lung, testes and ovaries. Absence of enzymatic activity causes Wolman's disease; a residual 3% of enzyme activity is enough to extend the life of a LAL-deficient patient into adulthood. Over 20 mutations of the *LIPA* gene have been reported in subjects from different countries including Austria, Croatia, Canada, France, Japan, Italy, Germany, Norway, Spain and Turkey and of different ethnic origins including Africans, Arabs, Caucasians, and Jews. A missense mutation in exon 8 has been reported in as many as 75% of cases of CESD with about 5% residual LAL activity. This common mutation, a G934→A exchange, results in the skipping of exon 8 from the mRNA transcript and in the loss of the internal amino acids 254–277 from the mature enzyme. Symptoms may be induced at any age. Hepatomegaly may be the only sign but is often associated with splenomegaly and gastrointestinal symptoms. Affected individuals rarely live beyond the fifth decade, dying of liver failure or myocardial infarction. Kinetic studies have shown that the hypercholesterolemia is due to an overproduction of VLDL apoB-100 and an impaired LDL clearance. Lovastatin (10–80 mg/day) was shown to lower LDL-C without normalizing it and to reduce the hepatosplenomegaly substantially. It decreases the apoB production rate but paradoxically does not increase the fractional catabolic rate of LDL. According to studies in mice, this disease may be amenable to gene therapy.

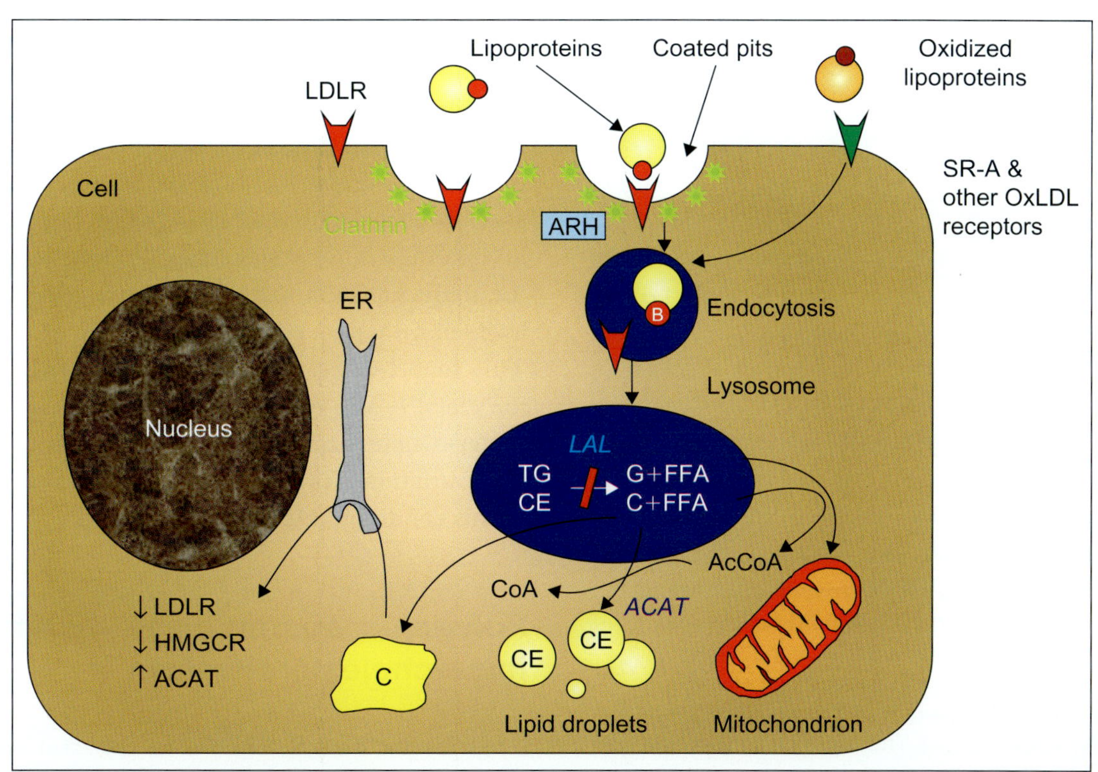

1.37 Site of enzymatic defect in Wolman's disease and cholesteryl ester storage disease (CESD). Cholesteryl esters (CE) and triglycerides (TG) carried by lipoproteins (LDL, VLDL, chylomicron remnants, IDL, oxidized LDL or modified LDL) are taken up by receptor-mediated endocytosis to reach the lysosome for processing. In the lysosome, the receptor is either broken down or exported for recycling. TG and CE are hydrolysed to their components: glycerol (G), free cholesterol (C), and free fatty acids (FFA) by lysosomal acid lipase (LAL). Normally, the free cholesterol is liberated into the cytoplasm where it is re-esterified with fatty acids by acyl-CoA:cholesterol acyl transferase (ACAT) for storage in lipid droplets or the FFA are directed towards mitochondria for β-oxidation. When LAL is mutated (red bar), the defective enzyme leads to accumulation of TG and CE in the lysosome and accounts for lipid infiltration of the liver, intestine, spleen, adrenals, testes and many other tissues. Macrophages, with their many cell surface receptors for oxidized LDL such as scavenger receptor A (SR-A), lectin-like oxidized LDL receptor (LOX-1), CD-36, scavenger receptor for phosphatidylserine and oxidized LDL (SR-PSOX) etc. will turn into lipid-laden foam cells (favouring the atherogenic process in the arterial wall). The free cholesterol pool of the cell (lower left) has important regulatory functions on LDL receptor activity (↓), HMG-CoA reductase (↓), and ACAT activity (↑). Its reduction in LAL deficiency promotes increased HMG-CoA reductase activity, increased LDL receptor (LDLR) expression in Wolman's disease but reduced LDLR expression in CESD (because of residual LAL activity in the latter), and reduced ACAT activity. Modified with permission from Assmann G, Seedorf U (2001). *Molecular Bases of Metabolic Disease.* McGraw Hill, New York.

A diagnosis of CESD in a hypercholesterolemic patient should be suspected if it is associated with the presence of hepatomegaly and splenomegaly, abnormal liver enzymes (alanine aminotransferase and aspartate aminotransferase elevation), absence of a family history of premature coronary artery disease (because of the recessive mode of inheritance), and absence of xanthomas that are seen in familial hypercholesterolemia. Other manifestations may include severe chronic diarrhea and weight loss (the only presentation in a recently reported case), recurrent abdominal pain, neurological complaints (headaches, vertigo, hypersomnia, loss of consciousness), gastrointestinal bleeding, hypoprothrombinemia, epistaxis and delayed puberty. Liver biopsy may assist in establishing the diagnosis and the extent of liver involvement. Light microscopy will demonstrate lipid droplets in parenchymal cells and in enlarged Kupffer's cells, septal fibrosis and periportal inflammation. Electron microscopy will reveal cytoplasmic inclusions limited by trilaminar membranes characteristic of lysosomes (**1.38**). The diagnosis is confirmed by measurement of acid lipase activity in lymphocytes or skin fibroblasts. Neutral lipid accumulation may be demonstrated in cultured skin fibroblasts taken from severe cases or in circulating leucocytes (**1.39**). Sequencing of *LIPA* is used in specialist clinics to determine the causal mutations.

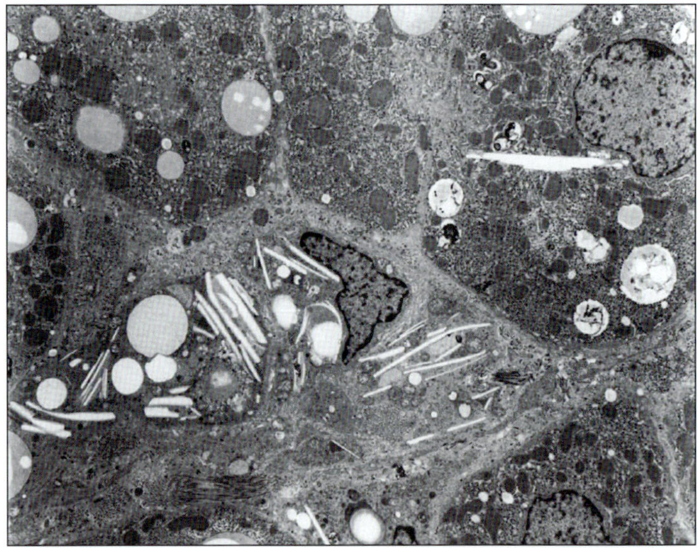

1.38 Electron micrograph of a liver biopsy in cholesteryl ester storage disease showing typical lipid inclusions. Ultrastructural features of the portal tract showing many vacuoles and empty clefts left by the fixation procedure of cholesteryl esters in the cytoplasm of parenchymal cells and of an enlarged Kupffer's cell (centre). The liver biopsy was obtained from a 5-year-old girl with hyperlipoproteinemia, severe diarrhea and hepatosplenomegaly. The membrane-lacking parenchymal droplets contained mostly triglycerides whereas the material in Kupffer's cells represented cholesteryl ester deposits frequently limited by cytomembranes. Reproduced with permission from Boldrini R *et al.* (2004). Wolman disease and cholesteryl ester storage disease diagnosed by histological and ultrastructural examination of intestinal and liver biopsy. *Pathol Res Prac*, **200**: 231–240.

The report of a serendipitous diagnosis of CESD in a 51-year-old man from a liver biopsy performed because of suspected liver cancer has raised important questions. This man had a long clinical history of combined hyperlipidemia (total cholesterol of 10.7 mmol/l; triglycerides of 3.8 mmol/l) and severe premature atherosclerosis but no hepatomegaly, liver dysfunction or splenomegaly. He was homozygous for the frequent G934→A mutation. He died aged 52 years of liver failure as a consequence of extensive tumour infiltration. This report indicates that CESD may remain undetected for years. It also raises the possibility that this condition is under-diagnosed and more common than anticipated. The wide variation of phenotypic expression also makes diagnosis of this condition difficult in adulthood.

Polygenic, sporadic and multifactorial hypercholesterolemias

These terms have been used loosely and sometimes interchangeably to describe hypercholesterolemias of undetermined etiology. These may occur in the absence of a family history (sporadic), may be associated with a familial component of imprecise genetic mode of inheritance or may be construed as being the result of the interaction of several genes with a small effect (oligogenic or polygenic). They may be the result of one or more environmental factors (e.g.

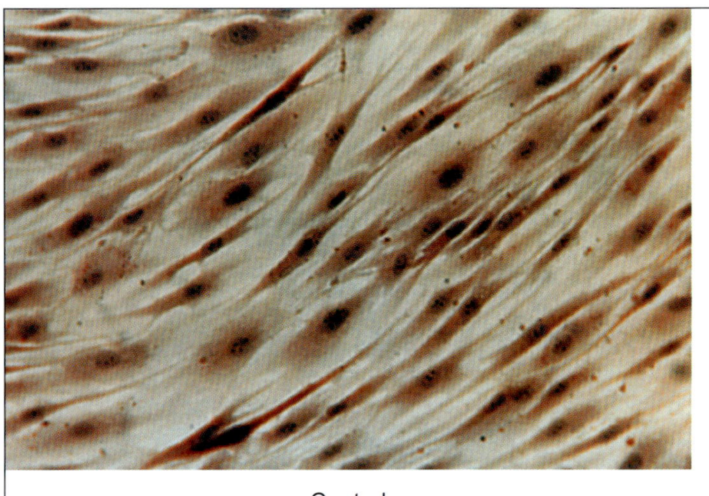

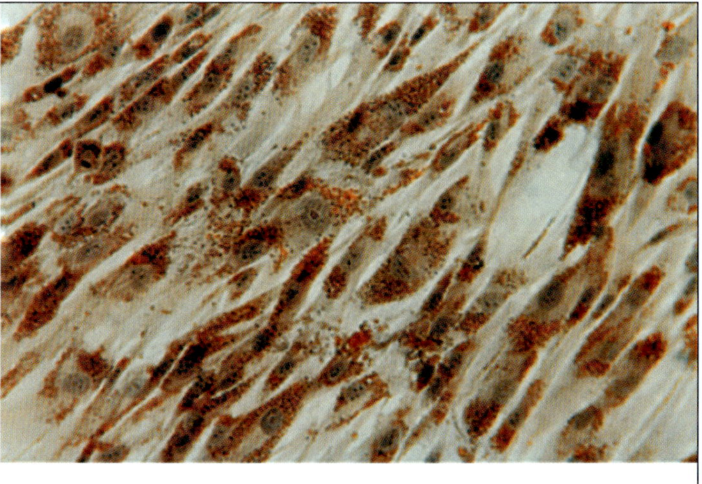

1.39 Neutral lipid accumulation in fibroblasts in Wolman's disease. Staining of neutral lipids with oil red O in a monolayer culture of fibroblasts from a normal subject and a patient with Wolman's disease (fetal death). The massive intracellular accumulation of orange-red droplets reflects the presence of trapped cholesteryl esters in lysosomal vesicles characteristic of acid lysosomal lipase deficiency. Reproduced with permission from Zschenker O *et al.* (2001). Characterization of lysosomal acid lipase mutations in the signal peptide and mature polypeptide region causing Wolman disease. *J Lipid Res*, **42**: 1033–1040.

high saturated fat – high cholesterol diet, obesity, caloric excess, stress, subclinical hypothyroidism, pregnancy, menopause) interacting (or otherwise) with a genetic predisposing factor or susceptibility gene (multifactorial). They apply also to hyperlipidemias generally. In the study of Goldstein and colleagues in 1973 on myocardial infarction survivors, which led to the notion of familial combined hyperlipidemia, 14% had isolated hypercholesterolemia and 17% had isolated

hypertriglyceridemia defined as 'sporadic or polygenic' with no definite etiology established (**1.40**). This work served as the basis for defining familial combined hyperlipidemia (see Chapter 2). The terms as currently used may be reflecting undetermined or non-established etiology or a combination of unrelated cholesterol- (or lipid-) raising factors (multifactorial).

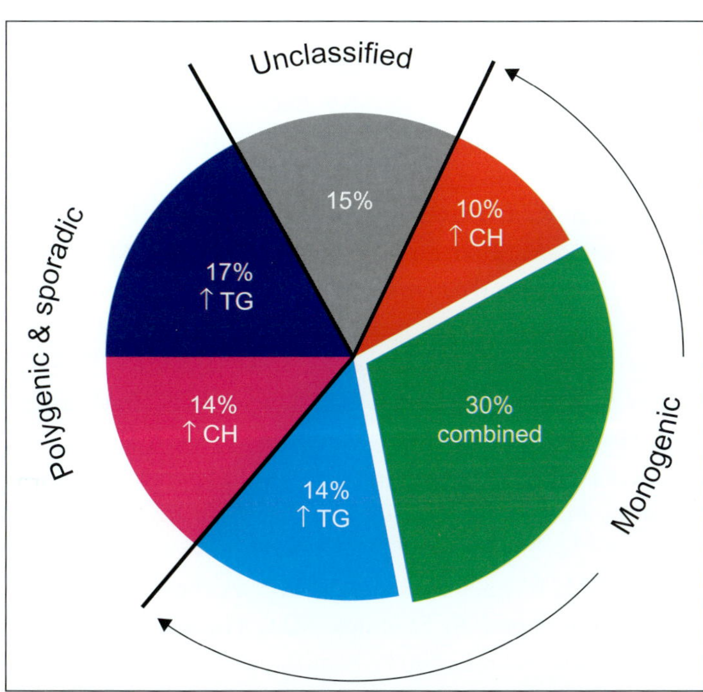

1.40 Genetic hyperlipidemia in 157 myocardial infarction survivors. From 500 individuals who survived a myocardial infarction, a family study was carried out in 157 (31%) who were hyperlipidemic and served as probands for genetic analysis. The 95th percentile was used as a cut-off point to separate normolipidemic from hyperlipidemic individuals. Those in the unclassified category represent survivors in whom a family study was not possible because fewer than three relatives were available. Four cases of type III dysbetalipoproteinemia (2.4% of these 157 subjects) are not included here. A 'monogenic' mode of inheritance included 10% with isolated hypercholesterolemia (CH), 14% with isolated hypertriglyceridemia (TG) and 30% who, along with their relatives, had either hypercholesterolemia, hypertriglyceridemia or both. This served to define 'familial combined hyperlipidemia'. In some of the 'polygenic' and 'sporadic' cases, no hyperlipidemia was found on re-testing in the absence of drug therapy. Redrawn with permission from Goldstein JL *et al.* (1973). Hyperlipidemia in coronary heart disease. II. Genetic analysis of lipid levels in 176 families and delineation of a new inherited disorder, combined hyperlipidemia. *J Clin Invest*, **52**: 1544–1568.

Further reading

Dominant monogenic forms
Familial hypercholesterolemia (FH)

Aalst-Cohen ES, Jansen AC, De Jongh S, Sauvage Nolting PR, Kastelein JJ (2004). Clinical, diagnostic, and therapeutic aspects of familial hypercholesterolemia. *Semin Vasc Med*, **4**: 31–41.

Brown MS, Goldstein JL (1986). A receptor-mediated pathway for cholesterol homeostasis. *Science*, **232**: 34–47.

Civeira F and Management Familial Int Panel (2004). Guidelines for the diagnosis and management of heterozygous familial hypercholesterolemia. *Atherosclerosis*, **173**: 55–68.

Hobbs HH, Russell DW, Brown MS, Goldstein JL (1990). The LDL receptor locus in familial hypercholesterolemia: mutational analysis of a membrane protein. *Annu Rev Genet*, **24**: 133–170.

Hopkins PN (2003). Familial hypercholesterolemia – improving treatment and meeting guidelines. *Int J Cardiol*, **89**: 13–23.

Morganroth J, Levy RI, McMahon AE, Gotto AMJ (1974). Pseudohomozygous type II hyperlipoproteinemia. *J Pediatr*, **85**: 639–643.

Schmidt HHJ, Stuhrmann M, Shamburek R, Schewe CK, Ebhardt M, Zech LA, Buttner C, Wendt M, Beisiegel U, Brewer HB Jr, Manns MP (1998). Delayed low-density lipoprotein (LDL) catabolism despite a functional intact LDL-apolipoprotein B particle and LDL-receptor in a subject with clinical homozygous familial hypercholesterolemia. *J Clin Endocrinol Metab*, **83**: 2167–2174.

Tremblay AJ, Lamarche B, Ruel IL, Hogue JC, Bergeron J, Gagne C, Couture P (2004). Increased production of VLDL apoB-100 in subjects with familial hypercholesterolemia carrying the same null LDL receptor gene mutation. *J Lipid Res*, **45**: 866–872.

Familial defective apolipoprotein B-100 (FDB)

Borén J, Ekström U, Ågren B, Nilsson-Ehle P, Innerarity TL (2001). The molecular mechanism for the genetic disorder familial defective apolipoprotein B100. *J Biol Chem*, **276**: 9214–9218.

Davignon J, Dufour R, Roy M, Betard C, Ma Y, Ouellette S, Boulet L, Lussier-Cacan S (1992). Phenotypic heterogeneity associated with defective apolipoprotein B-100 and occurrence of the familial hypercholesterolemia phenotype in the absence of an LDL-receptor defect within a Canadian kindred. *Eur J Epidemiol*, **8**(Suppl 1):10–17.

Innerarity TL, Mahley RW, Weisgraber KH, Bersot TP, Krauss RM, Vega GL, Grundy SM, Friedl W, Davignon J, McCarthy BJ (1990). Familial defective apolipoprotein B-100: a mutation of apolipoprotein B that causes hypercholesterolemia. *J Lipid Res*, **31**: 1337–1349.

Miserez AR, Muller PY (2000). Familial defective apolipoprotein B-100: a mutation emerged in the Mesolithic ancestors of Celtic peoples? *Atherosclerosis*, **148**: 433–436.

Schaefer JR, Scharnagl H, Baumstark MW, Schweer H, Zech LA, Seyberth H, Winkler K, Steinmetz A, Marz W (1997). Homozygous familial defective apolipoprotein B-100 – Enhanced removal of apolipoprotein E-containing VLDLs and decreased production of LDLs. *Arterioscler Thromb Vasc Biol*, **17**: 348–353.

Whitfield AJ, Barrett PHR, Van Bockxmeer FM, Burnett JR (2004). Lipid disorders and mutations in the *APOB* gene. *Clin Chem*, **50**: 1725–1732.

Autosomal dominant hypercholesterolemia (FH3)

Abifadel M, Varret M, Rabes JP, Allard D, Ouguerram K, Devillers M, Cruaud C, Benjannet S, Wickham L, Erlich D, Derre A, Villeger L, Farnier M, Beucler I, Bruckert E, Chambaz J, Chanu B, Lecerf JM, Luc G, Moulin P, Weissenbach J, Prat A, Krempf M, Junien C, Seidah NG, Boileau C (2003). Mutations in PCSK9 cause autosomal dominant hypercholesterolemia. *Nat Genet*, **34**: 154–156.

Benjannet S, Rhainds D, Hamelin J, Nassoury N, Seidah NG (2006). The proprotein convertase (PC) PCSK9 is inactivated by furin and/or PC5/6A: functional consequences of natural mutations and post-translational modifications. *J Biol Chem*, **281**: 30561–30572.

Chen SN, Ballantyne CM, Gotto AM Jr, Tan Y, Willerson JT, Marian AJ (2005). A common PCSK9 haplotype, encompassing the E670G coding single nucleotide polymorphism, is a novel genetic marker for plasma low-density lipoprotein cholesterol levels and severity of coronary atherosclerosis. *J Am Coll Cardiol*, **45**: 1611–1619.

Dubuc G, Chamberland A, Wassef H, Davignon J, Seidah NG, Bernier L, Prat A (2004). Statins upregulate PCSK9, the gene encoding the proprotein convertase neural apoptosis-regulated convertase-1 implicated in familial hypercholesterolemia. *Arterioscler Thromb Vasc Biol*, **24**: 1454–1459.

Lagace TA, Curtis DE, Garuti R, McNutt MC, Park SW, Prather HB, Anderson NN, Ho YK, Hammer RE, Horton JD (2006). Secreted PCSK9 decreases the number of LDL receptors in hepatocytes and in livers of parabiotic mice. *J Clin Invest*, **116**: 2995–3005.

Ouguerram K, Chetiveaux M, Zair Y, Costet P, Abifadel M, Varret M, Boileau C, Magot T, Krempf M (2004). Apolipoprotein B100 metabolism in autosomal-dominant hypercholesterolemia related to mutations in PCSK9. *Arterioscler Thromb Vasc Biol*, **24**: 1448–1453.

Rashid S, Curtis DE, Garuti R, Anderson NN, Bashmakov Y, Ho YK, Hammer RE, Moon YA, Horton JD (2005). Decreased plasma cholesterol and hypersensitivity to statins in mice lacking Pcsk9. *Proc Natl Acad Sci USA*, **102**: 5374–5379.

Timms KM, Wagner S, Samuels ME, Forbey K, Goldfine H, Jammulapati S, Skolnick MH, Hopkins PN, Hunt SC, Shattuck DM (2004). A mutation in *PCSK9* causing autosomal-dominant hypercholesterolemia in a Utah pedigree. *Hum Genet*, **114**: 349–353.

Varret M, Rabès JP, Saint-Jore B, Cenarro A, Marinoni JC, Civeira F, Devillers M, Krempf M, Coulon M, Thiart R, Kotze MJ, Schmidt H, Buzzi JC, Kostner GM, Bertolini S, Pocovi M, Rosa A, Farnier M, Martinez M, Junien C, Boileau C (1999). A third major locus for autosomal dominant hypercholesterolemia maps to 1p34.1-p32. *Am J Hum Genet*, **64**: 1378–1387.

Deficiency of cholesterol 7α-hydroxylase (CYP7A1)

Beigneux A, Hofmann AF, Young SG (2002). Human CYP7A1 deficiency: progress and enigmas. *J Clin Invest*, **110**: 29–31.

Pullinger CR, Eng C, Salen G, Shefer S, Batta AK, Erickson SK, Verhagen A, Rivera CR, Mulvihill SJ, Malloy MJ, Kane JP (2002). Human cholesterol 7α-hydroxylase (CYP7A1) deficiency has a hypercholesterolemic phenotype. *J Clin Invest*, **110**: 109–117.

Recessive forms

Autosomal recessive hypercholesterolemia

Canizales-Quinteros S, Aguilar-Salinas CA, Huertas-Vazquez A, Ordonez-Sanchez ML, Rodriguez-Torres M, Venturas-Gallegos JL, Riba L, Ramirez-Jimenez S, Salas-Montiel R, Medina-Palacios G, Robles-Osorio L, Miliar-Garcia A, Rosales-Leon L, Ruiz-Ordaz BH, Zentella-Dehesa A, Ferre-D'Amare A, Gomez-Perez FJ, Tusie-Luna MT (2005). A novel ARH splice site mutation in a Mexican kindred with autosomal recessive hypercholesterolemia. *Hum Genet*, **116**: 114–120.

Cohen JC, Kimmel M, Polanski A, Hobbs HH (2003). Molecular mechanisms of autosomal recessive hypercholesterolemia. *Curr Opin Lipidol*, **14**: 121–127.

Garcia CK, Wilund K, Arca M, Zuliani G, Fellin R, Maioli M, Calandra S, Bertolini S, Cossu F, Grishin N, Barnes R, Cohen JC, Hobbs HH (2001). Autosomal recessive hypercholesterolemia caused by mutations in a putative LDL receptor adaptor protein. *Science*, **292**: 1394–1398.

Harada-Shiba M, Takagi A, Miyamoto Y, Tsushima M, Ikeda Y, Yokoyama S, Yamamoto A (2003). Clinical features and genetic analysis of autosomal recessive hypercholesterolemia. *J Clin Endocrinol Metab*, **88**: 2541–2547.

Jones C, Hammer RE, Li WP, Cohen JC, Hobbs HH, Herz J (2003). Normal sorting but defective endocytosis of the low density lipoprotein receptor in mice with autosomal recessive hypercholesterolemia. *J Biol Chem*, **278**: 29024–29030.

Mishra SK, Keyel PA, Edeling MA, Dupin AL, Owen DJ, Traub LM (2005). Functional dissection of an AP-2 beta 2 appendage-binding sequence within the autosomal recessive hypercholesterolemia (ARH) protein. *J Biol Chem*, **280**: 19270–19280.

Naoumova RP, Neuwirth C, Lee P, Miller JP, Taylor KG, Soutar AK (2004). Autosomal recessive hypercholesterolemia: long-term follow up and response to treatment. *Atherosclerosis*, **174**: 165–172.

Soutar AK, Naoumova RP, Traub LM (2003). Genetics, clinical phenotype, and molecular cell biology of autosomal recessive hypercholesterolemia. *Arterioscler Thromb Vasc Biol*, **23**: 1963–1970.

Zuliani G, Vigna GB, Corsini A, Maioli M, Romagnoni F, Fellin R (1995). Severe hypercholesterolemia: unusual inheritance in an Italian pedigree. *Eur J Clin Invest*, **25**: 322–331.

Lysosomal acid lipase deficiency

Assmann G, Seedorf U (2001). Acid lipase deficiency: Wolman's disease and cholesteryl ester storage disease. In: Scriver CR, Beaudet AL, Sly WS, Valle D (eds) *The Metabolic and Molecular Bases of Inherited Disease*. McGraw-Hill, New York, pp. 3551–3572.

Boldrini R, Devito R, Biselli R, Filocamo M, Bosman C (2004). Wolman disease and cholesteryl ester storage disease diagnosed by histological and ultrastructural examination of intestinal and liver biopsy. *Pathol Res Pract*, **200**: 231–240.

Drebber U, Andersen M, Kasper HU, Lohse P, Stolte M, Dienes HP (2005). Severe chronic diarrhea and weight loss in cholesteryl ester storage disease: a case report. *World J Gastroenterol*, **11**: 2364–2366.

Du H, Heur M, Witte DP, Ameis D, Grabowski GA (2002). Lysosomal acid lipase deficiency: Correction of lipid storage by adenovirus-mediated gene transfer in mice. *Hum Gene Ther*, **13**: 1361–1372.

Levy R, Ostlund RE Jr, Schonfeld G, Wong P, Semenkovich CF (1992). Cholesteryl ester storage disease: complex molecular effects of chronic lovastatin therapy. *J Lipid Res*, **33**: 1005–1015.

Chapter 2

Hereditary Hypertriglyceridemias

Lipoprotein lipase deficiency (familial hyperchylomicronemia)

Lipoprotein lipase (LPL) deficiency (OMIM No. 238600) is a rare autosomal recessive disorder, which was first reported as a separate entity in Europe by Bürger and Grütz in 1932 (hepatosplenomegalic lipidosis with xanthomatosis, the Bürger–Grütz disease), and by Holt and co-workers at Johns Hopkins University in 1939 (idiopathic familial lipemia) when the recessive mode of inheritance was recognized. The link with defective clearance of triglyceride-rich lipoproteins was made in the early 1960s by Havel and Gordon. It was also called familial fat-induced hyperlipemia because dietary fat markedly worsened the hypertriglyceridemia, and familial hyperchylomicronemia or type I hyperlipoproteinemia in the Fredrickson classification (referring to the selective accumulation of chylomicrons in fasting plasma). It was given a name related to its etiology when it was shown to be secondary to LPL gene (*LPL*) mutations. The word chylomicronemia is sometimes used instead of hyperchylomicronemia because in normal fasting plasma, chylomicrons are usually absent or barely measurable. The term 'chylomicronemia syndrome' has a more general meaning, referring to the presence in plasma of large lipoprotein particles that originate from dietary fat. This occurs in many forms of hereditary or acquired hypertriglyceridemia.

LPL is a key enzyme in lipid metabolism. It is expressed in various tissues, primarily adipocytes, skeletal muscle cells and the heart. Its primary function is to hydrolyse the triglyceride-rich lipoproteins (TRL), chylomicron and very-low-density lipoproteins (VLDL) in the vessel lumen to liberate monoglycerides and free fatty acids (FFA) for tissue utilization. In the process, smaller cholesteryl ester enriched remnant lipoproteins are formed for clearance by the liver and surface remnants carrying apolipoprotein AI (apoAI) are transferred to high-density lipoproteins (HDL). When this enzyme is deficient there is reduced formation of chylomicron remnants, fewer FFA reaching the liver to contribute to VLDL formation with fewer apoAI surface remnants for HDL, which results in high triglyceride, low low-density lipoprotein-cholesterol (LDL-C) and low HDL-C (**2.1**). The major co-factor and activator of LPL is apoCII present in HDL, VLDL and chylomicrons. FFA are the main energy source of skeletal muscle, and are stored in human adipose tissue if not used immediately for energy. The remnants of these TRL are eventually taken up by the liver through receptor-mediated endocytosis where LPL, apoE and proteoglycans contribute to ligand binding (**2.2**). The LDL receptor (LDLR) and the LDL receptor-related protein (LRP) are the main receptors for remnant lipoprotein uptake in the liver. The VLDL receptor appears to be involved in other tissues (heart, skeletal muscle, fat, brain and macrophages) and the apoB-48 receptor located on macrophages may take up chylomicron remnants and favour foam cell formation. The existence of LPL was first recognized by Paul Hahn in 1943 when he noticed that an intravenous injection of heparin could clear postprandial lipemia in dogs. It was therefore given the name 'heparin-releasable clearing factor' because LPL, which is attached to the endothelium by membrane-bound heparan sulphate proteoglycan chains (**2.2**), is displaced by heparin that competes for binding to HSPG and released for massive action. Post-heparin lipolytic activity is used to demonstrate low or absent LPL activity in familial hyperchylomicronemia. The contribution of the two components, LPL and hepatic lipase (HL) can also be determined individually.

The human LPL gene is located on chromosome 8 (8p22), spans ~30 kb, comprises 10 exons and encodes a

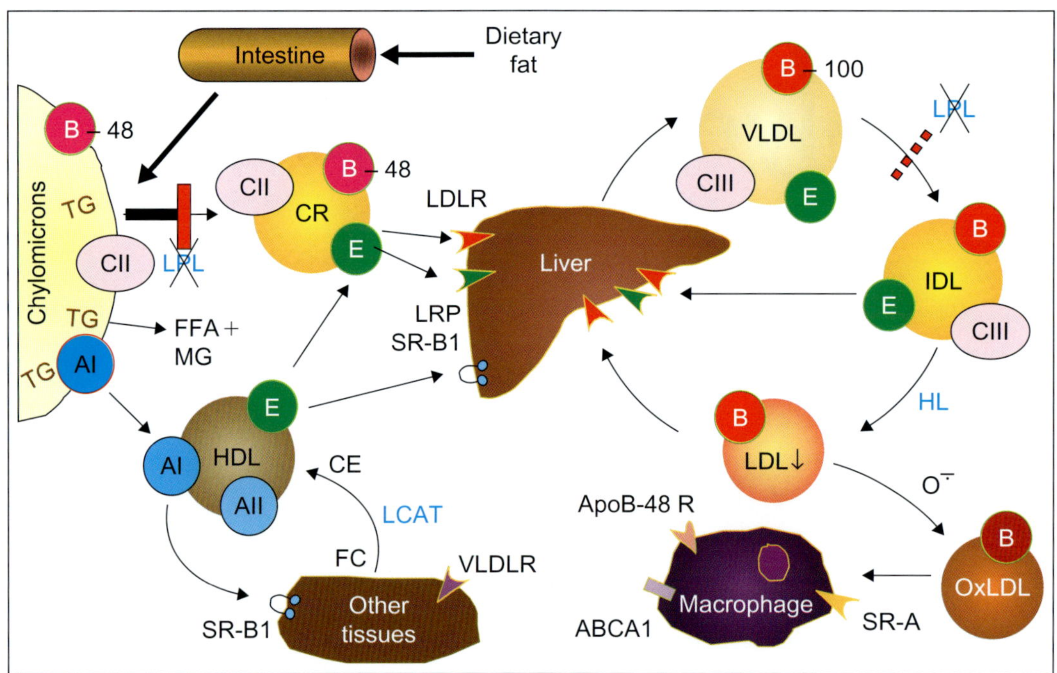

2.1 Metabolic defect in lipoprotein lipase (LPL) deficiency. Dietary fat is processed into micelles and absorbed in the intestine where it is packaged by the enterocytes into chylomicrons. These very large lipoprotein particles (>75 nm) are rich in triglycerides (TG) and maintained in 'solution' in plasma by their surface apolipoproteins, mainly apoB-48, apoAI and apoCs. ApoCII is an activator of LPL, surface apoAI is transferred to high-density lipoproteins (HDL) and apoB-48 serves to interact with receptors once these particles are broken down by LPL and acquire apoE from HDL to become chylomicron remnants (CR). This transformation is the result of the action of LPL bound to the endothelium that hydrolyses triglycerides into free fatty acids (FFA) – also referred to as non-esterified fatty acids (NEFA) – monoglycerides, and glycerol as the particles travel in the blood stream.

The remnant particles are taken up by the liver through receptor-mediated endocytosis; essentially via the LDL receptor and the LDL receptor-related protein (LRP). LPL contributes to this receptor uptake. In LPL deficiency (shown by the red vertical bar) there is reduced formation of chylomicron remnants, less FFA reaching the liver to contribute to VLDL formation, and less apoAI surface remnants for HDL, which results in high triglycerides, low low-density lipoprotein-cholesterol (LDL-C) and low HDL-C. There is an apoB-48 receptor on macrophages that can take up chylomicron remnants and contribute to the formation of foam cells and therefore to atherogenesis. In LPL deficiency, fewer CM particles reach the macrophage apoB-48 receptor which may account for the rarity of atherosclerosis reported in this disease. LPL also contributes to the lipolysis of very-low-density lipoproteins (VLDL) and it is a paradox (still unexplained) that familial hyperchylomicronemia is usually not associated with an increase in VLDL. VLDL production can increase for other reasons, however; in this case the lipoprotein phenotype includes both an excess of chylomicrons and an excess VLDL (type V pattern) (see **2.7**). The VLDL receptor (VLDLR) is not present in the liver and has been claimed to contribute to the uptake of lipoprotein remnants. See **1.2** for abbreviations and further information.

475 amino acid protein containing 5 domains including a 27-amino acid signal peptide. Nearly 100 different mutations have been found in the LPL gene, most located in exons 5 and 6, some of which affect the function of the enzyme. The most common mutations are the $Asp_9 \rightarrow Asn$ (D9N), $Gly_{188} \rightarrow Glu$ (G188E), $Asn_{291} \rightarrow Ser$ (D291S) and $Ser_{447} \rightarrow Ter$ (S447X) substitutions (**2.3**). One mutation, $Ser_{447} \rightarrow Ter$ (S447X), is associated with a gain of function of LPL activity, reduced triglycerides and increased HDL-C. LPL deficiency occurs with a frequency of about 1 in 1 000 000 worldwide. The frequency of the disease may be higher in areas where a founder effect exists.

Homozygosity and compound heterozygosity for mutations in the LPL gene resulting in loss of enzyme function are the major causes of familial hyperchylomicronemia. Although LPL is bound to the capillary endothelium, LPL mRNA is not found in the endothelial cells but rather in the adjacent cells (i.e. hepatocyte, adipocyte, cardiomyocyte, or macrophage) from where it is secreted.

LPL deficiency usually starts in childhood with symptoms of severe abdominal pain, acute pancreatitis, and hepatosplenomegaly, and failure to thrive. In adults, other typical manifestations include eruptive xanthomas (**2.4**), lipemia retinalis (**2.5**), memory loss, and sensory peripheral

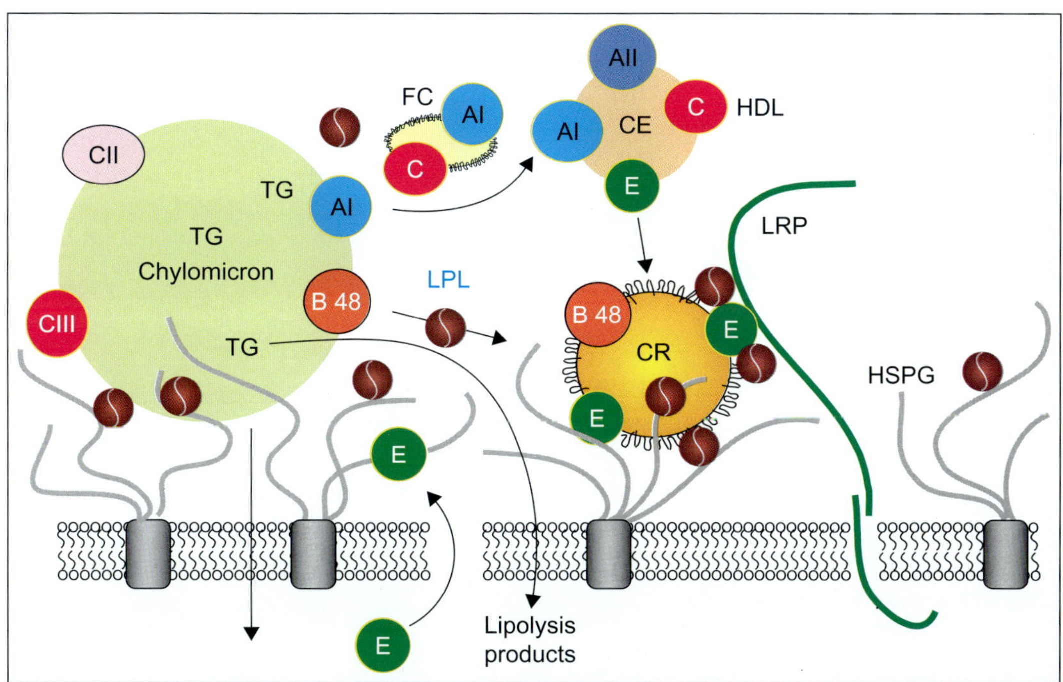

2.2 A model of chylomicron remnant uptake. The lipoprotein lipase (LPL) homodimers (dark red circles) can bind simultaneously to heparan sulphate proteoglycan (HSPG) (grey chains anchored to integral membrane proteins), to lipoproteins, and to other proteins such as apoE and receptors. This allows contact of several LPL molecules with the large chylomicrons for their effective hydrolysis. Lipolysis occurs through a series of attachment and detachment events. The products of lipolysis diffuse in the subendothelial space. ApoE (green circles) is secreted by the hepatocytes into the space of Dissé and reaches the endothelium surface to link with the remnants. LPL, because of its non-catalytic bridging function, facilitates apoE ligand binding to LDL receptor-related protein (LRP) and other receptors, thereby enhancing their clearance by the underlying hepatocytes. HSPG and apoE play a critical role in the sequestration and capture of the remnants. As the large particles shrink down into the remnant size, their surfaces become redundant (frills on CR) and surface components including free cholesterol (FC) and apoAI split off and are transferred to HDL. Chylomicron remnants (CR) gain apoE mostly from HDL, lose apoCII, and are taken up by LRP for endocytosis. It seems that hepatic lipase also secreted by the hepatocytes has a similar role to that of LPL. A direct uptake by HSPG has also been postulated. Composite diagram redrawn from Olivecrona T, Bengtsson-Olivecrona G (1993). Lipoprotein lipase and hepatic lipase. *Curr Opin Lipidol*, **4**: 187–196. Ji ZS, Fazio S, Lee YL, Mahley RW (1994). Secretion-capture role for apolipoprotein E in remnant lipoprotein metabiolism involving cell surface heparan sulfate proteoglycans. *J Biol Chem*, **269**: 2764–2772 and Mahley RW, Ji ZS (1999). Remnant lipoprotein metabolism: key pathways involving cell- surface heparan sulfate proteoglycans and apolipopprotein E. *J Lipd Res*, **40**: 1–16.

neuropathy. It is also characterized by severe fasting hypertriglyceridemia, usually greater than 11.3 mmol/l (1000 mg/dl); a large increase in chylomicrons, giving a milky appearance to plasma, which is topped by a creamy layer on standing; low HDL-C levels; and small dense LDL particles (**2.6**). These patients generally do not seem to be at increased cardiovascular risk.

The frequency of heterozygosity for the four most common mutations of the LPL gene in population-based studies ranges from 0.04% to 22%. The reduction in post-heparin plasma LPL activity also varies greatly depending on the mutation, from –53% for $Gly_{188} \rightarrow Glu$ to +4% for $Ser_{447} \rightarrow Ter$ substitutions. Consequently, the average change in plasma triglycerides of heterozygous carriers ranges from +78% to –8% and the change in HDL-C from –0.25 to +0.04 mmol/l. The odds ratio for ischemic heart disease in heterozygous carriers of the $Gly_{188} \rightarrow Glu$ mutation is 4.9, and only 0.8 for those bearing the $Ser_{447} \rightarrow Ter$ mutation. Most of the heterozygous subjects do not have the typical clinical manifestations of the homozygotes, unless a secondary cause of hypertriglyceridemia (such as obesity, alcohol consumption, diabetes mellitus, pregnancy) or other hyperlipidemia-inducing gene defects that contribute to increased TRL synthesis are present.

Diagnosis of LPL deficiency is based essentially on the typical clinical picture, in particular eruptive xanthomas in adults, and hepatosplenomegaly and abdominal pain in children, evidence of consanguinity in the family and

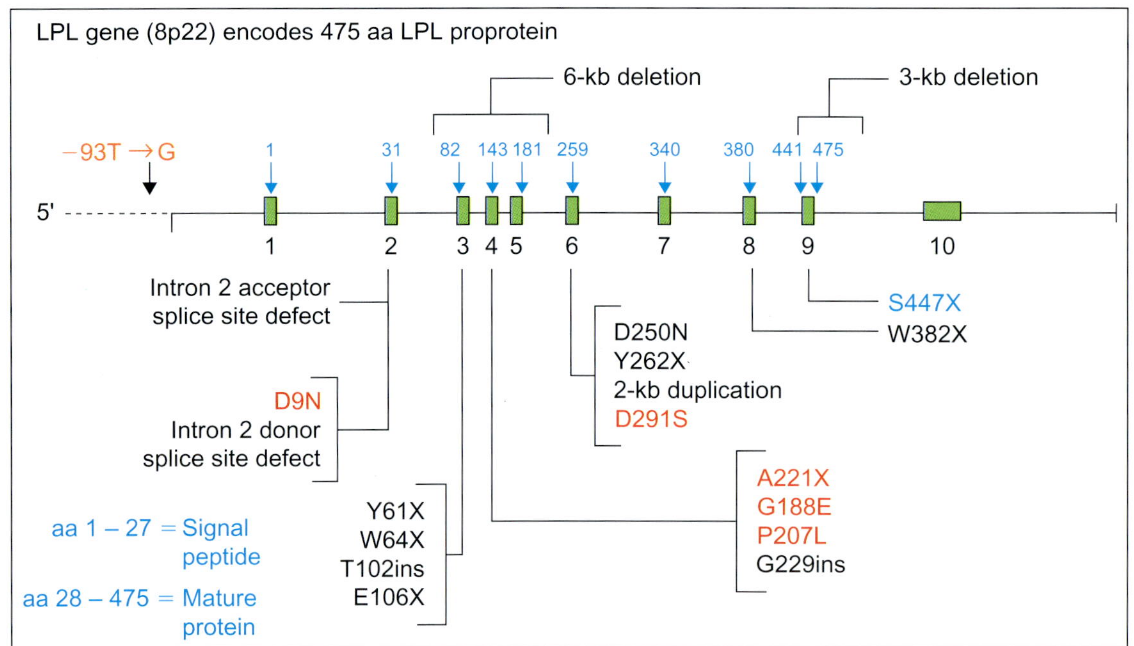

2.3 Major mutations of the lipoprotein lipase (LPL) gene. This diagram provides the gene location of a few of nearly 100 different reported mutations. The most common mutations of the LPL gene are depicted in red. Gilbert and co-workers ([2001]. *Ann Génét*, **4**: 25–32) indexed all publications on *LPL* mutations and noted that one of them, G188E, was observed in 52 cases from 17 articles. These mutations are all associated with the chylomicronemia phenotype except S447X (blue), which is associated with an increased activity of LPL, reduced triglycerides, and increased high-density lipoprotein-cholesterol (HDL-C), and D291S, which has a modest effect on plasma lipoproteins. *LPL* mutations are distributed widely in the world. The promoter variant −93T→G represents 76% of *LPL* mutations in African blacks. The most common mutations among French-Canadians in the Province of Quebec where a founder effect exists are P207L, G188E, and D250N. Diagram partially updated from Santamarina-Fojo S (1992). Genetic dyslipoproteinemias: role of lipoprotein lipase and apolipoprotein C-II. *Curr Opin Lipidol*, **3**: 186–195.

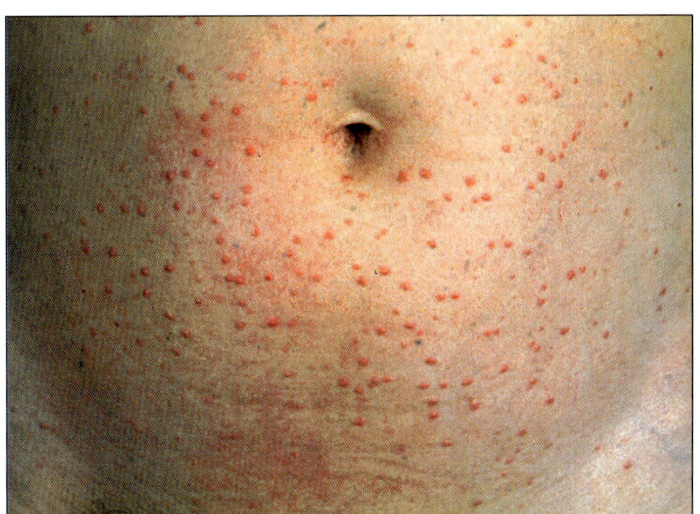

2.4 Eruptive xanthomas of the abdomen in lipoprotein lipase (LPL) deficiency. Eruptive xanthomas are usually yellowish to whitish, often with a reddish base. They are frequently found on the arms, back, thorax and buttocks. They appear in clusters, crops or as a few sparse lesions on hands or other parts of the body. They may develop within a few days and are often mistaken by the affected individual for a rash or an infection. They supervene in about 50% of subjects with LPL deficiency.

demonstration of fasting chylomicronemia. The exquisite sensitivity of plasma triglycerides to dietary fat is another clue (**2.7**), but a fat load test is usually unnecessary and should be done with caution, if at all, as it has the potential to provoke an attack of pancreatitis. The diagnosis may be confirmed by measuring the post-heparin plasma LPL lipolytic activity, measuring post-heparin plasma LPL mass, or by more specifically identifying the causal mutation in the LPL gene, as may be done in several lipid clinics. Other primary and secondary causes of chylomicronemia should be excluded. The latter includes: acute alcohol misuse, primary acute pancreatitis with secondary hyperlipidemia, uncontrolled diabetes, hyperlipemia of pregnancy, plasma sample taken after a fatty meal, and mixed hypertriglyceridemia (type V lipoprotein phenotype) without LPL abnormality. Importantly, familial chylomicronemia may present on occasion as mixed hypertriglyceridemia, i.e. high exogenous and endogenous triglycerides (lipoprotein phenotype V), if one of these other conditions is present (**2.7**). This may happen in familial combined hyperlipidemia (see

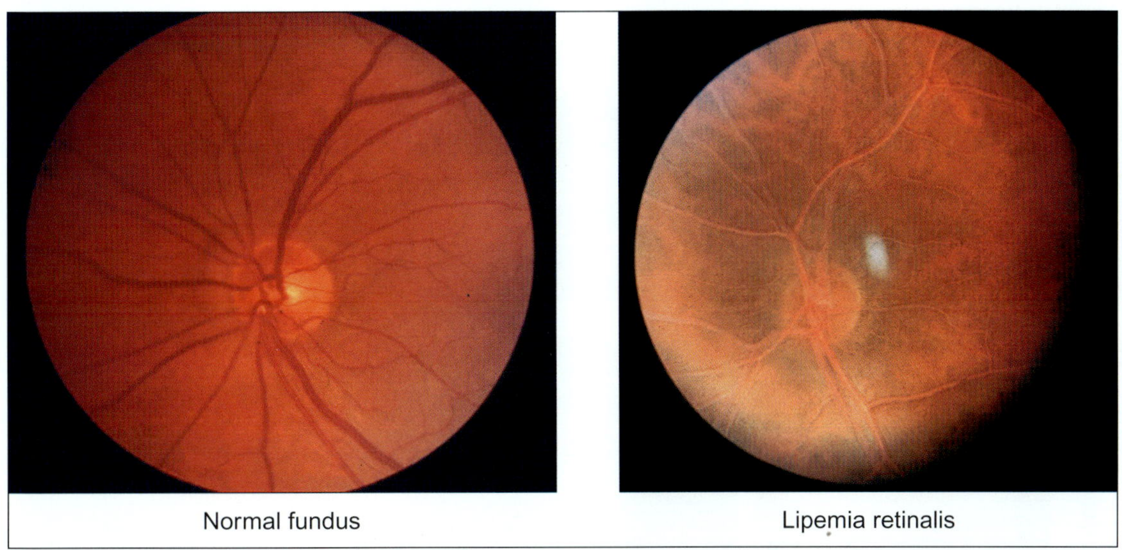

2.5 Lipemia retinalis in lipoprotein lipase (LPL) deficiency. In the normal fundus (left), it is easy to differentiate the pale arteries from the red veins. In contrast, in the lipemic fundus (right) there is virtually no difference in colour between the two. The entire retina and vessels have a pale salmon-pink discoloration. This is the fundus of a young woman with familial hyperchylomicronemia who is homozygous for the G188E mutation. Her lipoprotein electrophoreses are shown in **2.7**. At the time this picture was taken she was hospitalized for acute pancreatitis and her plasma triglyceride level was 90.4 mmol/l (8000 mg/dl). The lipemic aspect of the retinal vessels proceeds from the periphery towards the centre gradually as triglycerides increase. The threshold for these changes is around 22.6 mmol/l (2000 mg/dl).

below). Interference with normal LPL activity is responsible for the other primary causes of hyperchylomicronemia, apoCII deficiency and familial hyperchylomicronemia, due to a circulating inhibitor of lipoprotein lipase.

ApoCII deficiency (OMIM No. 207750) is secondary to a mutation in *APOC2* (**2.8**), the gene on chromosome 19q13.2 that encodes apoCII, the activator of LPL. Breckenridge reported the first cases of apoCII deficiency in Canada in 1978, finding that a transfusion for anemia providing normal apoCII improved the associated severe hypertriglyceridemia. ApoCII deficiency essentially mimics the clinical and biochemical features of familial LPL deficiency except that affected subjects tend to be detected at a later age than the former (13–39 years of age, but as early as 6 years and as late as 60 years) and the phenotype is generally milder, probably depending on the level of residual apoCII in plasma. One case in infancy presented as a lipid encephalopathy. In patients with the disease, apoCII is reduced or absent on isoelectric focusing (IEF) gel electrophoresis of delipidated VLDL (**2.9**). The LPL defect is corrected *in vitro* by addition of plasma from the patient compared with that of a normal subject to activate lipase in the skim-milk lipase assay. Specialized laboratories can determine the specific mutation if necessary.

Familial hyperchylomicronemia due to a circulating inhibitor of lipoprotein lipase (OMIM No. 118830), has been reported in 1983 by Brunzell and co-workers, found in a mother and son. The mother had a clinical phenotype similar to that of LPL deficiency, with eruptive xanthomas, massive hypertriglyceridemia (20.4 mmol/l or 1813 mg/dl of chylomicron triglycerides), no diabetes and a history of unexplained abdominal pain in childhood. Her apoCII was normal. Unlike LPL deficiency, however, LPL was present in adipose tissue at 30-fold and two-fold greater levels than in normal subjects in mother and son, respectively. Their plasma contained an unidentified inhibitor of LPL capable of inhibiting post-heparin plasma lipolytic activity. Present in the non-lipoprotein fraction, the inhibitor was heat-stable, non-dialysable, and sensitive to repeated freezing and thawing. Inheritance did not appear to be recessive as the son and a grandson had marked hypertriglyceridemia. This anomaly remains an enigma.

Treatment of familial hyperchylomicronemia relies on drastic reduction of dietary lipids to less than 10–15% of total calories. This will reduce the triglyceridemia in a few days or weeks (**2.7**). Alcohol intake is contraindicated. Medium-chain triglycerides (MCT) are used to provide a source of fat that does not contribute to chylomicron

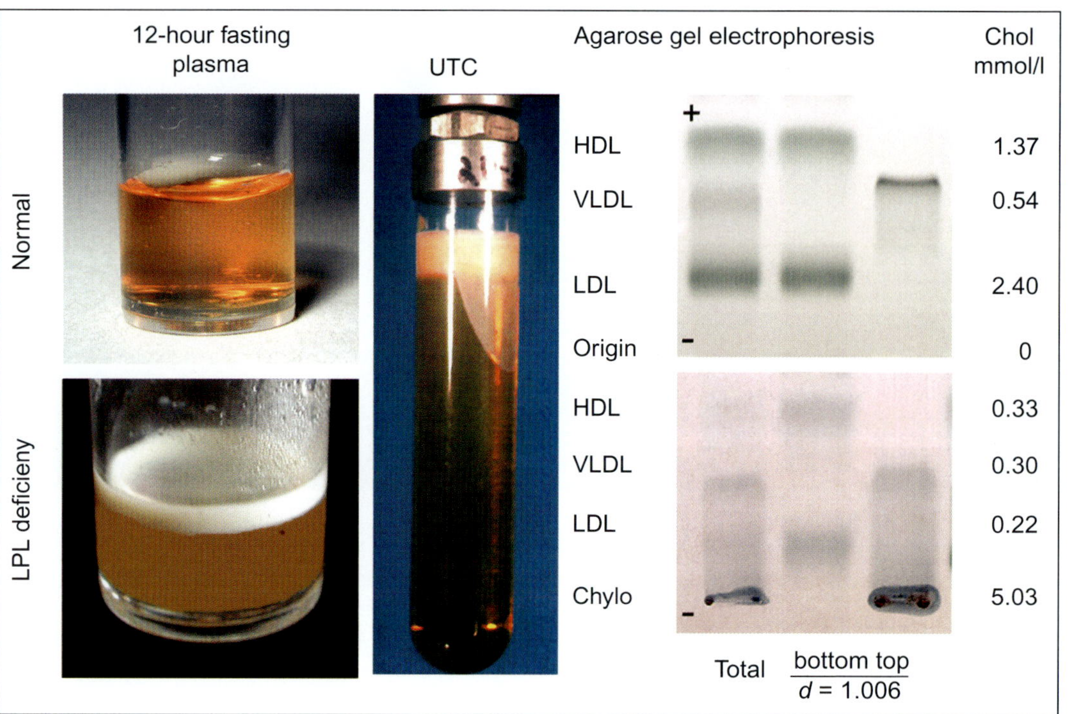

2.6 Demonstration of hyperchylomicronemia in lipoprotein lipase (LPL) deficiency. The left panel compares normal plasma and plasma from an LPL-deficient patient which were left to stand overnight in a refrigerator. The blood samples were obtained after a 12-hour fast. The floating creamy supernatant is typical of hyperchylomicronemia. The plasma before standing is turbid and whitish. The 'refrigerator test' is the simplest way to demonstrate the presence of chylomicrons for the practitioner. Ultracentrifugation at the aqueous density of plasma (d = 1.006), 50 000 rpm in a 50.4 Ti Beckman rotor for 8 hours developing 312 000 $\times$ g, separates chylomicrons and very-low-density lipoproteins (VLDL) at the top of the tube from the other plasma lipoproteins which sink to the bottom (centre panel). The creamy layer is chylomicrons; the white part adhering to the wall downward represents smaller particle size triglyceride-rich lipoproteins (TRL), mostly VLDL.

This is the original preparative ultracentrifugation procedure developed by Havel *et al.* ([1955]. *J Clin Invest*, **35**: 1345.) which separates lipoproteins according to their relative buoyancy. Total plasma and separated lipoproteins (top and bottom of the tube) can then be further separated according to charge by agarose gel electrophoresis as seen in the right panel. The migration is from the origin (–) upward towards the anode (+). The upper electrophoresis is that of a normal plasma, the lower one, that of a patient with LPL deficiency. In the latter, chylomicrons stay at the origin, and the low-density lipoproteins (LDL) (β-lipoproteins), VLDL (preβ-lipoproteins) and high-density lipoproteins (HDL) (α-lipoproteins) are very discrete bands (cholesterol values for these different fractions are given on the right). There are no chylomicrons in normal fasting plasma. The same amount of plasma was deposited at the origin in both cases. Chylomicrons are buoyant and separate readily without having to resort to prolonged ultracentrifugation. Centrifugation at 58 450 $\times$ g will allow their separation from plasma in 30 minutes.

formation. The latter are made in the intestinal wall from absorbed long chain fatty acids ($\geq$16 carbon chains) and reach the circulation via lymphatics; MCT (12–14 carbon chains), in contrast, gain access to the liver via the portal vein and are metabolized differently. Lipid-lowering medications are ineffective in homozygous subjects. In the impending pancreatitis state, stopping food intake and maintaining hydration with water only for 1–2 days will alleviate abdominal pain and may avert an acute pancreatitis. Chylomicronemia syndromes are further discussed below (see Familial mixed hypertriglyceridemia).

Familial endogenous hypertriglyceridemia (familial hypertriglyceridemia)

Familial endogenous hypertriglyceridemia (FEHTG), also called primary, essential or familial hypertriglyceridemia (FHTG), carbohydrate-induced hypertriglyceridemia, or type IV hyperlipoproteinemia is characterized by elevation of fasting plasma triglycerides associated with increased VLDL-C, normal to moderately low LDL-C in smaller, denser more numerous lipoprotein particles and decreased

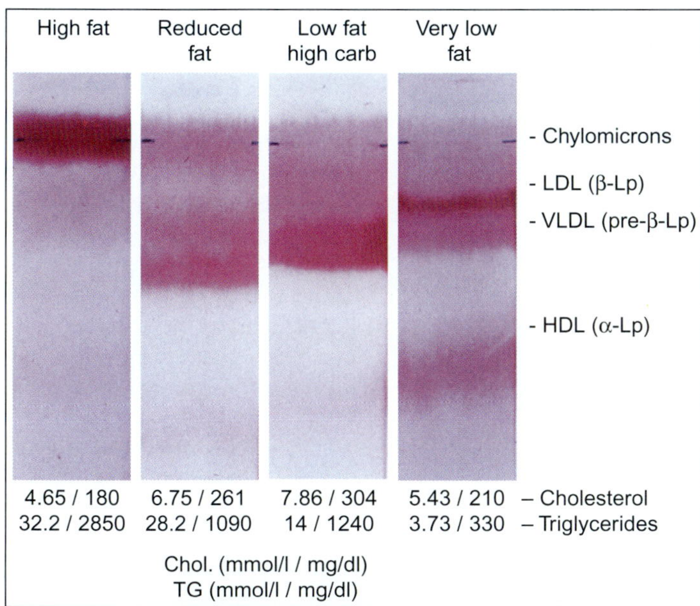

2.7 Diet may change the lipoprotein profile in lipoprotein lipase (LPL) deficiency. The lipoprotein profile is revealed here by paper electrophoresis of total plasma after a 12-hour period of fasting in the same patient with LPL deficiency (homozygous for the G188E mutation) at different times after dietary modifications were made. This is the original method in albumin containing buffer with lipids stained by oil red O developed by Lees and Hatch for the phenotyping of dyslipoproteinemias according to Fredrickson and co-workers (1967). *N Engl J Med* **276**: 34, 94,148, 215, 273. As fat is reduced and carbohydrate (carb) is reciprocally increased in the diet, the hyperchylomicronemia recedes, and the very-low-density lipoproteins (VLDL), low-density lipoproteins (LDL) and high-density lipoproteins (HDL) increase. On the right, on a diet of 15 g of fat per day, there is only a residual hypertriglyceridemia of 3.73 mmol/l. The Fredrickson lipoprotein phenotype evolves from type I to types V, IV and IIb. It is noticeable that very high triglyceride (TG) level due to chylomicronemia is associated with a lower level of total cholesterol (Chol; 4.65 mmol/l) than when the severe hypertriglyceridemia is due to endogenous TG (7.86 mmol/l). In the 'Fredrickson era' the phenotyping was used to diagnose separate disease entities. When used now, it has mostly a descriptive value to report on the lipoprotein distribution, except for type III (familial dysbetalipoproteinemia) which can be strongly suspected on the basis of lipoprotein electrophoresis alone (broad beta band), see Chapter 3.

HDL-C levels. This profile corresponds to Fredrickson's type IV lipoprotein phenotype – this is why it is often referred to as 'type IV'. It has an apparent autosomal dominant mode of inheritance with age-dependent penetrance. Although not caused by conditions raising the level of plasma triglycerides, it can be amplified by them. These conditions include a diet rich in carbohydrate, abdominal obesity with or without

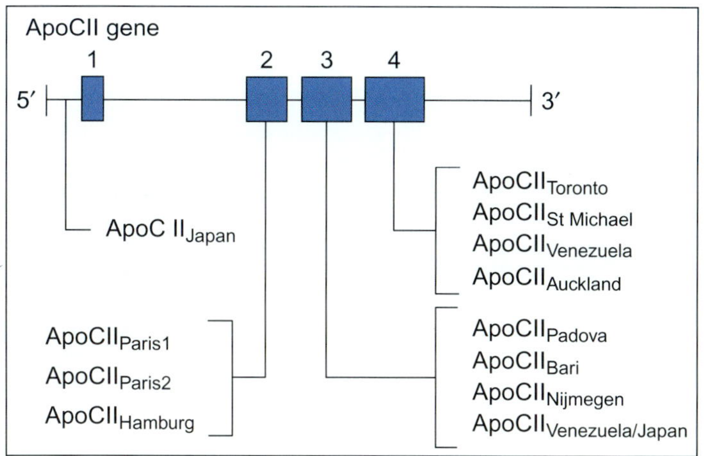

2.8 Mutations associated with apolipoprotein CII (apoCII) deficiency. The apoCII mutations are given by the name of the location where they were discovered rather than the specific DNA (or protein) defects. This illustrates the diversity of origin of the mutations causally related to apoCII deficiency. Redrawn from Santamarina-Fojo S (1992). *Curr Opin Lipidol* (1992). **3**: 186 and updated (Wilson C *et al.* [2003]. Apolipoprotein C-II deficiency presenting as a lipid encephalopathy in infancy. *Ann Neurol*, **53**: 807–810).

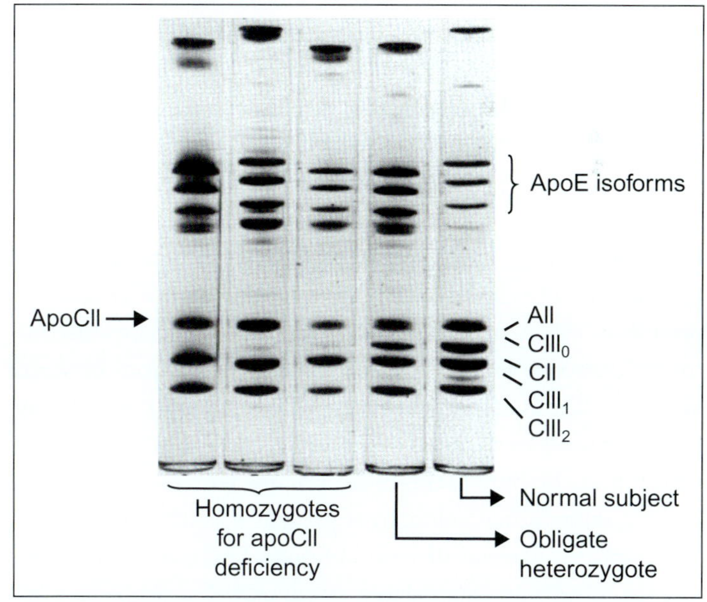

2.9 Isoelectric focusing of very-low-density lipoproteins (VLDL) apolipoproteins in apolipoprotein CII (apoCII) deficiency. Apolipoproteins of delipidated VLDL are separated on a pH gradient by isoelectric focusing. ApoCII is virtually absent from the first three tubes obtained from samples of three subjects homozygous for apoCII deficiency. ApoCII is present, albeit reduced, in an obligate heterozygote sample compared with a normal sample (extreme right). Reproduced from Breckenridge WC *et al.* (1982). Apolipoprotein and lipoprotein concentrations in familial apolipoprotein C-II deficiency. *Atherosclerosis*, **44**: 223–235.

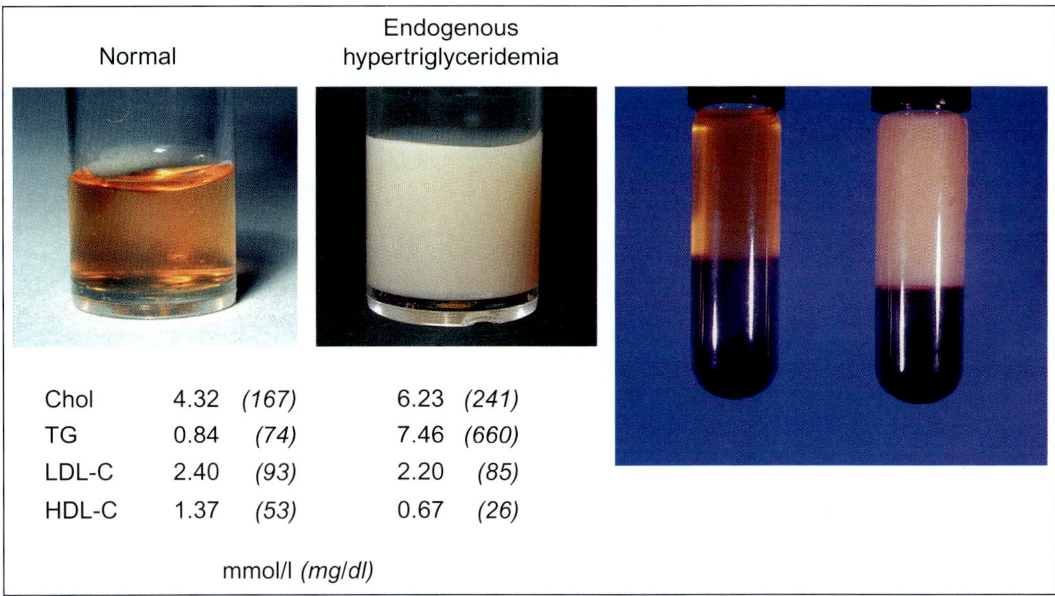

	Normal	Endogenous hypertriglyceridemia
Chol	4.32 (167)	6.23 (241)
TG	0.84 (74)	7.46 (660)
LDL-C	2.40 (93)	2.20 (85)
HDL-C	1.37 (53)	0.67 (26)

mmol/l *(mg/dl)*

2.10 Diffuse lactescence of plasma in endogenous hypertriglyceridemia. Discrete turbidity (cloudiness) of plasma seen with increased very-low-density lipoproteins (VLDL) (around 2.8 mmol/l or 250 mg/dl of triglycerides [TG]) in familial hypertriglyceridemia (FHTG) rapidly evolves towards diffuse lactescence as triglyceride levels increase. Chylomicrons are usually not present at the top as a creamy layer in a tube of fasting plasma left overnight in a refrigerator (left). The same picture is maintained when TG levels reach over 11.3 mmol/l (1000 mg/dl) (right).

insulin resistance, a lack of exercise, an increase in alcohol consumption, use of estrogens, glucocorticoids or any other causes of secondary hypertriglyceridemia. FEHTG is often accompanied by hyperuricemia, obesity and insulin resistance. Typically, triglycerides range between 2.3 mmol/l and 5.7 mmol/l (200–500 mg/dl), high levels imparting a diffuse lactescence to plasma (**2.10**). An increased postprandial triglyceridemia that may exceed 11.3 mmol/l (1000 mg/dl) is also part of the disease. It is rarely associated with clinical signs other than arcus corneae and/or xanthelasmas. However, in an occasional severe case with triglycerides ≥11.3 mmol/l (≥1000 mg/dl), that might result from the compounding effect of precipitating factors, especially uncontrolled diabetes, a more dramatic clinical picture may be seen. With or without associated elevation of chylomicrons, it may be manifested by hepatosplenomegaly, tuberous or eruptive xanthomas, lipemia retinalis and acute pancreatitis (**2.11**). Finally, when atherosclerosis is present it is often expressed as peripheral arterial disease although late coronary artery disease (CAD) and stroke may occur as well.

Kinetic studies have shown that the metabolic defect in FEHTG is an overproduction of VLDL by the liver with or without reduced VLDL catabolism (**2.12**). The increase in synthesis and secretion of large triglyceride-rich lipoproteins is associated with enhanced formation of small dense LDL deemed more atherogenic because of their small size, the fact that they carry lipoprotein-associated phospholipase A$_2$ (high levels constitute a CAD risk factor) and their greater propensity for oxidation. A prospective study by Austin and

co-workers has shown that in FEHTG families the cardiovascular risk is increased (relative risk of 1.70, not significant) and the baseline triglyceride level predicts the subsequent cardiovascular mortality among relatives (relative risk 2.7, *P* = 0.02, when adjusted for LDL-C) (**2.13**). In these families the mean fasting triglyceride level was 2.38 mmol/l (211 mg/dl). Even though the occurrence of endogenous hypertriglyceridemia in families is well documented, no single causal gene has yet been identified although many genes responsible for variation in triglyceride levels have been uncovered that may induce (or enhance) endogenous hypertriglyceridemia. The presence of atherosclerotic cardiovascular disease varies widely among FEHTG families. This probably relates to the relative contribution of genetic, metabolic, and environmental factors which determine the atherogenic potential of the disease. The amount of small dense LDL produced, the apoE genotype, the level of apoCIII or of apoAV are among the major determinants of plasma VLDL concentrations, their composition and their atherogenic effect.

Whether endogenous hypertriglyceridemia is inherited as a familial trait or secondary to diabetes, the following scenario may occur. Large triglyceride-rich VLDL-1 lead to the formation of slowly metabolized LDL particles that become enriched in triglycerides as they lose cholesteryl esters. These, in turn, are good substrates for hepatic lipase and their lipolysis will generate smaller, denser more readily oxidizable atherogenic LDL particles (**2.12**). A recent genome-wide scan for quantitative trait loci suggests that two separate loci may be determining the LDL particle size (chromosome 6)

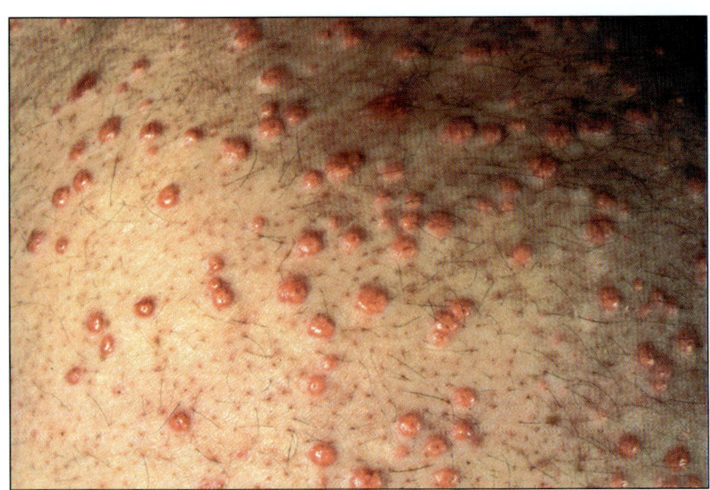

2.11 Eruptive xanthomas in crops with an inflammatory appearance. Eruptive xanthomas on the buttocks in a patient with severe endogenous hypertriglyceridemia. This 37-year-old chef was seen at the authors' lipid clinic a few weeks after his release from the hospital where he had been admitted for acute pancreatitis. He was obese (body mass index of 39), had type 2 diabetes, mild hypothyroidism, and essential hypertension. At the time this picture was taken, lipemia retinalis was present, his plasma triglycerides were 142 mmol/l (12 585 mg/dl) with a total cholesterol of 27.28 mmol/l (1055 mg/dl). He indulged in a high-caloric diet. His apoE phenotype was E3/3. No chylomicrons were found in the fasting state visually or by preparative ultracentrifugation or lipoprotein electrophoresis. Questions regarding the family history often do not reveal familial endogenous hypertriglyceridemia (FEHTG) as either triglycerides are not routinely measured in some areas or modest elevation of triglycerides are not considered worth mentioning.

To demonstrate that the underlying defect is FEHTG one has to obtain blood samples from first-degree relatives and document the fasting endogenous hypertriglyceridemia. This is a case in point that a combination of secondary causes of hypertriglyceridemia may induce a severe clinical and biochemical phenotype in FTGH. When this patient's diabetes was finally under control with oral hypoglycemic agents and later with insulin, with an appropriate diet and his hypothyroidism treated, there was a residual endogenous hypertriglyceridemia that yielded to the addition of a fibrate to the regimen. Sometimes pruritus is associated with this type of lesion.

and the plasma triglyceride levels (chromosome 15) even though these two traits are closely correlated.

ApoE is synthesized by the liver and incorporated into triglyceride-rich chylomicrons and VLDL. The catabolism of these lipoproteins is more or less efficient according to the apoE phenotype (determined by 3 alleles: ε2, ε3 or ε4). Subjects homozygous for the ε2 allele (E2/2 phenotype) have a propensity to develop dysbetalipoproteinemia (type III)

(see Chapter 3, Familial dysbetalipoproteinemia). But it has also been demonstrated by Dallongeville and colleagues, in a meta-analysis of 45 population samples from 17 different countries, that subjects with the E3/2, E4/3 or E4/2 phenotypes have significantly higher plasma triglyceride concentrations than the carriers of the most common phenotype (E3/3). In another study, interaction between apoE phenotype and sucrose intake was also documented. A high sucrose intake was associated with high triglyceride concentrations only in subjects bearing the ε2 allele. The authors have shown in their laboratory that the relative enrichment in ε2 allele frequency occurring in subjects with endogenous hypertriglyceridemia supervenes in the absence of hyper-apobetalipoproteinemia (LDL apoB ≤ 104 mg/dl) but not in its presence (LDL apoB ≥ 125 mg/dl), hyper-apoB serving as a marker of familial combined hyperlipidemia (FCH). The relative ε3 allele frequency was 0.153 and 0.091, respectively. Importantly, atherogenic remnant lipoproteins are formed more readily in the presence of the ε2 allele.

ApoCIII synthesized in the liver and the intestine is an essential constituent of triglyceride-rich lipoproteins. It plays an important part in determining their metabolic fate because it inhibits the hydrolysis of these particles by lipoprotein lipase and their apoE-mediated uptake by the liver. Also, plasma apoCIII is a predictor of risk for the development and progression of CAD. A close association between SstI polymorphism (3238C>G) in the untranslated region of the apoCIII gene (*APOC3*) and levels of plasma triglycerides has been reported by different investigators. A strong association between the S2 allele and high triglyceride levels (odds ratio: 9.95 vs. S1/S1) has been consistently observed in various populations. The rare S2 allele in Caucasians (0–11%) is more common in Asian Indians (31%). Other polymorphisms of *APOC3* (–455T>C; –482C>T) located within the insulin-responsive element in the promoter region have also been associated with elevated plasma triglycerides. Furthermore, patients homozygous for the –455C variant have higher apoCIII levels and are poorly responsive to the apoCIII-lowering effect of polyunsaturated fatty acids (PUFA).

Recently, a new member of the apolipoprotein family, apoAV has been identified. It is present in plasma in smaller concentrations than the other apolipoproteins (5–50 μg/dl) and is associated with VLDL, HDL and chylomicrons. Although its role in lipoprotein metabolism is not fully elucidated, apoAV is involved in triglyceride-rich lipoprotein assembly in the liver. The ApoAV gene (*APOA5*) is located

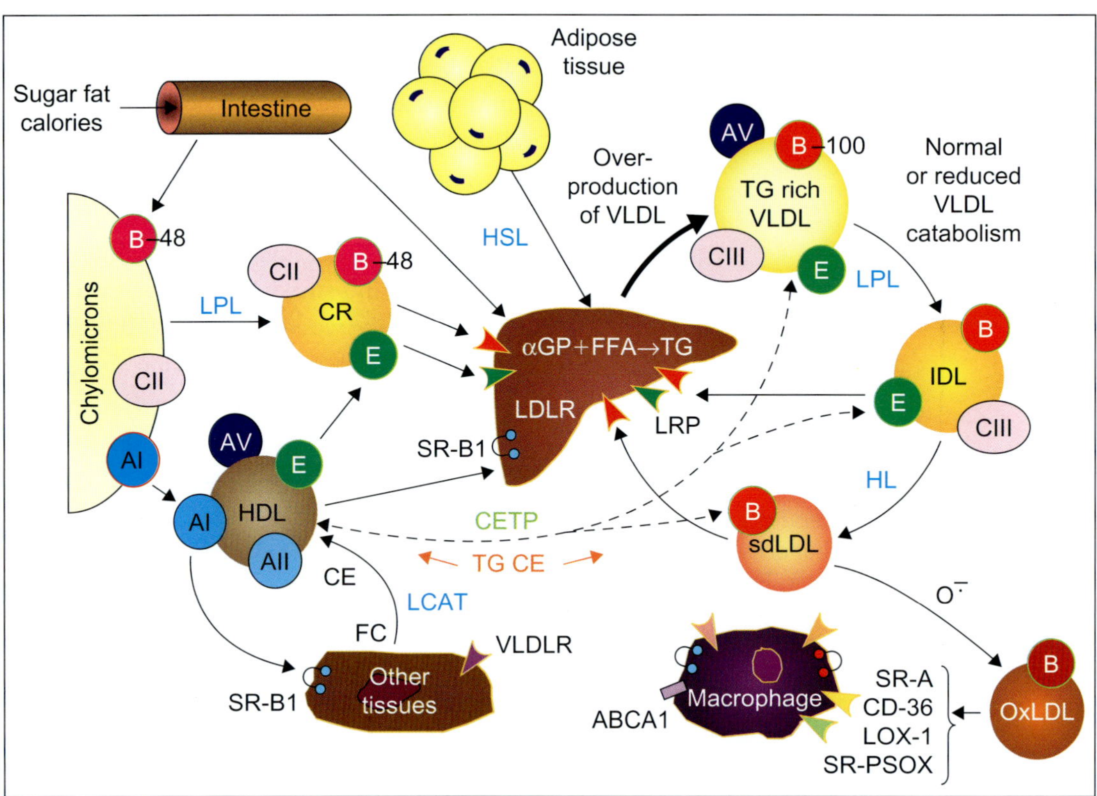

2.12 Metabolic defect in familial endogenous hypertriglyceridemia (FEHTG). The basic defect in FEHTG is an overproduction of unusually large triglyceride (TG)-enriched very-low-density lipoproteins (VLDL) that may or may not be associated with a reduced catabolism. The large VLDL-1 gives rise to a wide range of smaller and smaller lipoprotein particle sizes as triglycerides (TG) are replaced with cholesteryl esters (CE) in the lipolytic cascade under the action of lipoprotein lipase (LPL) and hepatic lipase (HL). Cholesteryl ester transfer protein (CETP) is shown for the first time in this figure; its role is to exchange triglycerides for CE between apoB-containing lipoproteins (dotted lines) and high-density lipoproteins (HDL). The process leads to formation of VLDL remnants (intermediate-density lipoproteins [IDL]) that may or may not be readily taken up effectively by the LDL receptor (LDLR) or LDL receptor-related protein (LRP). Eventually, normal LDL as well as a large number of small dense oxidizable LDL (sdLDL) are formed at the end of the cascade. HDL are reduced as triglycerides increase and cholesteryl esters are transferred to the VLDL of diminishing size. Oxidized LDL (OxLDL) induced by superoxide anions and other free radicals are atherogenic as they are readily taken up by the various OxLDL receptors on macrophages: scavenger receptor class A (SR-A); lectin-like oxidized LDL receptor-1 (LOX-1); CD36 – a class B scavenger receptor with many·functions, also called fatty acid translocase (FAT); and scavenger receptor for phosphatidyl serine and oxidized LDL (SR-PSOX), also called CXLC16, recently discovered by Shimaoka T, Kume N, Minami M, Hayashida K, Kataoka H, Kita T, Yonehara S (2000). Molecular cloning of a novel scavenger receptor for oxidized low density lipoprotein, SR-PSOX, on macrophages. *J Biol Chem*, **275**: 40663–40666.

Dietary sugars (top) provide the substrate for glycerol formation, *sn*-glycerol-3-phosphate (αGP), and adipose tissue via the action of hormone-sensitive lipase (HSL) provides the free fatty acids (FFA) for endogenous triglyceride synthesis and VLDL production. Endogenously, glycolysis and FFA from endothelial lipolysis will also provide substrates for triglyceride formation. Apo AV, present in small amounts in plasma and carried by HDL, VLDL and chylomicrons, is depicted as a reminder that reduced apoAV is associated with increased triglyceride levels. Low LPL activity (reduced lipolysis) and high apoCIII (reduced receptor uptake) will also increase plasma triglycerides. It is to be noted that changes in conformation of apoB on IDL and LDL derived from large triglyceride-rich VLDL will impede interaction with LDLR and increase the residence time of these particles in plasma, enhancing their likelihood of being oxidized. The triglyceride-enriched particles down the cascade are a good substrate for hepatic lipase which contributes to formation of small dense LDL. Any of these lipoprotein alterations may take place when triglycerides increase above the upper limit of their levels in adult of 1.7 mmol/l (150 mg/dl). Many of the findings illustrated in this figure have originated from work carried out in the laboratories of Packard and Shepherd in Glasgow from kinetic studies (see Packard CJ [2003]. Triacylglycerol-rich lipoproteins and the generation of small, dense low-density lipoprotein. *Biochem Soc Trans*, **31**: 1066–1069).

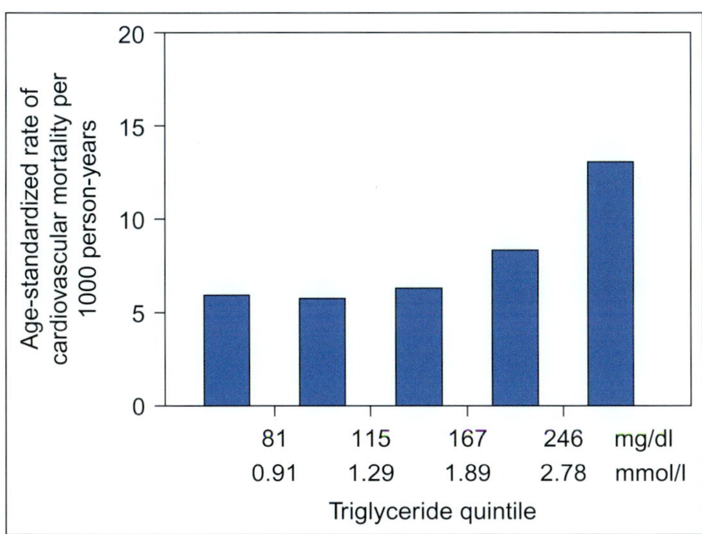

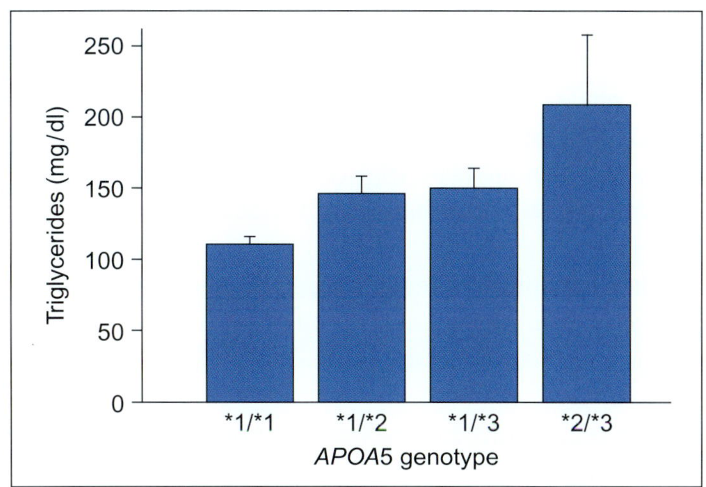

2.13 Baseline triglycerides predict 20-year cardiovascular mortality in familial endogenous hypertriglyceridemia and familial combined hyperlipidemia. This is part of a study that considered familial combined hyperlipidemia families (FCH) ascertained from probands surviving a myocardial infarction and familial hypertriglyceridemia (FHTG) families ascertained from hypertriglyceridemic subjects devoid of clinical evidence of coronary artery disease. Baseline triglycerides were predictive of subsequent cardiovascular mortality among all relatives in these hypertriglyceridemic families (relative risk of 1.9 for a 1 − log unit increase in triglycerides in mg/dl), and this result remained statistically significant after adjustment for total cholesterol. Separately, baseline triglycerides were not predictive of cardiovascular mortality in FCH (relative risk [RR] 1.7 [P = 0.06], but were in FHTG (RR 2.9; P <0.001). Interestingly, the adjusted relative cardiovascular risk was 1.70 in both FCH and FHTG, but this was significant only in FCH. Redrawn from Austin MA *et al.* (2000). Cardiovascular disease mortality in familial forms of hypertriglyceridemia: A 20-year prospective study. *Circulation*, **101**: 2777–2782.

2.14 Effect of variation at the *APOA5* locus on plasma triglycerides. Plasma triglyceride concentrations in a random sample of 500 normolipidemic Caucasian men and women as a function of their *APOA5* genotype demonstrate that variations at the *APOA5* locus affected plasma triglyceride levels in the Berkeley Lipid Study Population. This was found to be independent of the effect of *APOC3* Sst1 polymorphism on plasma triglycerides. Haplotypes APOA5*2 and *3 were defined by the −1131C and the c. 56G minor alleles, respectively. The c.56G single nucleotide polymorphism responsible for the S19W base change alone was found to be independently associated with increased triglyceride levels in several population samples. Redrawn from Pennacchio LA, Rubin EM (2003). Apolipoprotein A5, a newly identified gene that affects triglyceride levels in humans and mice. *Arterioscler Thromb Vasc Biol,* **23**: 529–534.

30 kb downstream and has become part of the previously well-defined *APOA1/C3/A4* gene cluster on chromosome 11q23. It contains 4 exons, encodes a protein of 366 amino acids and its expression is upregulated by agonists of the nuclear receptors peroxisome proliferator activated receptor-α (PPARα) and farnesoid X receptor (FXR) and down-regulated by insulin. Three common haplotypes of *APOA5* have been studied in humans (*APOA5*1; APOA5*2; APOA5*3*). These haplotypes were constructed from some of the known sequence variations of *APOA5* (−12,238T>C, −1131T>C, −3A>G, c.56C>G, 476G>A, and 1259T>C). (*Note*: The 'c.' in c.C56G stands for cDNA; the numbering is that of the cDNA, not that of the genomic DNA.) The two minor haplotypes (*A5*2/A5*3*) are found in 25–50%

of black, Hispanic or white people, and are associated with a 30% increase in plasma triglyceride concentration (**2.14**), an association that is independent of the apoCIII SstI polymorphism. In the Chinese population, individuals carrying a minor T-553 allele have an odds ratio of 11.73 for developing hypertriglyceridemia compared with individuals without that allele.

Polymorphism of other genes, involved in lipid metabolism or not, such as the genes coding for lipoprotein lipase, acyl-Co A synthetase or retinitis pigmentosa-1, have been reported to increase plasma triglyceride concentrations. Whether they act independently or in conjunction with poor lifestyle habits to promote hypertriglyceridemia still has to be determined for many of them. But certainly for the majority of affected individuals, endogenous hypertriglyceridemia results from a complex gene – environment interaction.

Although it exists as a separate well-defined inherited entity, the diagnosis of FEHTG is difficult to establish. This is because:

- its dominant mode of inheritance has not yet been resolved by the finding of a single culprit gene
- the phenotype can be mimicked by many conditions, including other genetically inherited disorders, especially the endogenous hypertriglyceridemia observed in FCH (see Chapter 3), diabetes, the metabolic syndrome and obesity
- other susceptibility genes, genetic polymorphisms, drugs and many environmental conditions – dietary factors in particular – may modulate its phenotype positively or negatively
- the family history may be negative from the cardiovascular standpoint
- its demonstration in families needs actual assessment of the lipoprotein profile in first-degree relatives

- cut-offs for 'normal' triglycerides have been set too high in the past
- concomitant pro-triglyceridemic factors may mask the underlying disease until the demonstration is made of a residual genetic hypertriglyceridemia (i.e. after control of diabetes, arrest of alcohol consumption, implementation of a low-calorie diet, etc.) or the source of enhancement is demonstrated (heterozygosity for an LPL defect and a diet high in simple sugars are common).

The diagnosis is made when these confounding factors have been dealt with (*Table 2.1*). The most common source of confusion in differential diagnosis is the endogenous hypertriglyceridemia associated with FCH in the absence of an increased LDL level. This can be resolved by showing the

---

Table 2.1 Confounding factors in the diagnosis of familial endogenous hypertriglyceridemia

- Failure to obtain a lipoprotein profile in first-degree relatives
- Few helpful clinical clues usually present
- Delayed expression of phenotype
- Family history of cardiovascular disease often discrete
- Confusion with the hypertriglyceridemia of familial combined hyperlipidemia
- Co-existence of primary and secondary causes of hypertriglyceridemia
- Spurious increase in triglycerides due to hyperglycerolemia (rare)
- No single gene defect yet identified as causal
- Failure to sort out secondary causes of hypertriglyceridemia:
  - *Dietary*: alcohol, simple carbohydrates, calories
  - *Hormonal*: estrogens, oral contraceptives, hormone replacement therapy, selective estrogen receptor modulators (tamoxifen)
  - *Drugs*: atypical antipsychotics, isotretinoin, antiretroviral therapy, corticosteroids, clomifene, thiazides, β-blockers
  - *Diseases*: diabetes, obesity, insulin resistance, pancreatitis, renal insufficiency, nephrotic syndrome, hypothyroidism, Cushing's syndrome, storage disorders
  - *Physiological conditions*: pregnancy, postprandial sample
- Variation in phenotype because other susceptibility genes for hypertriglyceridemia are present:
  - *LPL* mutations
  - *ApoCIII* polymorphisms
  - *ApoA5* polymorphisms or mutations
  - *HL* mutations
  - Retinitis pigmentosa-1 gene (*RP-1*) polymorphism
  - *MACS2* member of the acyl-CoA synthetase gene family (L513S polymorphism)
  - Triglycerides are context sensitive and fluctuate widely in the same individual from day to day
  - Failure to recognize triglycerides as a cardiovascular disease risk marker and, in some laboratories, not including it in the lipid profile
  - Conditions that lower triglycerides and may mask the hypertriglyceridemia on occasion (important weight loss, prolonged fasting, some cholesterol-lowering agents, etc.)

variation of lipoprotein phenotypes among the first-degree relatives in FCH not seen in FEHTG. Also, the VLDL triglyceride/apoB ratio is greater in VLDL of FEHTG (25.7 ± 8.9, $n = 14$) than in the hypertriglyceridemic FCH (9.6 ± 12.3, $n = 14$, $P < 0.001$) or normal subjects 9.7 ± 3.3 as shown by Brunzell and colleagues (**2.15**). This measurement may be carried out in most lipid clinics. FH and FEHTG may co-exist in the same family with disastrous cardiovascular consequences (**2.16**). Presence of tendon xanthomas and family evaluation will facilitate the diagnosis in this case. Demonstration of the endogenous hypertriglyceridemia is easy. Looking at a tube of plasma stored overnight in the refrigerator reveals a diffuse turbidity of plasma already visible at 3.4 mmol/l (300 mg/dl) that gets more opaque as triglycerides increase further (**2.10**). Lipoprotein electrophoresis combined with ultracentrifugation provides a full profile and allows measurement of major lipoprotein fractions (**2.17**) (see also Chapter 3, **3.12**). The presence of chylomicrons does not exclude FEHTG as other superimposed sources of variation may cause this added phenotype (type V). For example, on a background of what appears to be FCH or FEHTG, homozygosity for the *APOA5* c.433C>T (Q145X) mutation induces a chylomicronemia syndrome in the absence of LPL or apoCII deficiency (**2.18**).

The first approach to treatment is dietary restriction of refined sugars, and reduction of foods with a high glycemic index. (Glycemic index is defined as the incremental area under the glucose response curve after a standard amount of carbohydrate from a test food relative to that of a control food [either white bread or glucose]. High glycemic index foods have a high ratio of rapidly absorbable carbohydrates [simple sugars] to slowly absorbable ones [more complex carbohydrates].) Control of other factors that may induce endogenous hypertriglyceridemia is mandatory: caloric restriction for overweight and obesity, curbing the alcohol intake if it is alcohol inducible, and treating other causes of endogenous hypertriglyceridemia if present. If the dietary approach is not sufficient to normalize the hypertriglyceridemia, fibrates or nicotinic acid are indicated. Both will also raise HDL-C but some patients treated with fibrates may have an increase in LDL-C that must be attended to. Omega-3 fatty acid administration may also be helpful. A positive family or personal history of atherosclerosis should encourage treating aggressively.

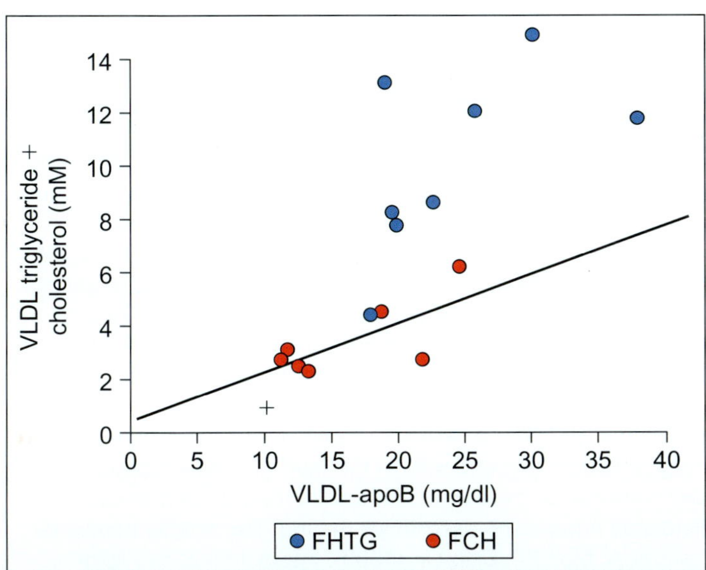

2.15 Very-low-density lipoproteins (VLDL) are more enriched in lipids in familial endogenous hypertriglyceridemia (FEHTG) than in familial combined hyperlipidemia (FCH). This figure shows a comparison of the relationship between VLDL triglyceride + cholesterol and VLDL-apoB in familial endogenous hypertriglyceridemia (FEHTG or FHTG) and familial combined hyperlipidemia (FCH). The regression line ($r = 0.70$) is for FCH and shows an increase in VLDL-apoB with increasing lipid content of VLDL particle, a situation similar to that observed in normal subjects. In FHTG, in contrast, the lipid content is disproportionately higher for similar concentrations of VLDL-apoB. In FHTG, the VLDL particles are larger in size and are triglyceride-enriched (VLDL-TG/apoB ratio is twice that of normal or of FCH VLDL), with a higher rate of triglyceride synthesis, stressing that these two conditions are metabolically distinct. Redrawn from Brunzell JD *et al.* (1983). Plasma lipoproteins in familial combined hyperlipidemia and monogenic familial hypertriglyceridemia. *J Lipid Res*, **24**: 147–155.

Familial mixed hypertriglyceridemia (type V, MHTG)

Familial mixed hypertriglyceridemia (type V, MHTG) refers to an excess of both plasma chylomicrons and VLDL (**2.19**) that aggregates in families. Type V shares the biological and clinical features of both type I and type IV hyperlipidemia (lipemic serum, hepatosplenomegaly, lipemia retinalis (**2.5**), eruptive (**2.4**, **2.11**) and tuberous or tubero-eruptive xanthomas). The very high plasma concentration of triglycerides, generally greater than 11.3 mmol/l (1000 mg/dl), is due to overproduction and decreased catabolism of both chylomicrons and VLDL particles. Turnover studies have shown similar increases in VLDL apoB synthesis in FEHTG (type IV) and MHTG (type V) patients but a greater reduction in fractional catabolic rate in type V subjects. Mixed

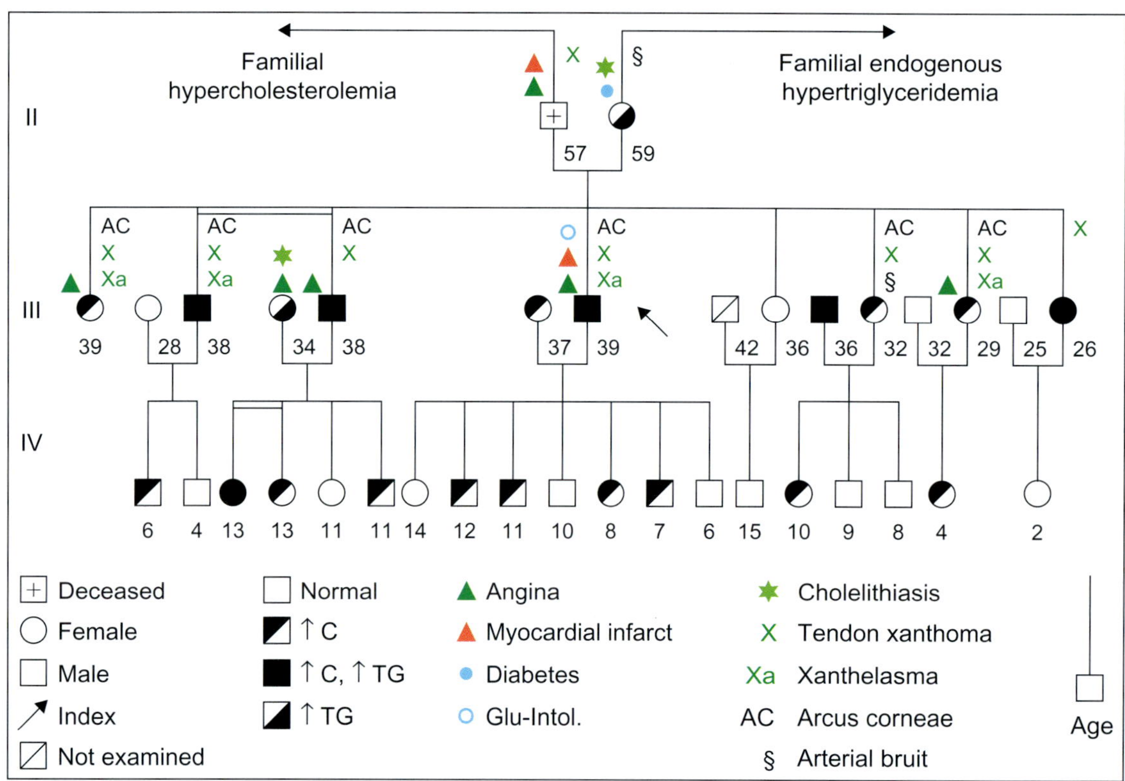

2.16 Co-segregation of familial endogenous hypertriglyceridemia (FEHTG) and familial hypercholesterolemia (FH) in the same family. In a 508-member pedigree, 375 living subjects were studied. Pedigrees were ascertained from a proband with FH and the presence of hypertriglyceridemia (therefore a type IIb lipoprotein phenotype). This pedigree was selected among 26 candidate families because of the large number of subjects on both parental sides and the large number of co-descendants. The objective was to assess the origin of the hypertriglyceridemia and the impact of two genetic disorders in co-descendants. As shown here, the inheritance of FEHTG from the maternal side and of FH from the paternal side was associated with deleterious clinical consequences before the age of 40 in generation III (that of the proband). Coronary artery disease was present in two siblings with combination of high triglyceride (↑TG) and cholesterol (↑C) levels.

Clinical manifestations of hyperlipidemia were present in all co-descendants. FEHTG was vertically transmitted as a dominant trait in generation II and III here and on the maternal side. However, the scarcity of hypertriglyceridemia in the third generation (ages 2–14) suggested delayed expression or incomplete penetrance of this trait. FEHTG tended to associate with insulin resistance and diabetes. Cholelithiasis aggregated on the maternal side. Many spouses had dyslipidemia suggesting assortative mating. The double horizontal bars are joining twins. Redrawn from Davignon J, Lussier-Cacan S, Gattereau A, Moll PP, Sing CF (1983). Interaction of two lipid disorders in a large French-Canadian kindred. *Arteriosclerosis*, **3**: 13–22, 1983.

hypertriglyceridemia does not seem to confer special predisposition to cardiovascular disease when adjusted for the other risk factors, but carries a significant risk of acute pancreatitis, which constitutes the most significant threat.

Unlike familial hyperchylomicronemia (FHC) (type I), MHTG is not a monogenic disease, the mode of inheritance is still undetermined and the plasma concentrations of post-heparin LPL and HL activities are usually normal. But one must remember, as mentioned earlier, that subjects with lipoprotein lipase deficiency (type I) can develop type V hyperlipidemia on stimulation of VLDL production by a diet rich in simple sugars (**2.7**). Similarly, subjects with type

IV, either associated with FEHTG or FCH may have some degree of fasting chylomicronemia, therefore exhibiting a type V lipoprotein phenotype (see Chapter 3, **3.9**, **3.10**). Early studies in the laboratory of Brewer at the National Institutes of Health showed an association with the apoE4 isoform (see Chapter 3 and **3.15** for apoE phenotyping). In two groups of type V patients from Finland and the US, the prevalence of apoE ε4 allele frequency was two to three times higher than in normal subjects; suggesting that apoE may have a role in the etiology of MHTG. On the other hand, Marçais and colleagues observed in a cohort of 176 patients with type 2 diabetes, that those who also had type

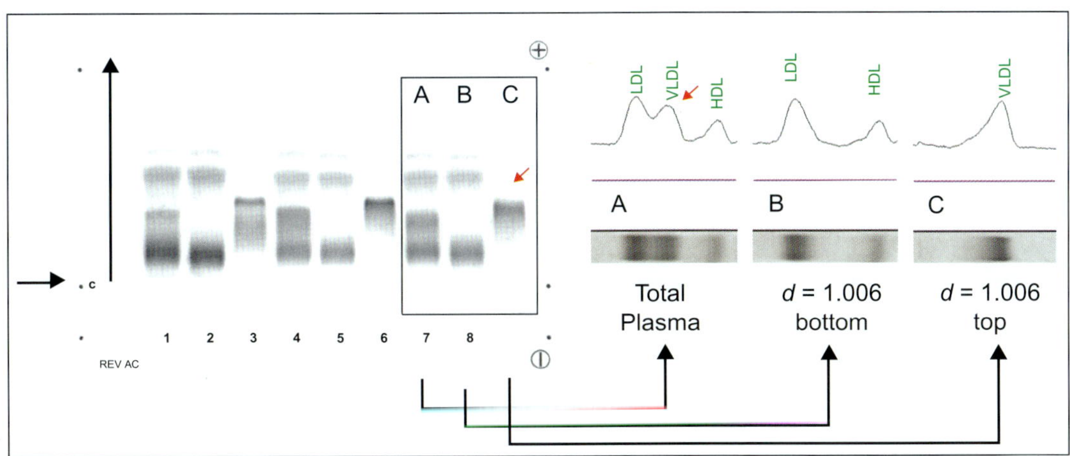

2.17 Standard method of separation of plasma lipoproteins demonstrating endogenous hypertriglyceridemia. Total plasma as well as the top and bottom fractions resulting from high-speed ultracentrifugation (see **2.6**) of plasma without additives other than EDTA at $d = 1.006$ (the effective aqueous density of separation 1.006 g/l is not the same as the density of plasma), are further separated by agarose gel electrophoresis. On the left panel three different samples are thus separated. The vertical arrow indicates direction of migration; the horizontal one, the point of origin of the migration. There are several agarose gel systems commercially available for lipoprotein separation by charge. Densitometric scanning of the separated bands provides a semiquantitative assessment of the major lipoprotein fractions (the three panels on the right). The red arrows indicate the pre-β migrating VLDL fraction typical of endogenous hypertriglyceridemia. This means of separation is commonly used in lipid clinics. Other more complex ultracentrifugation methods such as gradient density ultracentrifugation, use of zonal rotors or separation in an analytical ultracentrifuge are almost exclusively used in lipoprotein research laboratories. Ultracentrifugation is considered by some as a harsh treatment that may strip some lipoproteins from their apolipoproteins and alter their native state. A milder method to separate lipoproteins is by gel filtration on a superose column and elution in a fraction collector using a fast protein liquid chromatography (FPLC) system. Other methods are discussed in the following chapters.

V hypertriglyceridemia ($n = 32$) more often presented a genotype *E4/E2* (15% vs. 3%), an apoCIII S2 allele (50% vs. 15%) or a mutation of *LPL* (4/32 vs. 0). Overall, 68.7% of the diabetic people with MHTG were carriers of at least one mutation. Rare cases of autoimmune type V have also been reported, in one instance in association with a heterozygous LPL gene mutation (S172fsX179) and circulating antihuman LPL immunoglobulin G (IgG). In another instance, it was reported in combination with autoimmune hepatitis and systemic lupus erythematosus.

For most of the cases the exact cause of the disease is not well known, but it certainly often results from interactions between genes and environment. Many affected individuals share common features: diets rich in fat or simple sugars, obesity, poorly controlled diabetes (leading to severe xanthomatosis as in the patient illustrated in **2.20–2.22**), alcohol consumption, hyperuricemia, estrogen or oral contraceptive therapy. Clinical and biochemical features of severe hypertriglyceridemia are summarized in *Table 2.2*. Chait and Brunzell found that 110 out of 123 patients with triglyceride levels greater than 22.6 mmol/l (2000 mg/dl) had a secondary cause of hypertriglyceridemia. Unlike FHC, it is not present in childhood. But similarly, the diagnosis unfortunately is often made on the occasion of a first, unexplained attack of acute pancreatitis, when the fasting serum is found to be lipemic with a very high triglyceride level measured in the first 24–48 hours.

The subject of hyperlipidemic pancreatitis has been reviewed exhaustively by Yadav and Pitchumoni in 2003. The attack is often triggered by a secondary factor such as alcohol misuse, uncontrolled diabetes (both type 1 or type 2) or introduction of a new drug with the potential to increase plasma triglycerides. It is generally believed that a triglyceride level greater than 11.3 mmol/l (1000 mg/dl) is needed to precipitate an episode of acute pancreatitis, but some type V patients can tolerate very high levels of triglycerides (>56.5 mmol/l or >5000 mg/dl) without ever presenting acute pancreatitis. Others present recurrent episodes as soon as their triglyceride levels approach the critical 11.3 mmol/l. It is thus very difficult to predict which patient with MHTG will develop pancreatitis. Interestingly, serum pancreatic enzymes may be normal or only minimally elevated, but the clinical course is similar to that of pancreatitis due to other causes. This has been attributed to an interference of plasma

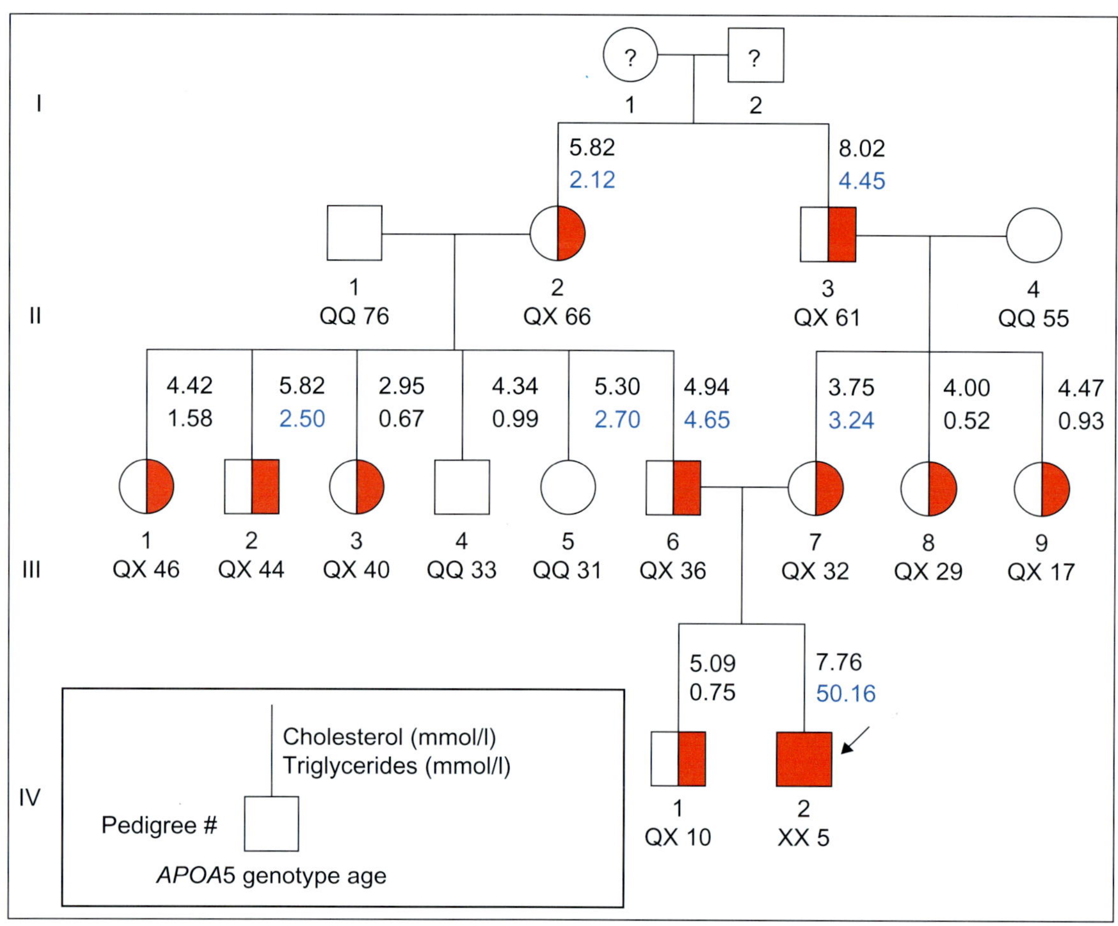

2.18 Homozygosity for the APOA5 Q145X mutation results in apoAV deficiency and a severe hyperchylomicronemia syndrome. The family tree demonstrates the consanguinity (generation I) allowing for homozygosity (XX) of a seemingly recessive trait, the APOA5 Q145X mutation. It also shows that hypertriglyceridemia (numbers in blue) does not segregate systematically with the presence of the heterozygous trait (male and female symbols half red and QX). The 61-year-old grandfather (II3) of the proband (arrow) has combined hyperlipidemia with a hypertriglyceridemic daughter and the 66-year-old grandmother (II2) has modest hypertriglyceridemia (no information on treatment) with three hypertriglyceridemic children, one of them not a carrier of the mutation. The hypertriglyceridemic subjects in generation III QX had an increase in very-low-density lipoproteins (VLDL) with no chylomicronemia (S Calandra, personal communication, 2006).This supports the notion that other transmitted forms of hyperlipidemia segregate in the family, FHTG on the II2 side and perhaps FCH on the II3 side, which might have contributed to the severe hypertriglyceridemia in the proband of 50.16 mmol/l (4478 mg/dl). The proband had both elevated chylomicrons and VLDL in the fasting state with a type V lipoprotein phenotype (S Calandra, personal communication, 2006).The 5-year-old proband had recurrent abdominal pain and eruptive xanthomatosis. His hypertriglyceridemia responded well to omega-3 fatty acids. The *Q145X* mutation (Gln$_{145}$→Ter; c.C433T) was predicted to encode a truncated non-functional 144-amino acid apoAV. This is the first report of severe hypertriglyceridemia ascribable in large part to homozygosity for an apoAV homozygous mutation. Redrawn and modified from Oliva CP, Pisciotta L, Volti GL, Sambataro MP, Cantafora A, Bellocchio A, Catapano A, Tarugi P, Bertolini S, Calandra S (2005). Inherited apolipoprotein A-V deficiency in severe hypertriglyceridemia. *Arterioscler Thromb Vasc Biol*, **25**: 411–417.

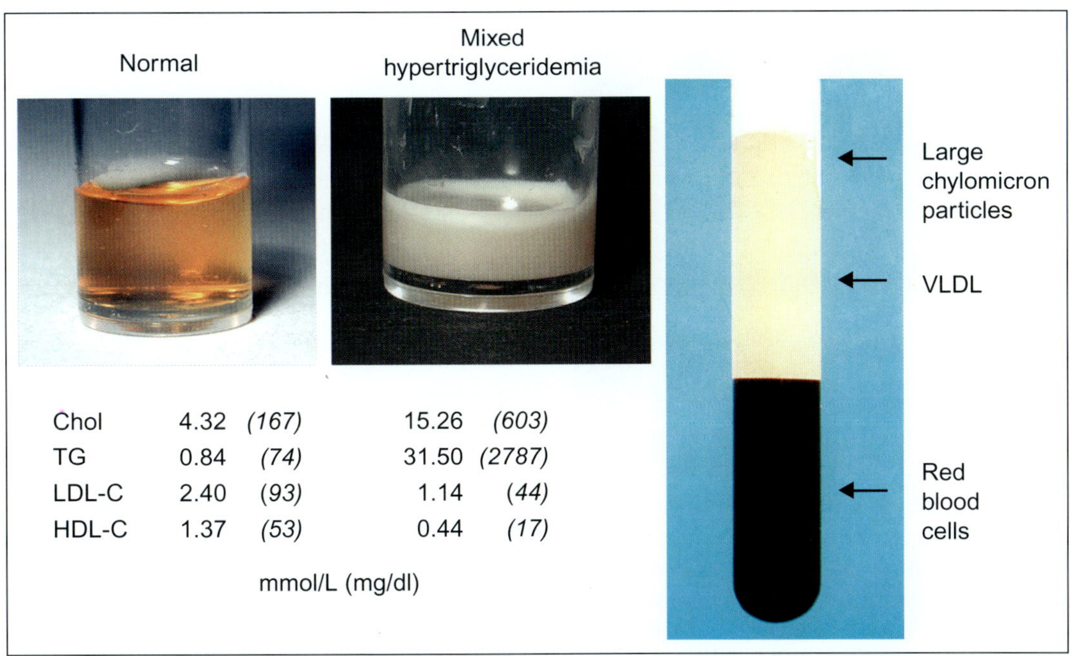

2.19 Diffuse lactescence and creamy layer in mixed hypertriglyceridemia. The standard procedure to measure the cholesterol content of the major lipoprotein fractions after a single ultracentrifugal run described in **3.12** was used here to obtain the lipoprotein profile in a normal subject (clear plasma) and in a patient with typical mixed hypertriglyceridemia (lactescent plasma with a creamy supernatant). Note the high total cholesterol (reflecting mostly very-low-density lipoproteins [VLDL]-C) and the low levels of LDL-C and HDL-C. The tube of blood on the right shows the clear separation of the creamy layer (chylomicrons) and the milky plasma (VLDL) after a short run in a standard centrifuge.

Table 2.2 Clinical features that may be associated with severe hypertriglyceridemia

- Lipemia retinalis
- Overweight, obesity, abdominal obesity
- Eruptive or tubero-eruptive xanthomas
- Recurrent acute pancreatitis
- Failure to thrive
- Episodes of severe abdominal pain
- Hepatosplenomegaly
- Hepatic steatosis
- Hypertriglyceridemic neuropathy (hyperesthesia or dysesthesia)
- Joint pain
- Mild transient cognitive impairment (loss of concentration or short-term memory)
- Symptoms of depression
- Signs of alcohol misuse
- Hyperuricemia
- Use of estrogen or glucocorticoids
- Symptoms of uncontrolled diabetes
- Milky serum or plasma with or without creamy supernatant
- High levels of total cholesterol and low levels of LDL-C and HDL-C

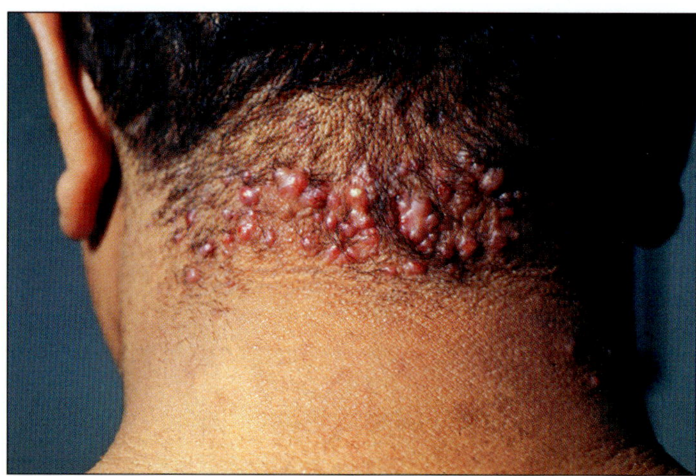

2.20 Tubero-eruptive xanthomas in a diabetic patient with a severe type V lipoprotein phenotype. This severe disseminated tubero-eruptive xanthomatosis developed in a 43-year-old patient with abdominal obesity and a severe mixed hypertriglyceridemia type V associated with untreated and uncontrolled type 2 diabetes mellitus. At the initial visit, his medical history did not reveal any cardiovascular event or episode of acute pancreatitis. He was complaining of typical polydipsia, polyuria and polyphagia. This was associated with a progressive itchy-inflammatory nodular skin eruption that had appeared 6 months before. He had hyperesthesia and paresthesia characterized by hypersensitivity and a burning sensation of the skin of both arms and thighs accompanied by sporadic cramps and weakness in his left calf (hypertriglyceridemic polyneuropathy). He was not following a diet or taking medication. His fasting lipid and lipoprotein profile was as follows: total cholesterol 21.70 mmol/l (839 mg/dl), triglycerides 82.66 mmol/l (7315 mg/dl), low-density lipoprotein-cholesterol 0.31 mmol/l (12 mg/dl), HDL-cholesterol 0.33 mmol/l (13 mg/dl) and chylomicron very-low-density lipoprotein-cholesterol 21.06 mmol/l (814 mg/dl). Fasting blood glucose was 19.8 mmol/l (356 mg/dl), HbA1c 9.6%, thyroid-stimulating hormone 1.99 mU/l, alanine aminotransferase 16 U/l, aspartate aminotransferase 22 U/l, and uric acid 471 µmol/l.

A few weeks after beginning appropriate dietary modifications (reduced calories, reduced intake of fat and simple sugars), intensive insulin therapy and gemfibrozil 1200 mg/day, the glucose level returned to normal, the fasting triglycerides decreased to 8.79 mmol/l and total cholesterol to 4.50 mmol/l, the polyneuropathy resolved completely and eruptive xanthomas started to regress, disappearing after 4 months of treatment. In the following years when the glycemic control for any reason temporarily deteriorated, the xanthomatosis and the neuropathic symptoms had a tendency to reappear. A residual hypertriglyceridemia in spite of controlled diabetes not yielding fully to dietary and fibrate therapy might reflect a genetic predisposition to hypertriglyceridemia.

lipids with the assay of pancreatic amylase and lipase or to the presence of an unknown inhibitor of the assay in plasma and urine. This interference or inhibition can be circumvented by serum dilution that will allow measuring amylase correctly.

The mechanism whereby hypertriglyceridemia causes pancreatitis is not fully understood. It has been ascribed to a combination of impeded capillary blood flow by chylomicrons causing local ischemia-acidosis and hydrolysis of triglycerides in the pancreas by pancreatic lipase resulting in high concentrations of unbound FFA that activate trypsinogen, are toxic and cause injury to the pancreatic cells. Whether hypertriglyceridemia can cause *chronic* pancreatitis remains controversial. Management of acute pancreatitis caused by hypertriglyceridemia is similar to that due to other causes, i.e. complete fasting, intravenous hydration, analgesia, etc. However, if parenteral nutrition is needed because of prolonged fasting, lipid infusions should be avoided to prevent resurgence of causal hypertriglyceridemia. Prevention of recurrent pancreatitis in type V patients relies on control of secondary factors such as alcohol abstinence, weight control, normalization of glycemia, maintenance of a healthy diet containing less than 50 g of lipids and less than 20 g of simple sugars and discontinuation of triglyceride-elevating drugs.

In the majority of type V subjects lipid-lowering treatment with a fibrate will also be necessary given the magnitude of the associated endogenous hypertriglyceridemia. Fibrates are the first line of treatment in type V; they are PPARα-agonists increasing the level of LPL and decreasing hepatic triglyceride synthesis. Fenofibrate and bezafibrate should be used in preference to clofibrate or gemfibrozil in type V because they are less likely to promote biliary tract lithiasis or sludge formation, another potential cause of acute pancreatitis. Fish oil can also be useful as an adjunct to therapy to normalize triglyceride levels, but they should be used with caution in the presence of significant chylomicronemia, because of the lipid load added. A minimum effective dose of 3–4 g/d of n-3 fatty acids is needed to reduce plasma triglycerides significantly (30–50%). Niacin can also be useful in treating type V patients because of its efficacy in lowering VLDL secretion, but close monitoring of glycemia, uricemia and HbA_{1c} is mandatory, especially in diabetic patients.

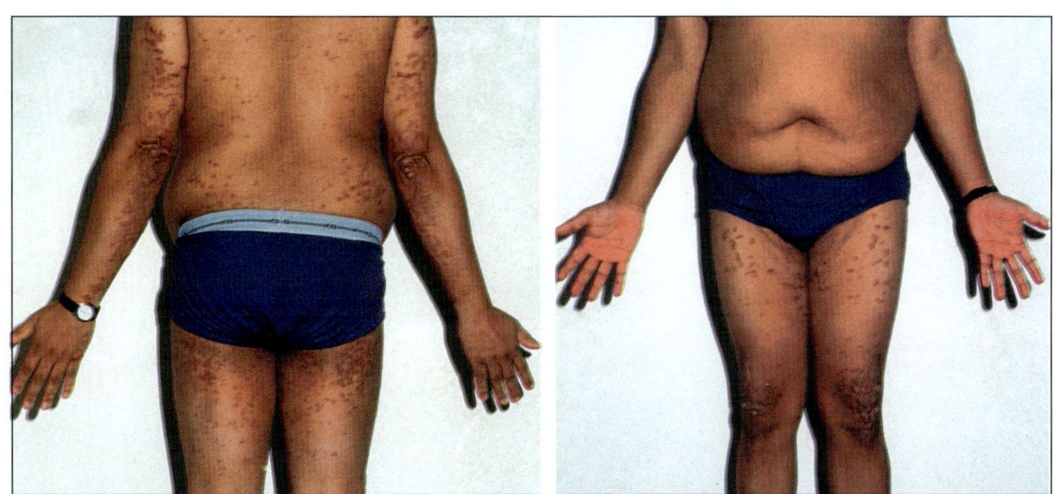

2.21 Widespread tubero-eruptive xanthomatosis in a diabetic patient with abdominal obesity and severe mixed hypertriglyceridemia (type V). This figure shows the widespread distribution of the eruptive and tubero-eruptive lesions in the patient in **2.20**. The redness of some of the lesions and their itchiness are compatible with an inflammatory component. The abdominal obesity is obvious.

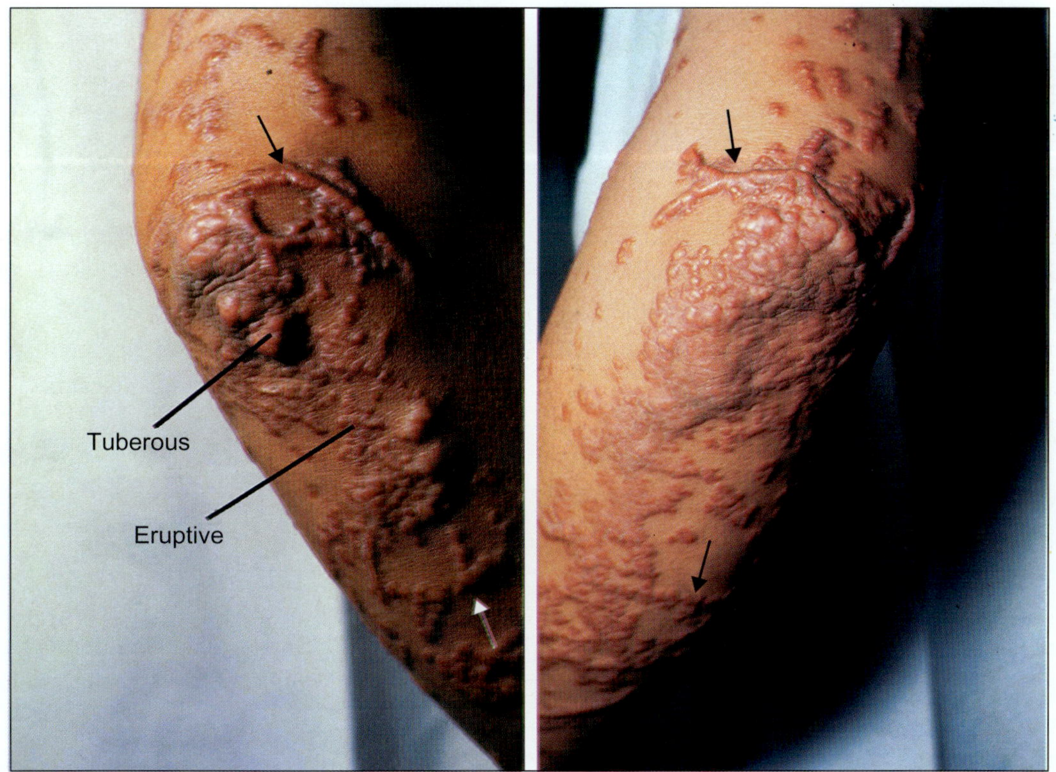

2.22 Extensive tubero-eruptive xanthomatosis of the elbows and evidence of Koebner phenomenon in a diabetic patient with severe mixed hypertriglyceridemia. Same patient as in **2.20** and **2.21**. In this close-up of the elbow lesions, it is noticeable that the eruptive lesions may be in clusters or follow a line (arrows). The latter is related to formation of lesions in areas where the patient scratched himself, injuring the skin. This is typical of the Koebner phenomenon often observed in severe mixed hypertriglyceridemia and in dysbetalipoproteinemia (type III). This phenomenon is explained in the legend of **3.29**.

Further reading

Lipoprotein lipase deficiency (familial hyperchylomicronemia)

Breckenridge WC, Alaupovic P, Cox DW, Little JA (1982). Apolipoprotein and lipoprotein concentrations in familial apolipoprotein C-II deficiency. *Atherosclerosis*, **44**: 223–235.

Evans V, Kastelein JJP (2002). Lipoprotein lipase deficiency – rare or common?. *Cardiovasc Drugs Ther*, **16**: 283–287.

Merkel M, Eckel RH, Goldberg IJ (2002). Lipoprotein lipase: genetics, lipid uptake, and regulation. *J Lipid Res*, **43**: 1997–2006.

Wilson CJ, Oliva CP, Maggi F, Catapano AL, Calandra S (2003). Apolipoprotein C-II deficiency presenting as a lipid encephalopathy in infancy. *Ann Neurol*, **5**: 807–810.

Wittrrup HH, Tybjaerg-Hansen A, Nordestgaard BG (1999). Lipoprotein lipase mutations, plasma lipids and lipoproteins, and risk of ischemic heart disease (a Meta-Analysis). *Circulation*, **99**: 2901–2907.

Familial endogenous hypertriglyceridemia (familial hypertriglyceridemia)

Austin MA, McKnight B, Edwards KL, Bradley CM, McNeely MJ, Psaty BM, Brunzell JD, Motulsky AC (2000). Cardiovascular disease mortality in familial forms of hypertriglyceridemia: a 20-year prospective study. *Circulation*, **101**: 2777–2782.

Brunzell JD, Albers JJ, Chait A, Grundy SM, Groszek E, McDonald GB (1983). Plasma lipoproteins in familial combined hyperlipidemia and monogenic familial hypertriglyceridemia. *J Lipid Res*, **24**: 147–155.

Chhabra S, Narang R, Krishnan L, Vasisht S, Agarwal DP, Srivastava LM, Manchanda SC, Das N (2002). Apolipoprotein C3 SstI polymorphism and triglyceride levels in Asian Indians. *BMC Genet*, **3**: 1–6.

Chhabra S, Narang R, Lakshmy R, Vasisht S, Agarwal DP, Srivastava LM, Manchanda SC, Das N (2004). Apolipoprotein C3 SstI polymorphism in the risk assessment of CAD. *Mol Cell Biochem*, **259**: 59–66.

Dallongeville J, Lussier-Cacan S, Davignon J (1992). Modulation of plasma triglyceride levels by apoE phenotype: a meta-analysis. *J Lipid Res*, **33**: 447–454.

Fujita Y, Ezura Y, Emi M, Ono S, Takada D, Takahashi K, Uemura K, Iino Y, Katayama Y, Bujo H, Saito Y (2003). Hypertriglyceridemia associated with amino acid variation Asn985Tyr of the RP1 gene. *J Hum Genet*, **48**: 305–308.

Iwai N, Mannami T, Tomoike H, Ono K, Iwanaga Y (2003). An acyl-CoA synthetase gene family in chromosome 16p12 may contribute to multiple risk factors. *Hypertension*, **41**: 1041–1046.

Olivieri O, Martinelli N, Sandri M, Bassi A, Guarini P, Trabetti E, Pizzolo F, Girelli D, Friso S, Pignatti PF, Corrocher R (2005). Apolipoprotein C-III, n-3 polyunsaturated fatty acids, and 'insulin-resistant' T-455C *APOC3* gene polymorphism in heart disease patients: Example of gene-diet interaction. *Clin Chem*, **51**: 360–367.

Packard CJ (2003). Triacylglycerol-rich lipoproteins and the generation of small, dense low-density lipoprotein. *Biochem Soc Trans*, **31**: 1066–1069.

Pennacchio LA, Rubin EM (2003). Apolipoprotein A5, a newly identified gene that affects triglyceride levels in humans and mice. *Arterioscler Thromb Vasc Biol*, **23**: 529–534.

Familial mixed hypertriglyceridemia (type V, MHTG)

Fallat RW, Glueck CJ (1976). Familial and acquired type V hyperlipoproteinemia. *Atherosclerosis*, **23**: 41–62.

Ghiselli G, Schaefer EJ, Zech LA, Gregg RE, Brewer HB, Jr (1982). Increased prevalence of apolipoprotein E4 in type V hyperlipoproteinemia. *J Clin Invest*, **70**: 474–477.

Greenberg BH, Blackwelder WC, Levy RI (1977). Primary type V hyperlipoproteinemia. A descriptive study in 32 families. *Ann Intern Med*, **87**: 526–534.

Marçais C, Bernard S, Merlin M, Ulhmann M, Mestre B, Rochet-Mingret L, Revol A, Berthezene F, Moulin P (2000). Severe hypertriglyceridemia in Type II diabetes: involvement of *apoC-III Sst-I* polymorphism, *LPL* mutations and *apo E3* deficiency. *Diabetologia*, **43**: 1346–1352.

Oliva CP, Pisciotta L, Volti GL, Sambataro MP, Cantafora A, Bellocchio A, Catapano A, Tarugi P, Bertolini S, Calandra S (2005). Inherited apolipoprotein A-V deficiency in severe hypertriglyceridemia. *Arterioscler Thromb Vasc Biol*, **25**: 411–417.

Yadav D, Pitchumoni CS (2003). Issues in hyperlipidemic pancreatitis. *J Clin Gastroenterol*, **36**: 54–62.

Chapter 3

Inherited Mixed Dyslipoproteinemias

Familial combined hyperlipidemia

The notion of familial combined hyperlipidemia (FCH, FCHL or multiple phenotype disease or multiple lipoprotein-type hyperlipidemia) evolved in the early 1970s from the work of Goldstein (who coined the term), Hazzard and Rose in the USA and from that of Nikkilä in Europe and their co-workers. Genetic analysis of lipid levels in families of survivors of myocardial infarction who had hyperlipidemia (**1.40**) revealed that, within a kindred, affected individuals (roughly 50% of the relatives) may have different lipoprotein phenotypes and that the phenotype may change over time within an individual. The lipoprotein phenotypes characterized according to the Fredrickson classification were either isolated hypercholesterolemia reflecting an increase in low-density lipoprotein-cholesterol (LDL-C) (type IIa), isolated hypertriglyceridemia due to increased very-low-density lipoproteins (VLDL) (type IV) or a combination of both (type IIb). Later, the presence of chylomicronemia was noted in some family members (type V) and it became clear that plasma apolipoprotein B (apoB) levels were elevated in this condition with a decrease in LDL particle size and an increase in LDL particle numbers (presence of atherogenic small dense LDL (sdLDL) prone to oxidation). This led Sniderman in Montreal to redefine FCHL as a *hypertriglyceridemic hyper-apoB state*. Hyper-apoB may be associated with normal cholesterol and triglyceride levels (referred to as 'NB' phenotype by the authors' research group). Originally, the lipoprotein pattern was deemed inherited as an autosomal dominant trait (**3.1**) with reduced penetrance and/or delayed expression, but today a polygenic mode of inheritance is favoured. The etiology is not fully established as efforts have been baffled by several confounding elements such as soft diagnostic criteria, differences in proband ascertainment, phenotypic overlap (metabolic syndrome, familial dyslipidemic hypertension, atherogenic lipoprotein phenotypes), heterogeneity of disease, genetic variations across populations, gene and environment interactions and lack of a specific marker. Controversial issues in FCH have been critically reviewed by Aguilar Salinas and colleagues recently. FCH bears OMIM No. 44250 (www.ncbi.nlm.nih. gov/entrez/dispomim.cgi?id=144250).

FCH is a common form of primary hyperlipidemia. Its prevalence ranges between 1:50 and 1:30 in Caucasians and it accounts for 15–20% of patients with angiographically documented coronary artery disease (CAD) before 60 years of age. It may account for 10–15% of myocardial infarctions in Caucasians. Its atherogenic potential is based on the presence of a large number of LDL particles of smaller size that are more prone to oxidation and promote foam cell formation. Elevated plasma apoB alone allows the separation of a subset of CAD patients with 'normal' LDL-C from subjects with normal coronary arteries (**3.2**). A case–control comparison in the National Heart, Lung and Blood Institute (NHLBI) Family Heart Study found that both FCH and familial endogenous hypertriglyceridemia (FEHTG) were associated with an odds ratio for CAD of 2.0 ($P = 0.003$ and $P = 0.002$, respectively). Furthermore, both were associated with an increased prevalence of the metabolic syndrome of 65% and 77%, respectively, compared with control families (19%, odds ratio 3.3 [$P < 0.001$]).

Several metabolic abnormalities have been reported in FCH including hepatic apoB overproduction resulting in high plasma levels of apoB and small dense LDL, delayed postprandial chylomicron remnant clearance and prolonged postprandial elevation of plasma free fatty acids and apoB-48 (**3.3**). It has been inferred that the heterozygous state for lipoprotein lipase (LPL) deficiency could contribute to

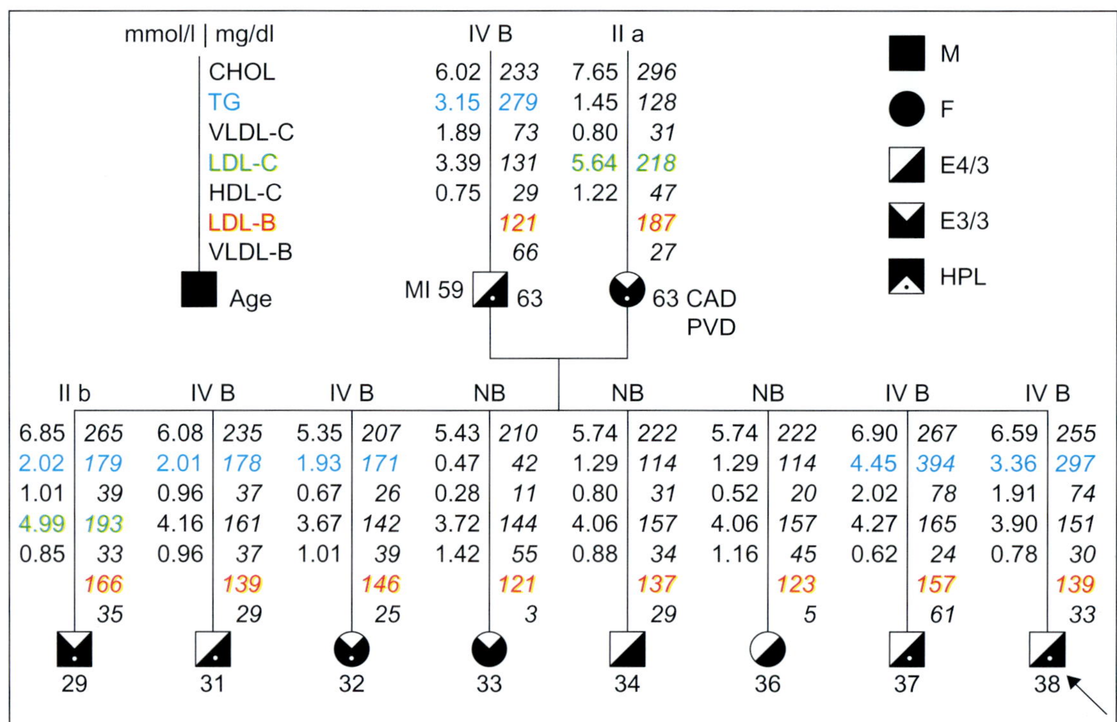

3.1 Apparent dominant mode of inheritance in a family with familial combined hyperlipidemia (FCH). This unique pedigree originates from a hyperlipidemic (HLP, marked by a dot on the diagram) father with the type IV phenotype and a hyperlipidemic mother with the type IIa phenotype (low-density lipoprotein cholesterol [LDL-C] in green >90th percentile). Both have elevated LDL-apoB (value of LDL-B in red) and both are presumed to originate from a familial combined hyperlipidemia family. At 63 years of age both have manifestations of atherosclerosis: myocardial infarction (MI), coronary artery disease (CAD) or peripheral vascular disease (PVD). The type IV is labelled B (IV B) because of the hyperapobetalipoproteinemia.

This putative FCH × FCH mating is further borne out as all descendants of this couple have hyper-apoB defined by levels of total apoB ≥120 mg/dl (LDL-B + VLDL-B) or LDL-apoB ≥100 mg/dl. Multiple phenotypes are present in first-degree relatives. Five subjects have hypertriglyceridemia, defined by a fasting plasma value ≥150 mg/dl (1.7 mmol/l) (figures in blue). Three normolipidemic descendants have only hyperapobetalipoproteinemia (NB). This is compatible with a dominant mode of inheritance (as opposed to a co-dominant mode) because none of the eight offspring has a more severe lipoprotein phenotype than the others although the likelihood of including a homozygote is high (1/4). The vertical transmission is obvious. Furthermore, the offspring range in age from 29 to 38 years of age, and there is a trend for the triglyceride levels to be higher in hypertriglyceridemics with ageing compatible with the reported delayed expression of this trait. The apoE phenotype is provided. It has been shown that the E4/3 phenotype (father and the four sons) may be associated with higher LDL-C levels than the E3/3 phenotype.

the FCH phenotype because reduced LPL activity has been observed in 30–50% of cases of FCH. A defective adipose tissue metabolism has also been postulated from several observations (**3.4**). These include a defect in the ability of insulin to suppress free fatty acid release from adipose tissue, impairment in insulin-mediated glucose disposal, an inefficient acylation stimulating protein (ASP)-mediated adipocyte triglyceride synthesis, and a defect in hormone-sensitive lipase-mediated lipolysis. Lowered plasma levels of adiponectin have also been linked to the pathogenesis of FCH (**3.4** and **3.5**). The atherogenic potential is attributed to the increased number of small dense LDL particles that are prone to oxidation and favour foam cell formation. Plasma

oxidized LDL are increased in FCH and there is a relative reduction in the cholesterol content of high-density lipoproteins (HDL). Triglyceride enrichment of HDL particles and enhanced hepatic lipase activity appear to be responsible for the reduction of HDL-C and HDL$_2$-C in FCH. Subjects with predominantly sdLDL show a hypertriglyceridemic, low HDL-C phenotype, with moderately elevated apoB and LDL-C levels. This associates with a ten times higher number of VLDL1 particles as well as smaller VLDL2 particles, in combination with increased plasma insulin concentration compared with the hypercholesterolemic phenotype with more buoyant LDL particles. It was also shown recently that, independently of the lipoprotein phenotype, a general

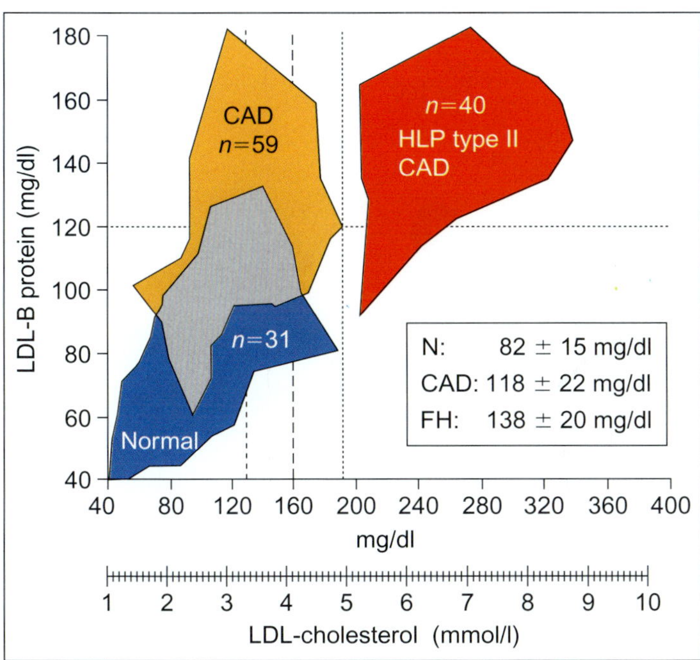

pattern of activated blood coagulation and impaired fibrino-lysis (elevated thrombin–antithrombin complex [TAT], activated factor XII [F XIIa], von Willebrand factor [vWF], plasminogen activator inhibitor-1 [PAI-1] and tissue derived plasminogen activator [t-PA] values) is present in FCH. An increase in PAI-1 and soluble thrombomodulin is especially associated with features of the metabolic syndrome. A state of endothelial activation is also observed in FCH. Interestingly, mean carotid intima-media thickness (IMT) correlates positively with the vWF antigen in FCH.

A large effort has been made to identify the genetic defect responsible for FCH. Genome-wide linkage studies indicate that more than three genes are responsible for the lipoprotein pattern. Three chromosomal regions have been proposed for the location of these genes with strong supportive evidence:

- 1q21–23: an association was found with FCH in Finnish, German, US, Mexican and Chinese families; this region includes the APOAII gene but a close association was established with the upstream transcription factor 1 (USF1 gene) in the same region which regulates several genes of glucose and lipid metabolism; a single nucleotide polymorphism (SNP) in an intronic response element of this gene (usf1s2) appears to relate with the cardiovascular risk associated with FCH
- 11p14.1–q12.1: this region associates with the cholesterol and triglyceride traits. Recent combined linkage and association analyses point strongly to two separate alleles

3.2 Hyper-apoB discriminates for coronary artery disease beyond low-density lipoprotein-cholesterol (LDL-C). This study was carried out in consecutive patients undergoing diagnostic cardiac catheterization for coronary artery disease (CAD). Thirty-one were 'free of CAD' (<25% stenosis) (blue cohort marked Normal) and 59 had CAD (≥50% stenosis; blinded evaluation, orange group). The mean ± SD for LDL-C was 2.9 ± 0.8 mmol/l (112 ± 30 mg/dl) and 3.46 ± 0.7 mmol/l (134 ± 27 mg/dl), respectively. A third group of 40 CAD subjects with 'type II hyperlipoproteinemia' representing essentially patients with familial hypercholesterolemia (FH) and an LDL-C ≥4.91 mmol/l (190 mg/dl) was used for comparison; the mean LDL-C in this group was 6.65 ±1.4 mmol/l (250 ± 55mg/dl, red). Although there is an overlap (grey zone) between normal and CAD subjects, discriminant analysis showed that LDL-apoB (LDL-B) most clearly separated the two groups compared with cholesterol, LDL-C or triglycerides.

Although assessment of disease severity has the limitations of angiographic evaluation, this work supports the importance of plasma LDL-apoB to separate patients at risk for CAD in the presence of 'normal' LDL-C. Among the hyper-apoB patients most would fit the definition of familial combined hyperlipidemia (FCH). LDL-B levels in these patients reached values observed in familial hypercholesterolemia (FH) with much higher LDL-C concentrations. The upper limit of normal for LDL-C when this work was published was 4.91 mmol/l (190 mg/dl). Afterwards it was brought down to 4.18 mmol/l (160 mg/dl), and later to 3.36 mmol/l (130 mg/dl). Even with these new cut-offs, part of the CAD sample remains in the upper left quadrant of hyper-apoB without hypercholesterolemia. Setting the limit of LDL-C in secondary prevention of CAD to 2.6 mmol/l (100 mg/dl) may include most of these hyper-apoB subjects and also most of the normal subjects. The apoB level is particularly important to know when identifying subjects at risk in an FCH family when triglycerides and total or LDL-C are normal (NB phenotype). The mean levels of LDL-B are given for the three different groups of patients illustrated on the left side of the graph. This figure was constructed from figures in the article by Sniderman AD *et al.* (1980). *Proc Natl Acad Sci USA*, **77**: 604, linking the data point at the extremes of the distribution for each sample.

at the *APOA1/C3/A4/A5* gene cluster on chromosome 11q23 to account for the transmission of FCH (Marc R *et al.* [2004] *Circ Res*, **94**: 993–999)
- 16q22–24.1: this region associates with the low HDL-C trait. Other loci with weaker evidence include 1p31, 1q41, 6q16.1–16.3 and 8p23.3–22.

At present, the evidence supports the notion that FCH is an oligogenic disease with a complex pattern of inheritance involving a number of modifying genes.

The diagnosis of FCH is based on the demonstration in the patient's family of the various lipoprotein phenotypes

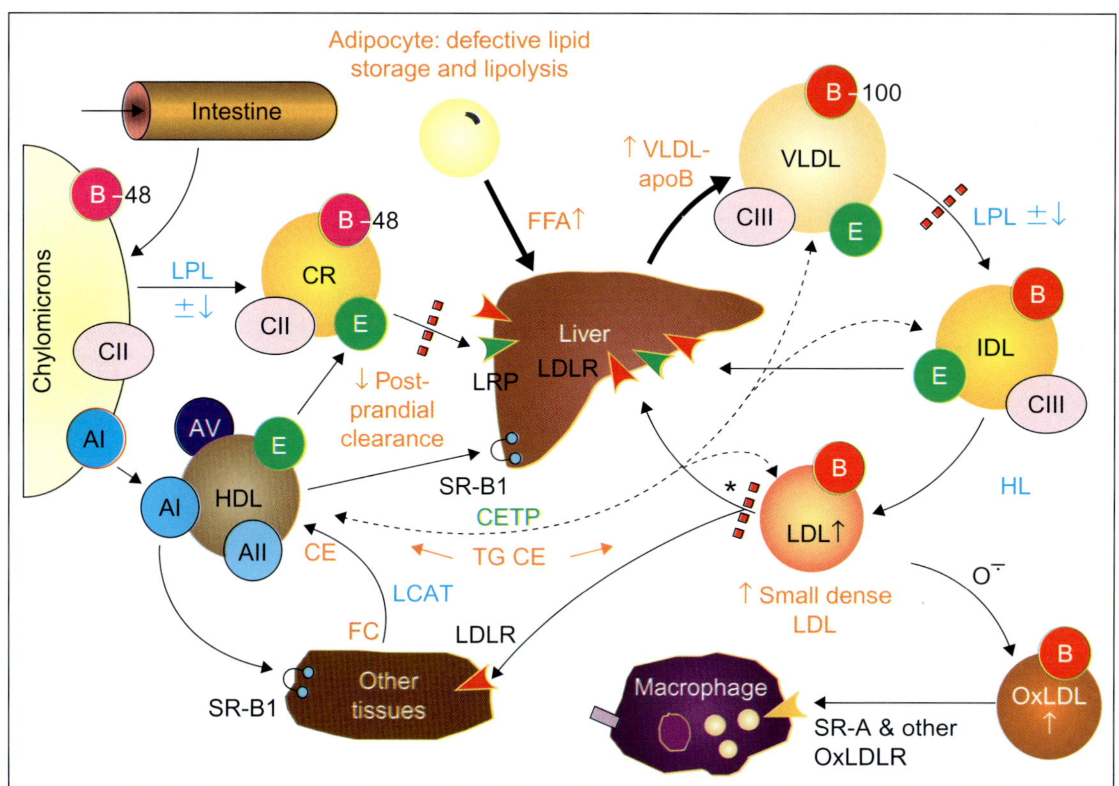

3.3 Metabolic defect in familial combined hyperlipidemia (FCH). In FCH there is a delayed clearance of postprandial chylomicron remnants (dotted red line on the left), with increased circulating levels of free fatty acids (FFA) and apoB-48. There is also reduced triglyceride synthesis from FFA in adipose tissue (see **3.4**) resulting in an enhanced flux of FFA to the liver for triglyceride synthesis. The major metabolic defect in FCH is an overproduction of very-low-density lipoprotein (VLDL)-apoB by the liver leading to increased plasma VLDL and apoB concentrations. The VLDL particle size and lipid content are smaller than in familial endogenous hypertriglyceridemia (FEHTG). The increase in VLDL may account for the hypercholesterolemia as well as for the hypertriglyceridemia (IIb) but the final lipoprotein phenotype may depend on variations in the fate and or composition of the VLDL particles.

Effective lipolysis coupled with reduced clearance of LDL may result in isolated hypercholesterolemia (IIa). In contrast, reduced lipoprotein lipase (LPL) activity (LPL ± ↓, dotted red line on the top right) – which occurs in as many as 50% of cases of FCH – with effective LDL clearance may favour the hypertriglyceridemic phenotype (IV), sometimes with traces of chylomicrons (type V). Phenotype variation over time may result from the transient effect of modulating environmental or genetic factors. The LDL particles formed tend to be small, dense and numerous. This is determined in part by the concentration and size of triglyceride-rich lipoproteins as there is an inverse relationship between triglycerides and LDL particle size ($r = -0.71$, $P < 0.001$, Vakkilainen J, Jauhiainen M, Ylitalo K, Nuotio IO, Viikari JSA, Ehnholm C, Taskinen MR [2002]. LDL particle size in familial combined hyperlipidemia: effects of serum lipids, lipoprotein-modifying enzymes, and lipid transfer proteins. *J Lipid Res*, **43**: 598–603. Small dense LDL (sdLDL) particles are made with the concerted action of cholesteryl ester transfer protein (CETP) and hepatic lipase (HL). Although an impaired LDL removal may be a secondary component in FCH pathophysiology (* with dotted red line), one family has been reported in which the FCH clinical and biochemical phenotype was essentially associated with a defect at this step in the absence of VLDL-apoB overproduction. For more details regarding the metabolic scheme and abbreviations, see **1.2** and **2.12**.

(IIa, IIb, IV, VB and NB, B indicating increased plasma apoB) which may change with time in an affected subject. Clinical features are usually discrete and non-specific such as xanthelasma and arcus corneae (**3.6–3.8**), until the manifestations of atherosclerosis, especially CAD, appear in the fifth and sixth decades in men, or the sixth and seventh decades in women. Cholesterol and/or triglycerides are elevated above the 90th percentile. Plasma apoB levels are usually ≥120 mg/dl in affected individuals. There is evidence that using apoB criteria for diagnosis may improve assignment to affected or non-affected. A nomogram based on values for total cholesterol, triglycerides and apoB adjusted for age and sex has been proposed by Veerkamp and co-workers for the diagnosis of FCH when at least one family member exhibits the phenotype and one family member has premature CAD. Until a clear genetic marker is available, however, a degree

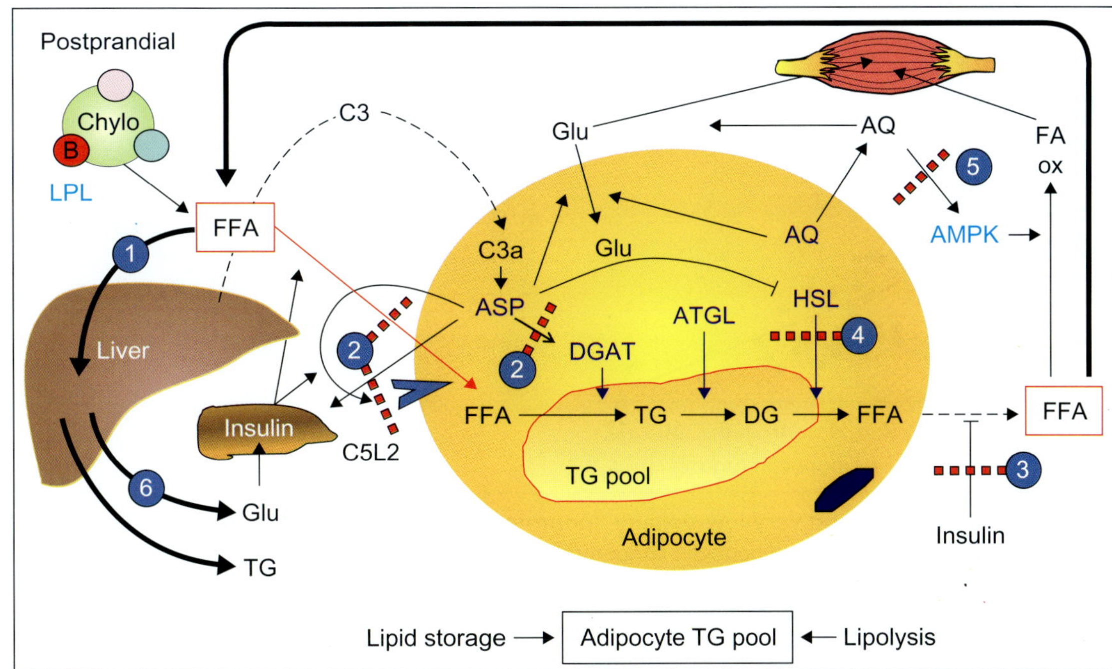

3.4 Putative involvement of adipose tissue in familial combined hyperlipidemia (FCH). In healthy subjects, there is a fine balance between free fatty acid (FFA) uptake and release by adipose tissue which reflects lipid storage and lipolysis, respectively, two physiologically important components of energy balance. In FCH, impairment of both lipid storage and lipolysis have been postulated. (1) After a fat meal in FCH, there is no major change in lipoprotein lipase (LPL) activity but increased serum free fatty acid (FFA) levels and flux to the liver with a transient increase in ketone bodies (0–8 hours). In the post-absorptive period (8–24 hours), FFA and ketone bodies rapidly decrease in subjects with FCH compared with normal subjects. This was ascribed by Meijssen *et al.* (2000), from Erasmus University, to inadequate incorporation of FFA into triglycerides in adipocytes coupled with a diminished release of FFA by hormone-sensitive lipase (HSP). This scenario is supported by other lines of evidence. (2) *Acylation-stimulating protein* (ASP), a complement C3a derivative, C3a-des-Arg, made in adipose tissue (with the concerted action of adipsin [factor D], complement factors C3 and B), promotes triglyceride (TG) synthesis by stimulating acyl-CoA:diacylglycerol acyl-transferase (DGAT), inhibits hormone-sensitive lipase (HSL) and favours glucose uptake in adipocytes. ASP is a lipid-storage hormone. Some of its autocrine and paracrine effects are mediated by its receptor C5L2 (an orphan G protein-coupled receptor) and enhanced by insulin. ASP activity is impaired in FCH and ASP-mediated triglyceride synthesis is reduced in adipose cells from FCH subjects as shown by Cianflone and co-workers in Montreal. They have also shown that in fibroblasts from FCH patients (patients with 'hyperapobetalipoproteinemia') the specific binding of ASP to a single class of surface receptors was reduced in proportion to reduction in triglyceride synthesis (apart from evidence of reduced receptor number, it is not established whether there is impaired receptor-ligand interaction or ASP resistance in FCH). This results in a diversion of FFA from lipid storage to liver uptake for triglyceride and very-low-density lipoproteins (VLDL) synthesis. The major source of C3, the precursor of ASP, is the liver. An increase in circulating C3 has been reported in FCH. (3) There is also a defect in the ability of insulin to suppress free fatty acid release from adipose tissue in FCH. (4) This adds to the problem of impaired activity of HSL leading to impaired lipolysis as reported by Reynisdottir and co-workers, from Huddinge Sweden, in 1995 in work carried out with subcutaneous adipose tissue from FCH patients, (although, in contrast, there has been no demonstration of reduced HSL gene expression nor linkage with the HSL gene in affected Finnish subjects). An inhibition of ASP receptor by an expanding triglyceride pool was postulated. (5) Adiponectin (AQ) is another hormone formed in adipose tissue with protective effects against atherosclerotic cardiovascular disease. van der Vleuten and colleagues in Nijmegen, the Netherlands, found that adiponectin is decreased in FCH independent of waist circumference and insulin resistance. It is an independent predictor of the atherogenic lipoprotein profile of FCH, including high triglyceride levels, low HDL-C levels and amount of circulating small dense LDL. Several properties of adiponectin may account for this. Adiponectin enhances fatty acid oxidation (FA ox) in the circulation and in skeletal muscle, through activation of AMP-activated kinase (AMPK). There is also a strong relationship between adiponectin levels and LPL activity. This is consistent with the fact that plasma apoB concentrations are inversely related to adiponectin levels and that adiponectin correlates positively with apoB catabolism (but not with apoB production) (**3.5**). Furthermore, adiponectin increases glucose (Glu) uptake by skeletal muscle and enhances insulin sensitivity. Therefore a reduction in adiponectin would enhance insulin resistance, which may occur in FCH. (6) Finally, FFA may also promote insulin resistance by increasing gluconeogenesis in the liver. Increased glucose production stimulates the pancreas to secrete more insulin, which may lead to increased fasting insulin and insulin resistance coupled with defective insulin action (see point 3). This can lead to reduced FFA trapping and further increase in circulating FFA thereby creating a vicious cycle.

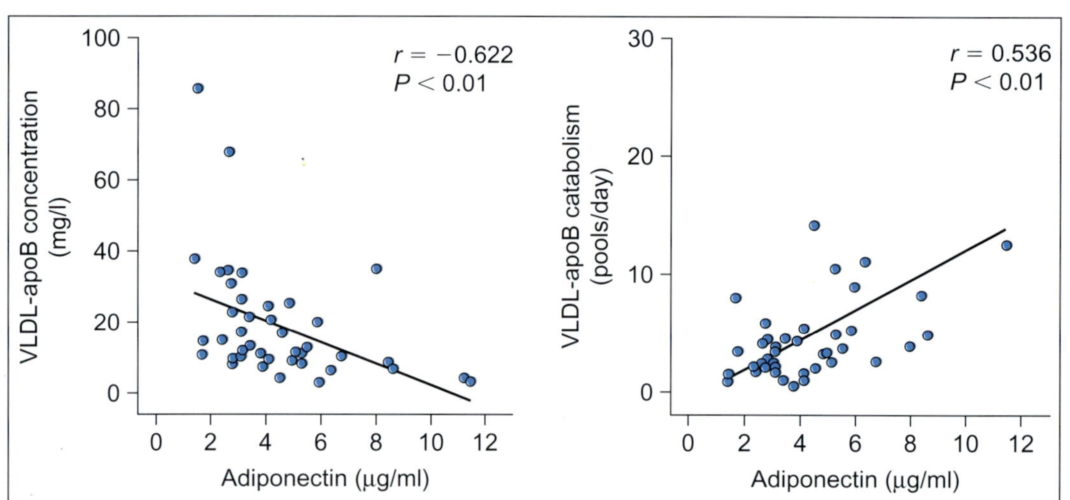

3.5 Relationship between adiponectin and very-low-density lipoprotein (VLDL)-apoB levels or catabolism. Ng and co-workers (2005) investigated the relationship of plasma adiponectin concentrations with VLDL-apolipoprotein B (apoB)-100 kinetics in men using stable isotopes. They showed that in multivariate analysis, plasma adiponectin concentration was the most significant predictor of plasma VLDL-apoB concentration ($P = 0.001$) and, with total or subcutaneous adipose tissue mass, was an independent predictor of VLDL-apoB catabolism ($P < 0.001$). The associations using a stepwise regression model including HOMA (homeostasis model assessment) score, age and total adipose tissue mass as co-variates are depicted in the left panel for apoB levels and the right panel for apoB catabolism ($n = 41$). There was no association of adiponectin with apoB production. In contrast with adiponectin, insulin resistance, measured with the HOMA, was a significant predictor of apoB production ($P < 0.05$). Interestingly, leptin, resistin, interleukin-6 and tumour necrosis factor α were not associated with any of the measured variables. Reproduced with permission from Ng TWK *et al.* (2005). Adipocytokines and VLDL metabolism: independent regulatory effects of adiponectin, insulin resistance, and fat compartments on VLDL-apolipoprotein B-100 kinetics? *Diabetes*, **54**: 795–802.

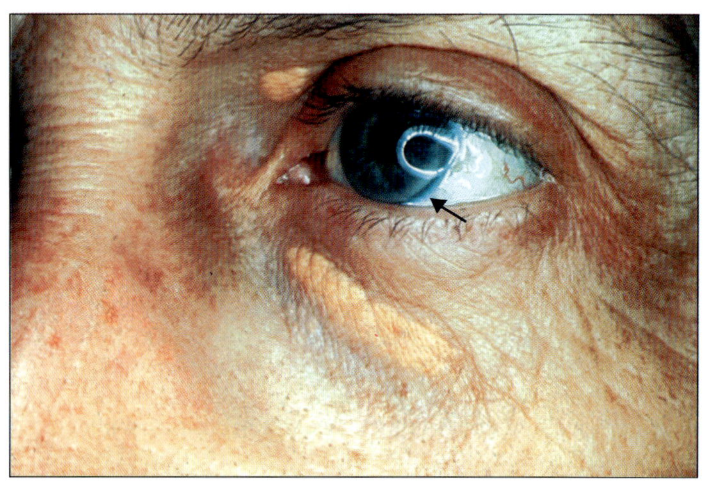

3.6 Discrete clinical signs in familial combined hyperlipidemia (FCH): xanthelasma and arcus corneae. Clinical signs when present tend to be discrete in FCH. Besides manifestations of atherosclerosis that might emerge eventually, such as arterial bruits, angina pectoris, transient ischemic attacks or other forms of expression of tissue ischemia, xanthelasma of the eyelids or arcus corneae may be the only clinical clue to the existence of FCH. This figure (the arrow is pointing to the arcus) is of a 46-year-old patient with hypercholesterolemia (phenotype IIa).

of uncertainty will remain in separating affected from non-affected individuals.

Using current criteria, a diagnosis of FCH may not be made unless a family survey is carried out. Therefore, 'combined hyperlipidemia' or 'mixed hyperlipidemia', referring to the co-existence of hypercholesterolemia and hypertriglyceridemia in a patient, are not synonymous with 'familial combined hyperlipidemia'. This combination could be due to a large number of causes including familial hypercholesterolemia (see **2.16**) or polygenic hypercholesterolemia with inheritance of familial hypertriglyceridemia from one of the parents, dysbetalipoproteinemia type III, secondary causes of hypertriglyceridemia or hypercholesterolemia associated with or superimposed on an inherited form of dyslipidemia, etc. Tendon xanthomas are not present in FCH, unless FH co-segregates in the same family. As discussed in Chapter 2, FEHTG differs from FCH in that the VLDL of FEHTG are more enriched in lipids and of larger size than VLDL of FCH (see **2.15**). Several risk factors seem to associate readily with FCH, such as obesity, hypertension and insulin resistance. Some degree of overlap may be seen with other conditions including the metabolic syndrome,

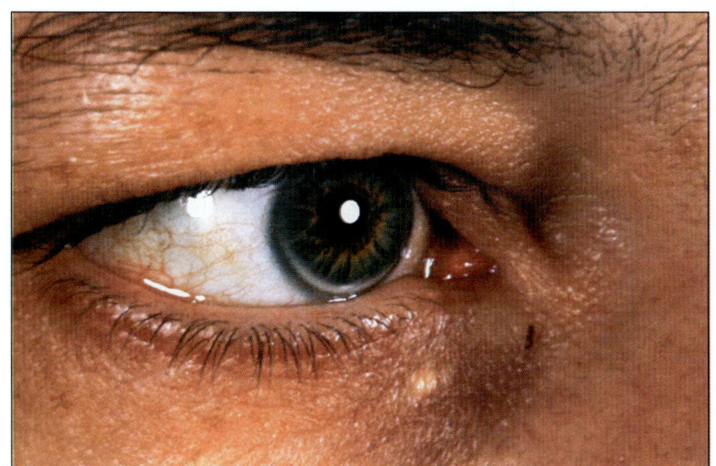

3.7 Discrete manifestations of familial combined hyperlipidemia (FCH): arcus corneae and xanthelasma. Corneal arcus and xanthelasma are not always as obvious as in **3.6**. Instead of fully encircling the cornea (see **1.3**), FCH is often manifested by a discrete lower (as above) or upper corneal crescent, always leaving a rim of clear cornea between the lipid deposit and the sclera. It may be easily missed if it is not looked for in particular using a light, especially for upper crescents, which are masked readily by the upper eyelid. They tend to occur more frequently in the elderly. In the past a distinction was made between arcus juvenilis and arcus senilis, the latter considered a degenerative ocular manifestation. In black people, arcus corneae are routinely seen in the absence of dyslipidemia. In this figure, a unique small xanthelasma is also present. Half of the subjects with xanthelasma also have dyslipidemia. Presence of either of these is an excellent clue for dyslipidemia.

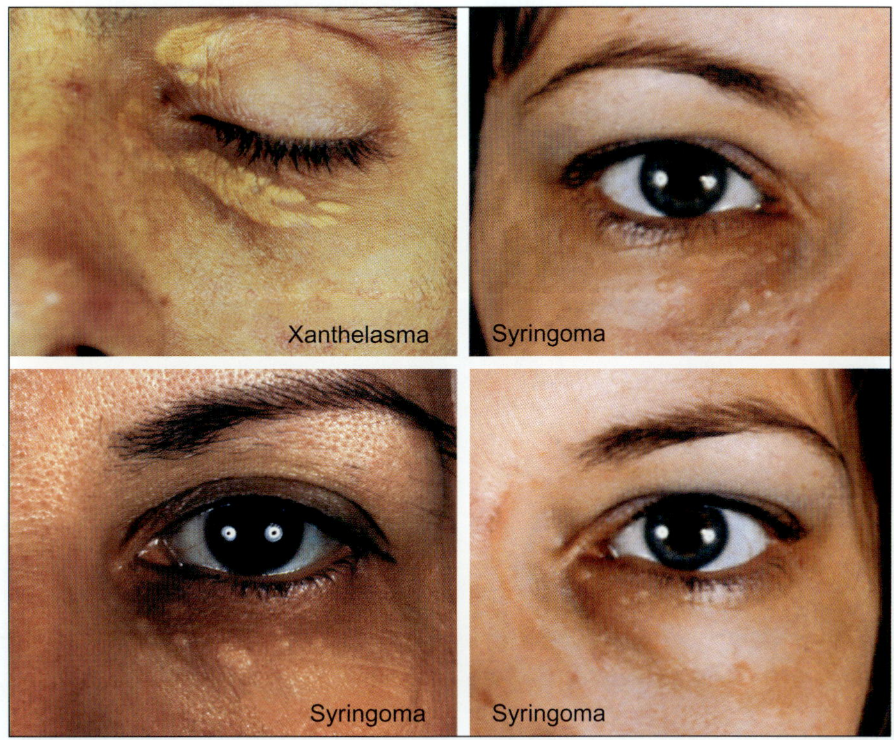

3.8 Syringoma is often mistaken for xanthelasma associated with dyslipidemia. The top left panel shows typical xanthelasmas of the eyelids and of the loose skin under the lower eyelid in a 38-year-old patient with familial combined hyperlipidemia (FCH; type IIa phenotype). They are typically planar, slightly raised, occurring in patches of various sizes, coalescing with a yellow to yellow-orange discoloration. The other three panels represent syringomas which, in contrast, are puncta of smaller sizes, are not found in patches or coalescing, and are more pinkish than yellow. These are small tumours, usually benign, of the sweat glands. The lower left panel shows typical syringomas in a 51-year-old woman, referred for hypercholesterolemia and xanthelasma of the eyelids. In fact she had histologically confirmed syringomas of the eyelids and not xanthelasma and hyperalphalipoproteinemia. Twenty-two years later her lipoprotein profile had changed very little: total cholesterol 5.98 mmol/l (231 mg/dl), low-density lipoprotein-cholesterol (LDL-C) 3.41 mmol/l (132 mg/dl), triglycerides 0.93 mmol/l (82 mg/dl), and HDL-C 2.15 mmol/l (83 mg/dl). She never developed clinical manifestations of atherosclerosis. The two panels on the right show a 33-year-old women who was referred to the authors' lipid clinic in 1972 for 'xanthelasma' and hyperlipidemia discovered fortuitously during a routine clinical examination. Further evaluation revealed that she had syringoma of the eyelids and not xanthelasma. The modest rise in cholesterol levels to 6.85 mmol/l (265 mg/dl) and triglycerides to 2.74 mmol/l (243 mg/dl) was not due to a familial diathesis but was secondary to oral contraceptives (norethindrone 1 mg/mestranol 50 μg). Lipids normalized on withdrawal and the dyslipidemia recurred on rechallenge. The positive family history of a premature death at the age of 45 of a maternal aunt due to coronary causes, which had suggested a familial disease turned out to be that of an unrelated spouse of a family member. Correct interpretation of the clues suggestive of dyslipidemia is a key element of the diagnostic process.

familial dyslipidemic hypertension (FDH) and the athero-genic lipoprotein pattern B. It is not clear at present if FDH constitutes a separate clinical entity from FCH. As LPL mutations may segregate in FCH families especially in areas where a founder effect may have occurred, a mixed hypertri-glyceridemia (type V) may be seen in patients homozygous for LPL deficiency as observed on occasion at the authors' lipid clinic (**3.9**). This occurrence probably explains early reports of type V as one of the multiple phenotypes of FCH (**3.10**).

There is evidence that FCH may be heterogeneous. Aguilar Salinas and co-workers in 1997 reported a family in which the clinical phenotype is indistinguishable from that of FCH but instead of observing an overproduction of VLDL apoB, the metabolic defect was an impaired apoB catabolism (**3.3**).

The treatment of FCH is a function of the lipid abnor-mality using dietary measures that would be appropriate for hypertriglyceridemia, hypercholesterolemia or both and for associated cardiovascular risk factors. The same attitude applies for drug treatment when goals of therapy are not attained, which is often the case, with lifestyle changes alone: statins for hypercholesterolemia and fibrates for hypertriglyceridemia. The combined phenotype may need a combination of both drugs applied with caution and monitoring for potential side effects. Nicotinic acid and its sustained release forms may be effective in monotherapy if well tolerated.

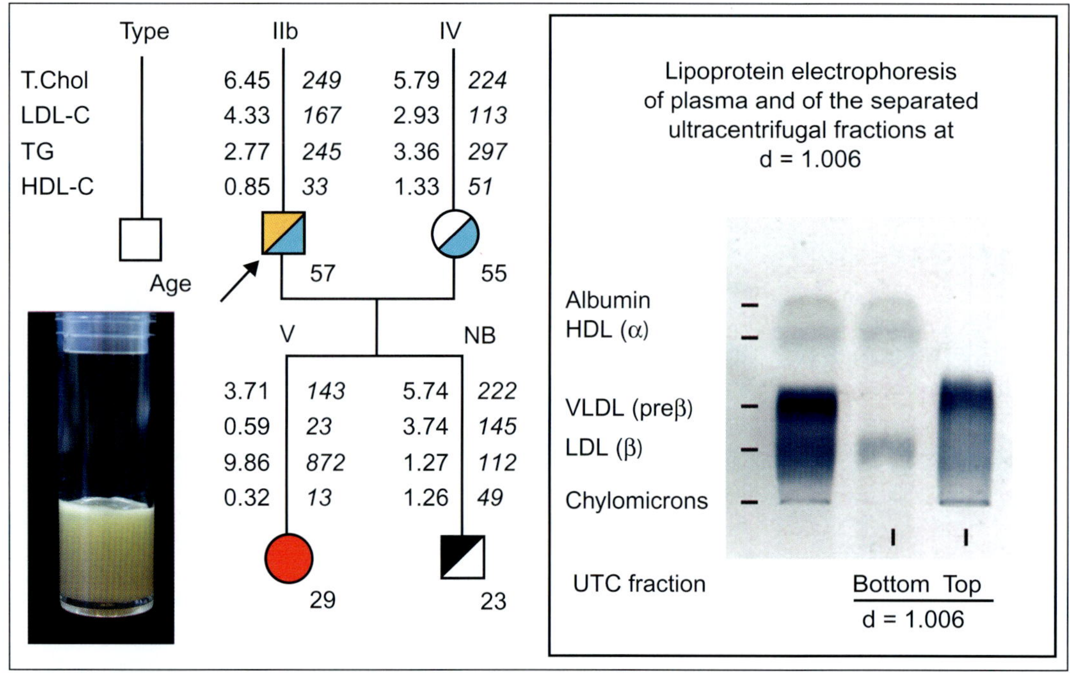

3.9 Type V secondary to the P207L LPL mutation in a familial combined hyperlipidemia (FCH) family. In this family the proband is a 57-year-old man with FCH. On the paternal side, four of his relatives had had a myocardial infarction and/or a cerebrovascular accident between the ages of 45 and 79. He himself had a cerebral thrombosis following a left carotid endarterectomy at the age of 44 after a few episodes of amaurosis fugax. His 55-year-old spouse was found to have hypertriglyceridemia (type IV). His daughter first consulted at the age of 21 years, five years after her father's first visit to the authors' lipid clinic. A diagnosis of familial hyperchylomicronemia had been made at the age of 8 months. She was followed regularly thereafter and was on a very low fat/no alcohol diet. Thus, she was able to avoid having pancreatic complications or developing eruptive xanthomas. Homozygosity for the P207L mutation of the LPL gene was established at the age of 19. At the authors' lipid clinic her lipoprotein phenotype was found to be type V. Chylomicrons ranged from traces on lipoprotein electrophoresis to a typical creamy layer on top of a diffusely milky plasma (image on the left). Her triglycerides tended to increase over seven years of follow-up and fluctuated widely from 3.83 mmol/l to 21.7 mmol/l. The recent lipoprotein analysis given above shows the phenotypic profile of type V in which the very-low-density lipoproteins (VLDL) fraction predominates (right panel). Her 23-year-old brother is normolipidemic, but his total plasma apoB is 121 mg/dl, which is compatible with the presence of an FCH susceptibility gene at this age (type NB). Red, mixed hypertriglyceridemia; yellow, hypercholesterolemia; blue, hypertriglyceridemia; black, hyperapobetalipoproteinemia.

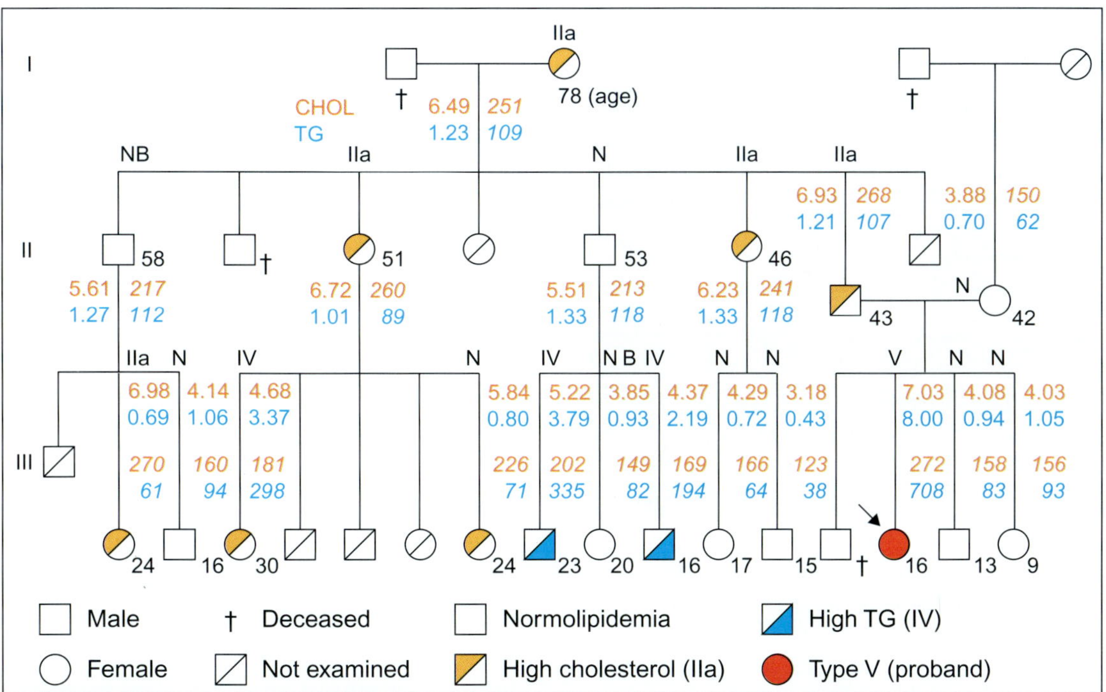

3.10 Mixed hypertriglyceridemia (type V) in a familial combined hyperlipidemia (FCH) family. There have been several reports of mixed hypertriglyceridemia (lipoprotein phenotype V) occurring in FCH families. This figure concerns one of the early reports (Kobori *et al.* 1986). The proband (arrow) was a 16-year-old girl with recurrent episodes of abdominal pain. As is often the case, laparotomy was carried out, which revealed that the pain was secondary to pancreatitis. Later on, the plasma was noted to be milky, which revealed the cause and she was referred to a lipid clinic where the family survey was done. This case is interesting because, first, the diagnosis of FCH was supported by raised levels of apoB in all hyperlipidemic cases, including the proband and the other hypertriglyceridemic subjects; there were two different phenotypes in the family (IIa and IV); there were discrete clinical manifestations (19 relatives were examined; there were no tendon xanthomas but corneal arcus was present in the father) and the presence of two normolipidemic subjects with hyper-apoB (NB phenotype). There was no overt coronary artery disease in this family with relatively young members (the oldest in generation II was 58 years and in generation III was 30 years). Second, there was a reduction in post-heparin lipolytic activities in the proband: LPL of 0.8 μM FFA/h/ml (normal: 2.5 ± 0.9) and HL 3.2 μM FFA/h/ml (normal: 6.9 ± 3.1), which is compatible with the authors' experience and that of others that mutations of the LPL gene may segregate independently in some FCH families. Secondary causes of dyslipidemia were excluded and there was no apoCII deficiency. The proband had the common E3/3 apoE phenotype. Her lipoprotein profile indicated endogenous hypertriglyceridemia (type IV) when her plasma triglycerides were lowered. There were no cases of dysbetalipoproteinemia (type III) in the family. Total cholesterol (dark orange figures, orange-yellow shading) and triglycerides (blue figures, blue shading) are given in mmol/l and in *mg/dl*. They are given in mg/dl in the original article. The lipoprotein phenotype is given at the top of the line of each pedigree member; note that 'NB' phenotype is the authors' interpretation, the plasma apoB was 116 mg/dl for the 58-year-old and 90 mg/dl for the 20-year-old relative. The age is given in the lower right corner of the square for males and the circle for females. Redrawn and modified from Kobori S *et al.* (1986). A kindred of familial combined hyperlipidemia (FCHL) with proband showing type V hyperlipoproteinemia. *Jpn J Med*, **25**: 306–312.

Familial dysbetalipoproteinemia and remnant excess

Classical dysbetalipoproteinemia type III

Although uncommon, the importance of this disease stems from the following points:

- it is a major diagnostic challenge (it is often missed)

- it has distinct clinical features, some of them pathogno-monic, which when present allow the clinician to make a conclusive diagnosis at bedside
- complex interactions determine its expression
- failure to make a diagnosis exposes the subject to premature CAD
- treatment is effective and avoids catastrophic consequences.

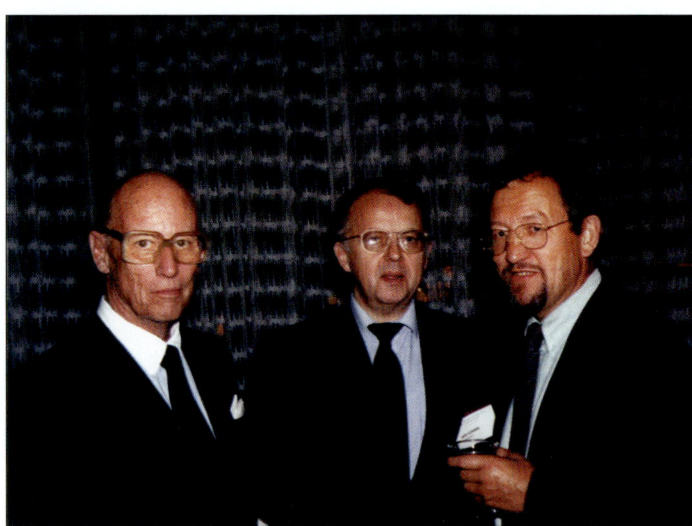

3.11 Three pioneers in lipidology. From left to right: Donald S Fredrickson, who developed the classification of hyperlipoproteinemia based on the lipoprotein phenotype; Gerd Assmann, who conducted the PROCAM epidemiological study; and Gerd Utermann, head of one of the two groups that unraveled the apoE polymorphism. This photograph was taken in October 1994 at the Xth International Symposium of Atherosclerosis in Montreal.

Familial dysbetalipoproteinemia (type III hyperlipoproteinemia, type III, broad beta disease, remnant removal disease, floating β lipoprotein disease) is a relatively rare condition (frequency of about 1–5/5000; 1–5/10 000 in Japan). It was first recognized in the early days of lipoprotein separation by analytical ultracentrifugation by Gofman and co-workers in 1952, at the Donner Laboratory in California, as a distinct lipoprotein profile (increase in the Sf 12–20 and Sf 20–100 fractions) associated with tuberous xanthomas. However, it was not until 1967 that it was identified as a separate nosological entity by Fredrickson (**3.11**) and his group at the National Institutes of Health (NIH). Many tools were available at the time to study plasma lipoprotein metabolism (**3.12**). The diagnosis then was essentially based on the clinical findings coupled with the appearance of a 'broad beta band' on electrophoresis of plasma lipoproteins migrating where β-lipoproteins (LDL) migrate (**3.13** and **3.14**), and reflecting an increase in cholesteryl ester enriched particles. These are partially degraded normal VLDL and chylomicrons, referred to as remnants (or intermediate-density lipoproteins [IDL]), forming large buoyant particles, depleted in apoC and enriched in apoE. Although they float with the VLDL fraction when separated by ultracentrifugation, they migrate at the level of β-lipoproteins on lipoprotein electrophoresis (hence the term 'floating β-lipoprotein' or β-VLDL) (**3.13**). The accumulation of plasma remnants results in high levels of cholesterol, triglycerides and apoE, low LDL-C concentrations and normal or low HDL-C. Because remnants are enriched in cholesteryl esters, the VLDL-C/triglyceride ratio is typically high (>0.3, if mg/dl is the unit used, or >0.7, if mmol/l is the unit used). This abnormal ratio was a major diagnostic clue in the past, before the role of apoE polymorphism was uncovered in the 1970s in the laboratories of Breslow and Zannis in the USA and Utermann (**3.11**) in Germany, and the association with the apoE2/2 phenotype established in Utermann's laboratory (1977). Thereafter, demonstration that the affected subject carries the E2/2 phenotype (**3.15**) or genotype (**3.16**) became a prerequisite to establish the diagnosis of type III.

The major metabolic defect in type III (**3.17**) is an impaired remnant lipoprotein clearance secondary to a reduced affinity of apoE2 for its receptor, the only apoE present on the remnant surface in subjects with the E2/2 phenotype. ApoE2 has 1% of the affinity of apoE3 or apoE4 for the LDL receptor (also called 'apoB-E receptor'). The apo E*2/2* phenotype in the presence of a second factor interfering with triglyceride-rich lipoprotein (TRL) metabolism (a 'second hit', **3.18**), results in delayed chylomicron remnant and VLDL-remnant (IDL) removal by the liver, impaired conversion of IDL into LDL and an overproduction of VLDL and of VLDL apoCIII. Plasma fasting apoB-48, a marker of chylomicron remnants, is increased ten-fold in type III compared with normal subjects (56.4 ± 7.9 µg/ml vs. 5.2 ± 3.8 µg/ml),an increase similar to the one observed in familial hyperchylomicronemia. Plasma levels of apoE are also elevated because remnant lipoproteins are rich in apoE. Among apoE2 homozygotes, men are more susceptible than women to type III. Animal studies have shown that estrogens affect both LDL receptor expression and lipolytic processing, explaining the resistance of women to this disorder until after menopause. Recent evidence indicates that changes in the carboxy-terminal end of the apoE2 molecule may contribute to the severity of the lipoprotein abnormality, favour the production of triglyceride-enriched VLDL that resist lipolysis, and are associated with a reduced LPL activity.

The inheritance of type III remained confusing until the role of apoE polymorphism was unravelled. In humans, apoE is coded by three alleles (ε2, ε3, ε4) of a modulator gene at the apoE locus on chromosome 19 (19q13.2) which

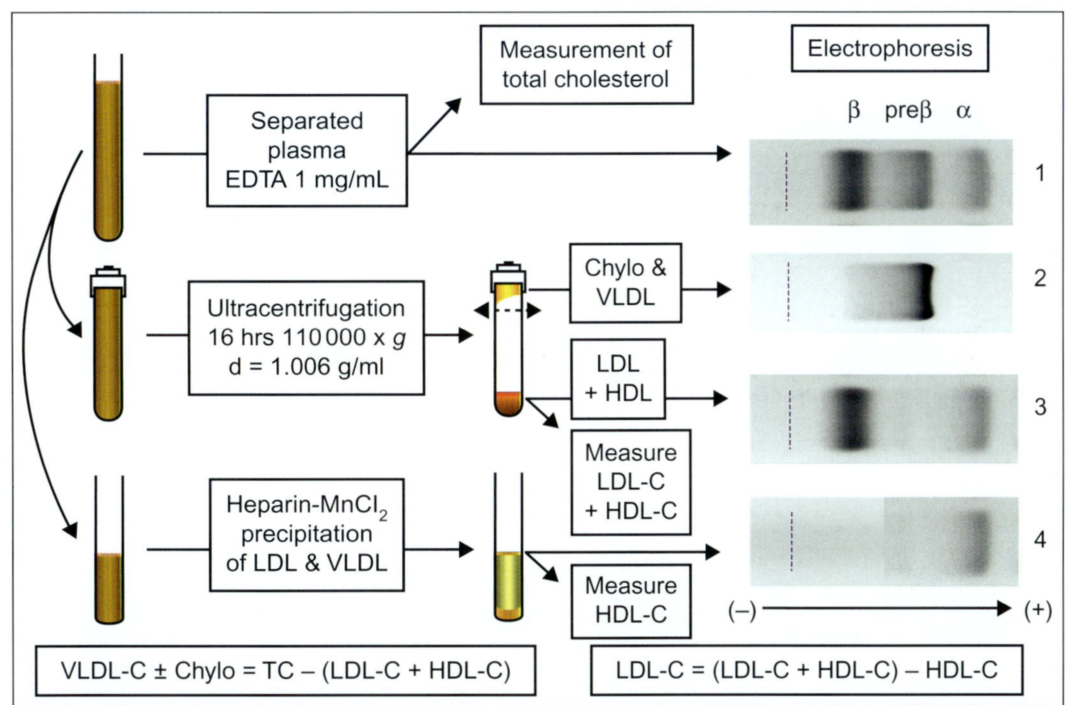

3.12 Lipoprotein-cholesterol determination. This figure depicts the standard procedure used to assess the cholesterol content of the major lipoprotein fractions by combining a single ultracentrifugal run with measurement of cholesterol in plasma, in the low-density lipoprotein (LDL) + high-density lipoprotein (HDL) fraction (bottom fraction, d > 1.006) and in the supernatant after precipitation of the apoB-containing lipoproteins with a combination of heparin and manganese chloride (or dextran sulphate and calcium chloride or other). The double arrowhead indicates where the ultracentrifuge tube is cut to separate the top and bottom fractions. Afterwards a simple calculation provides the VLDL + chylomicron-cholesterol fraction (bottom left box). Except for types I and V, there are no or few chylomicrons in fasting plasma. Therefore, this corresponds to VLDL-C in most instances, especially because the cholesterol content of chylomicrons is of the order of 2–6%. The lipoprotein electrophoresis of total plasma or of the top d < 1.006 fraction (lane 2 on the right) will indicate if chylomicrons are present. Chylomicrons stay at the origin, which is marked on the electrophoreses by a dotted line (see **3.9**). The LDL-C is calculated by subtracting HDL-C in the supernatant of the precipitate from the cholesterol measured in the LDL + HDL fraction (1.006 bottom fraction, d > 1.006) (bottom right box). Ultracentrifugation separates lipoproteins on the basis of their buoyancy at a given density, whereas electrophoresis separates them according to their charge. The other plasma proteins are present in the bottom fraction; because they contain virtually no cholesterol this does not interfere with the evaluation of the lipoprotein fractions. Similarly, all plasma proteins are still present in the lipoprotein electrophoresis. However, the staining technique uses a dye that stains only lipids (Oil red O or Sudan black) so that lipoprotein migration can be followed. Staining with Coomassie blue, a non-specific protein stain, will show all plasma proteins grossly separated according to their charge. Lipoproteins are classified as α or β depending on their migration to the position where α- or β-globulins would migrate, repectively. The 'gamma' globulins would move in the opposite direction towards the cathode (−). Very-low-density lipoproteins (VLDL) move in the preβ position (in front of β).

Much of the practical use of preparative ultracentrifugation for the study of lipoproteins stems from the work of Havel and co-workers at the NIH (Havel RJ *et al.* [1955]. *J Clin Invest*, **34**: 1345). They developed sequential preparative ultracentrifugation which allows further separation of lipoprotein fractions to measure their lipid and apolipoprotein composition. This is achieved by repeated ultracentrifugation after progressively raising the solvent density with potassium bromide. After floating and removing VLDL at plasma aqueous density (d = 1.006 g/ml), a second ultracentrifugation at d = 1.019 allows flotation of intermediate-density lipoproteins (IDL), and a third one at 1.063 g/ml allows flotation of LDL and HDL left in the bottom fraction. These notions are useful to understand the lipoprotein abnormalities in type III. The ultracentrifugation time mentioned for the separation of the fractions corresponds to a rotor spinning at 40 000 rpm; shorter times are used with rotors with higher speeds. The combined procedure described in this figure is the gold standard, and in the USA it is often referred to as the beta-quant procedure (βQ or BQ-LDL, see Maitra A *et al.* 1997). It can also be used for the measurement of apoB in the major lipoprotein fractions, using a specific anti-human apoB antibody in a enzyme-linked immunosorbent assay (ELISA). There are several simplified adaptations of this procedure and more direct methods are also commercially available. A critical review of these methods can be found in Nauck M *et al.* (2002). Methods for measurement of LDL-C: a critical assessment of direct measurement by homogeneous assays versus calculation. *Clin Chem*, **48**: 236–254.

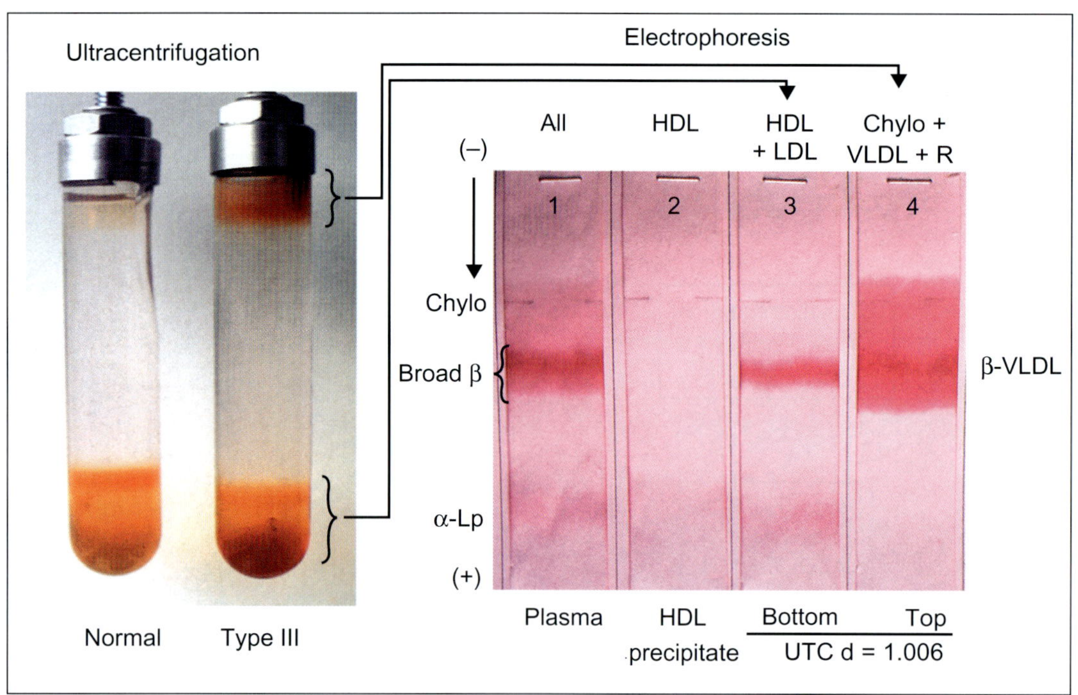

3.13 Demonstration of the 'floating' β-lipoprotein (β-VLDL) in type III. One of the unique characteristics of type III is the presence of a cholesteryl ester- and triglyceride-rich VLDL with a beta mobility on lipoprotein electrophoresis, thus the term β-VLDL. Normally, the LDL fraction is found at the bottom of the tube after ultracentrifugation at d = 1.006 g/ml. Because it is rich in carotene it is has a typical orange-yellow coloration (ultracentrifugation tube on the left). In type III, some of this orange colour is floating at the top (right tube) and, when this fraction is further separated by electrophoresis, a band with beta migration appears (strip 4), hence the expression 'floating β-lipoprotein'. In the bottom fraction, in contrast, only the β band typical of LDL and the α band typical of HDL is seen (strip 3). This patient had the full clinical phenotype III (see **3.22** and **3.24A**), her total cholesterol was 14.4 mmol/l (556 mg/dl) and her triglycerides 7.0 mmol/l (621 mg/dl). Lipoprotein electrophoresis of unfractionated plasma in type III (strip 1) often shows a large band in the β position referred to as a 'broad beta band'. This band was once deemed typical of this condition; however it is observed in only 50% of patients, hence the usefulness of demonstrating the presence of a β-VLDL. The lipoprotein electrophoresis on paper illustrated here carried out with an albumin-containing buffer was one of the first practical methods to separate plasma lipoproteins and was developed by Lees and Hatch ([1963]. *J Lab Clin Med*, **61**: 518). Its combination with ultracentrifugation was widely used in the lipoprotein phenotyping era. It has now been replaced by agarose gel electrophoresis (**2.17**) or electrophoresis on cellulose acetate (**3.14**) or similar techniques. Non-denaturing polyacrylamide gradient gel electrophoresis has also been used effectively.

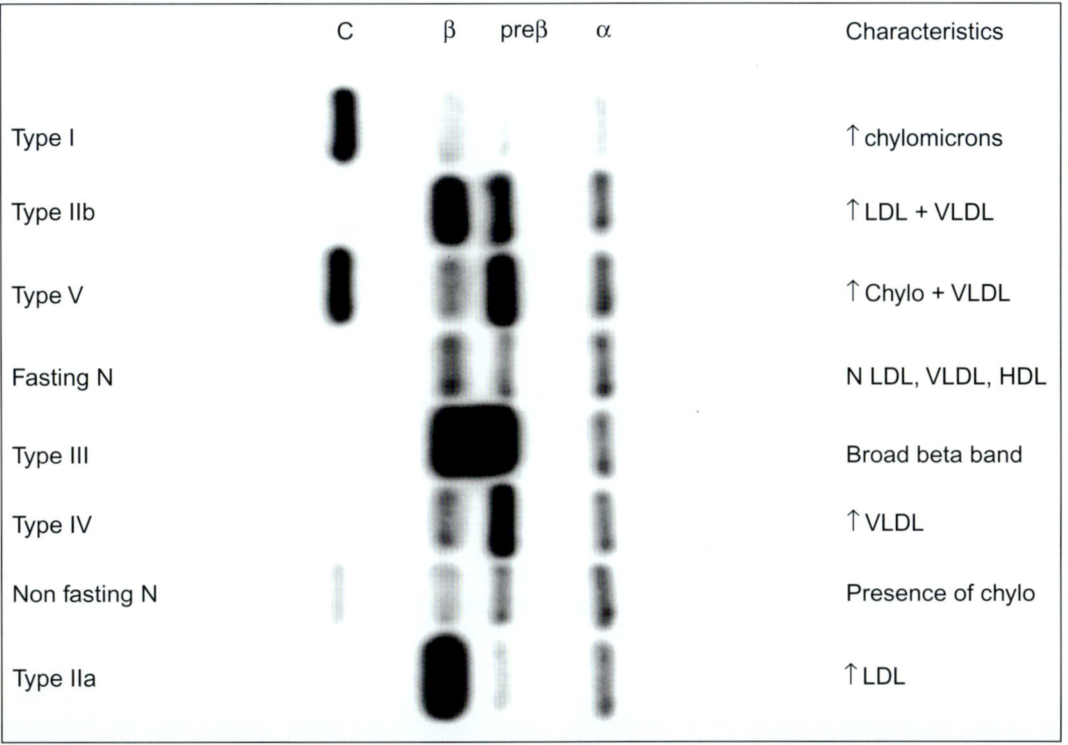

3.14 Lipoprotein phenotyping by electrophoresis on cellulose acetate. Lipoprotein phenotyping was developed by Fredrickson and his group at the National Institutes of Health and focused the attention of the clinician on the importance of the various lipoprotein fractions in health and disease. It helped the evaluation of metabolic abnormalities in lipid disorders: presence of chylomicrons of exogenous origin, of very-low-density lipoproteins (VLDL) of endogenous origin, high levels of low-density lipoproteins (LDL), and low levels of high-density lipoproteins (HDL). In particular, it advanced the diagnosis and characterization of type III dysbetalipoproteinemia. However, the test failed when the lipoprotein phenotype started to be equated with a specific disease entity: type IIa was used for familial hypercholesterolemia, type IV for familial hypertriglyceridemia and type I for familial lipoprotein lipase (LPL) deficiency. The overlap in lipoprotein phenotypes among specific lipoprotein disorders made this impractical, especially when the notion of familial combined hyperlipidemia was put forward in cases where the lipoprotein phenotype varied among individuals in a family and changed with time in a given individual. It has remained, nevertheless, a useful descriptive tool for identifying the types of lipids and lipoproteins accumulating in given subjects with dyslipoproteinemia. It is still used for this purpose and in situations when the etiology cannot be established. Type III has remained a useful shorthand term for dysbetalipoproteinemia. The lipoprotein phenotypes determined by electrophoresis on cellulose acetate according to a current commercial procedure (Helena Electrophoresis Procedure, Helena Laboratories, Beaumont, Texas) are depicted in this figure. N, normal. (www.helena.com/procedures/Pro003%20Rev7.pdf).

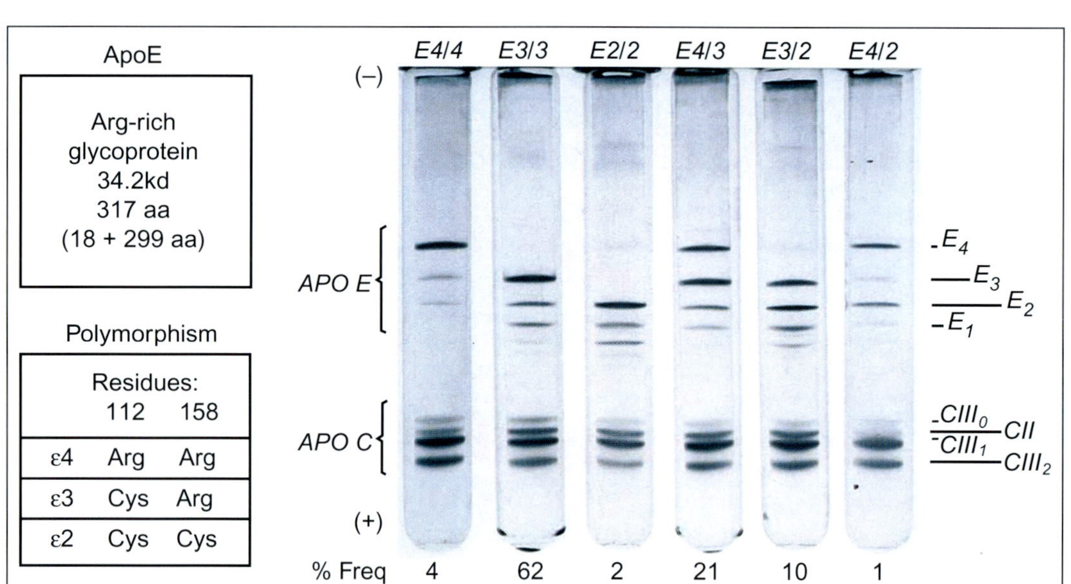

3.15 The six common apoE phenotypes determined by isoelectric focusing. A common protein polymorphism at residues 112 and 158 of the APOE gene is determined by three different alleles at the apoE locus, designated ε4, ε3 and ε2. ApoE is a 34.2 kD arginine-rich glycoprotein of 299 amino acid residues after removal of an 18-amino acid signal peptide. Isoelectric focusing (IEF) of delipidated very-low-density lipoproteins (VLDL) on polyacrylamide gel allows determination of the six apoE protein phenotypes, as illustrated here. The method used was developed in the authors' laboratory (Bouthillier D *et al.* [1989]. *J Lipid Res,* **24**: 1060) as a modification of the original technique of Warnick *et al.* ([1979]. *Clin Chem,* **25**: 279). The separation is driven by the relative charge of each isoform. Each arginine residue confers an added positive charge, hence apoE4, which is the most basic of the three isoforms, has the strongest positive charge. The lower bands in the apoE zone seen with each isoform are sialylated derivatives of the main isoforms. The common isoform, apoE3, has a cysteine at residue 112 and an arginine at residue 158, whereas arginines in apoE4, and cysteines in apoE2 are present at both sites (left lower box). This polymorphism results in six apoE phenotypes in the population: E2/2, E4/4 and E3/3 in homozygotes, and E3/2, E4/2 and E4/3 in heterozygotes. The frequency (Freq) in per cent is given for each phenotype in a typical Caucasian population sample. E3/3 is the most common; E4/4, E2/2 and E4/2 are the least common. Thus, 26% have the E4 isoform and 13% have the E2 isoform. The corresponding allele frequencies for this Canadian sample were 0.152 for ε4, 0.770 for ε3 and 0.078 for ε2. Reliable methods for apoE phenotyping on unfractionated plasma are also available. ApoE genotyping may be used as a substitute, but it does not provide exactly the same information for uncommon phenotypes (**3.16**). Reproduced from Bouthillier D, Sing CF, Davignon J (1983). Apolipoprotein E phenotyping with a single gel method: application to the study of informative matings. *J Lipid Res,* **24**: 1060–1069.

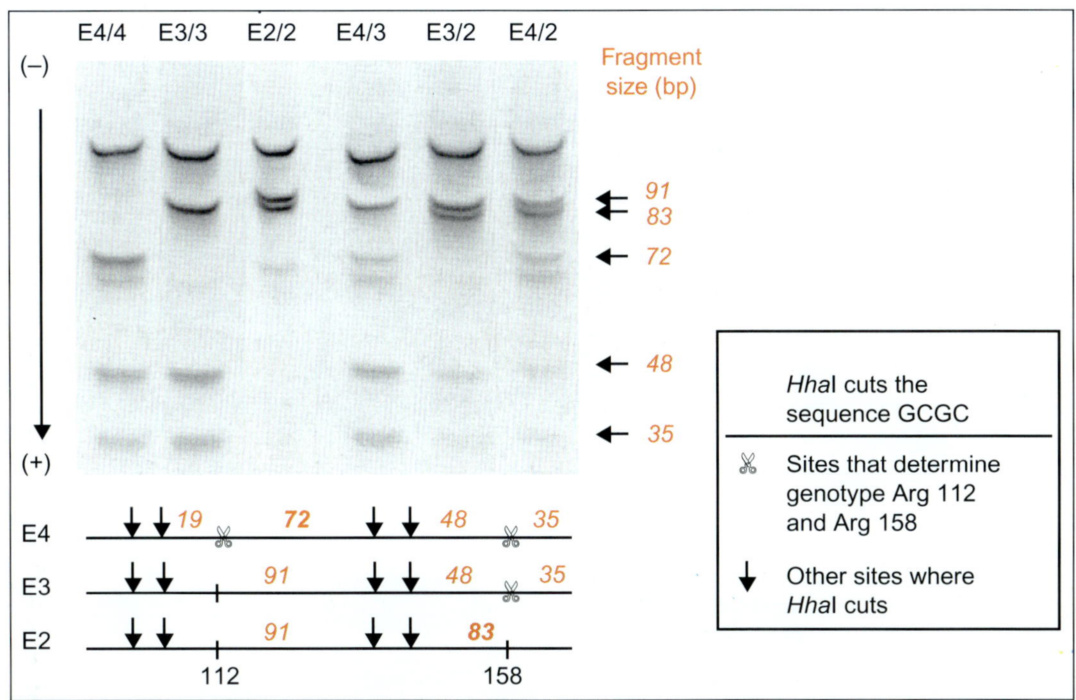

3.16 ApoE genotyping using gene amplification and cleavage with *Hha*I. Hixson and Vernier ([1990]. *J Lipid Res*, **31**: 545–548) used amplification of the APOE gene sequences coding for residues 112 and 158, digestion of the amplified products with the restriction enzyme *Hha*I (pronounce HaHa one) and separation of the cleaved fragments by polyacrylamide 15% gel electrophoresis to genotype apoE. This restriction isotyping (or restriction enzyme isoform genotyping) allows the identification of unique combinations of fragment sizes which provide an unambiguous typing of all six common genotypes. The principle is simple. The restriction enzyme *Hha*I cleaves at GCGC encoding Arg_{112} (E4) and Arg_{158} (E3, E4) determinant sites, but does not cut at GTGC encoding Cys_{112} (E2, E3) and Cys_{158} (E2) sites (see **3.15**). Depending on the apoE isoform, fragments of different lengths are formed as shown at the bottom of the figure: E4/4 (72, 48, 35 base pairs); E3/3 (91, 48, 35 bp) and E2/2 (91, 83 bp) or some combination of those in the heterozygotes (see gels for E4/3, E3/2 and E4/2). Note that a 72 bp fragment is typical of E4 and an 83 bp fragment indicates the presence of E2.

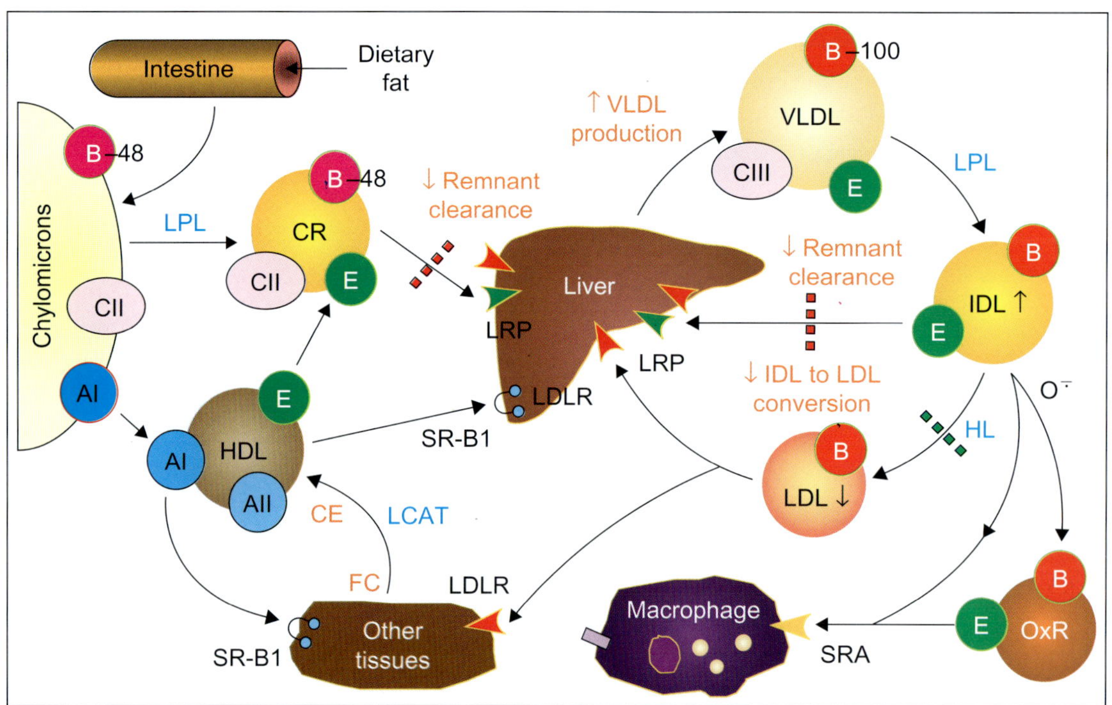

3.17 Metabolic defect in dysbetalipoproteinemia type III. Because of the reduced affinity of apoE2 for its receptors (LDL receptor, LDLR, and LDL receptor-related protein, LRP) there is delayed chylomicron (CR) and very-low-density lipoproteins (VLDL) remnant (IDL) clearance in type III (dotted red line). The presence of apoE2 as the sole apoE isoform (E2/2 phenotype) is not sufficient to cause this phenomenon as 95% of E2/E2 subjects are normolipidemic. A second factor must intervene to provoke VLDL and remnant accumulation (see **3.18**). This is usually a condition that increases VLDL production. Reduced conversion of intermediate-density lipoproteins (IDL) to low-density lipoproteins (LDL) (dotted green line) also contributes to this accumulation. It has not been established whether reduced activity of hepatic lipase (HL) is responsible for this, but there is reduced chylomicron remnant (CR) removal in the HL knockout mouse. In addition, HL deficiency in humans mimics type III. The resulting lipid and lipoprotein profile is characterized by elevated total cholesterol, triglycerides, VLDL-C, remnant cholesterol, apoE and apo CIII, and low LDL-C and HDL-C levels in plasma. Remnant concentration is independently predictive of coronary artery disease and remnant particles are atherogenic whether oxidized (OxR) or not, inducing the transformation of macrophages into foam cells *in vitro*. They are taken up by the aortic wall as efficiently as LDL. Also, remnant-like particles containing apoE have been isolated from human aortic intima and atherosclerotic plaques and remnants from type III patients induce endothelial plasminogen activator inhibitor-I (PAI-I) thereby contributing to a prothrombotic state. Chylomicron remnant accumulation accounts for the high levels of apoB-48 in type III. In this disease postprandial lipemia is markedly increased after a fat load.

determine six apoE genotypes (DNA) (**3.16**) or plasma phenotypes (protein) (**3.15**). The large majority of dysbetalipoproteinemia cases are associated with the E2/2 phenotype (not with a single normal, i.e. non-mutated–ε2 allele [E3/2 or E4/2]). Therefore, dysbetalipoproteinemia segregates in families with a recessive mode of inheritance. However, most E2/2 subjects (about 95%) are normolipidemic or even hypolipidemic. The type III phenotype (biochemical and clinical) is expressed especially when a second factor intervenes to promote remnant accumulation; the phenotype is context-dependent. Conditions that promote overproduction of triglycerides may be responsible for this expression (**3.18**). These include dietary changes, alcohol misuse, obesity, pregnancy, ageing, estrogen withdrawal, hormone administration, hypothyroidism, nephrosis, diabetes, glucose intolerance and co-inheritance of other genes determining hyperlipidemia.

Type III has many typical clinical features that facilitate the diagnosis when present. The frequency of the clinical manifestations in an early series of patients is presented in *Table 3.1*. These include planar xanthomas of the palmar creases (*xanthoma striata palmaris*) (**3.19**), which may subtly vary among patients (**3.20–3.23**), orange or brownish pigmentation of the palmar or plantar creases (**3.21**), and orange–yellow tubero-eruptive xanthomas of elbows, knees or buttocks (**3.24**), which are virtually pathognomonic of the disease. Eruptive xanthomas are not always markedly raised and may be discrete or occur in crops, even on the palmar face of the tip of the fingers (**3.25**). Corneal crescents or rings, xanthelasmas, tuberous xanthomas (**3.26–3.28**) and

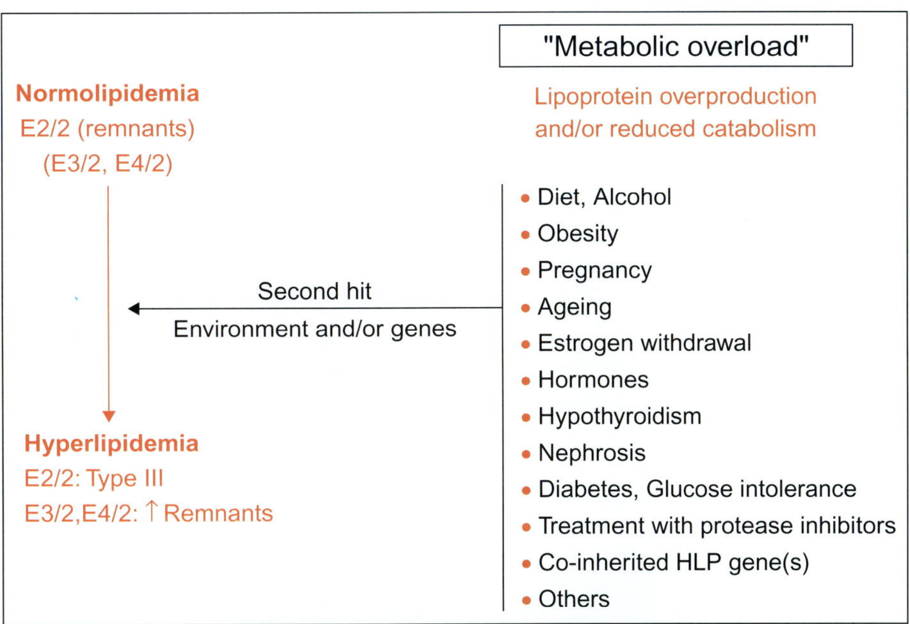

3.18 Complex interactions determining the type III phenotype. Presence of the E2/2 phenotype constitutes a genetic predisposition to type III hyperlipoproteinemia characterized by remnant lipoprotein accumulation. Environmental or genetic conditions that might result in an increase in triglyceride or VLDL production (or their reduced catabolism) could lead to development of type III. This is the 'second hit' hypothesis proposed by Utermann (**3.11**) and co-workers. Some of these conditions – dietary, physiological, genetic or pathological – are listed here. Virtually all secondary causes of hypertriglyceridemia could be included. Correction of the underlying problem may improve or correct the hyperlipidemia. This is typical of pregnancy-associated type III which disappears in a few weeks after delivery, and of hypothyroidism, the most insidious second hit in practice, which yields to thyroxin replacement. However, in some E2/2 subjects remnant lipoproteins may be identified in plasma even when they become normolipidemic (see **3.32**).

Table 3.1 Clinical data on 185 (54 female) patients aged 16–95 years with familial dysbetalipoproteinemia type III

	Subjects (%)
Tuberous and tubero-eruptive xanthomas	64
Xanthoma striata palmaris	55
Tendon xanthomas	13
Arcus corneae	11
Xanthelasma	7
Coronary artery disease	28
Peripheral vascular disease	21
Cerebrovascular disease	4
Gout	4
Diabetes (clinical)	4
Hypothyroidism	4

From Mahley RW, Rall SC Jr (1995). In: Scriver CR, *et al.* (eds) *The Metabolic and Molecular Bases of Inherited Disease.* Pooled data, mean cholesterol 11.6 mmol/l (450 mg/dl); triglycerides 6.4 mmol/l (570 mg/dl).

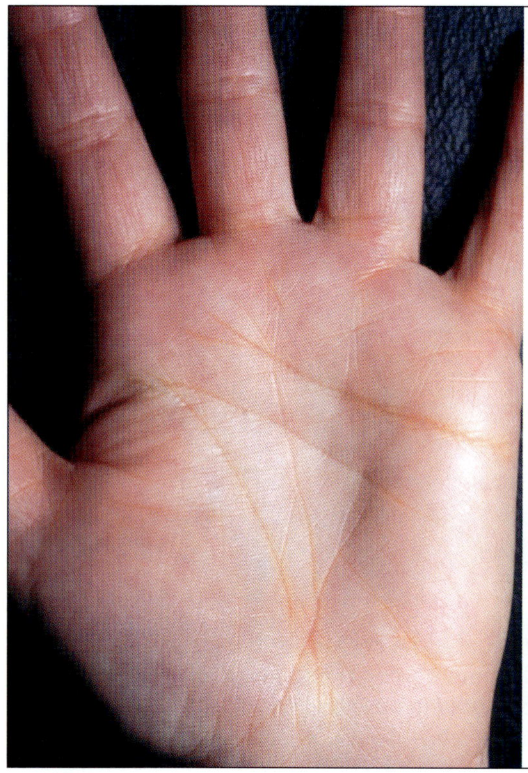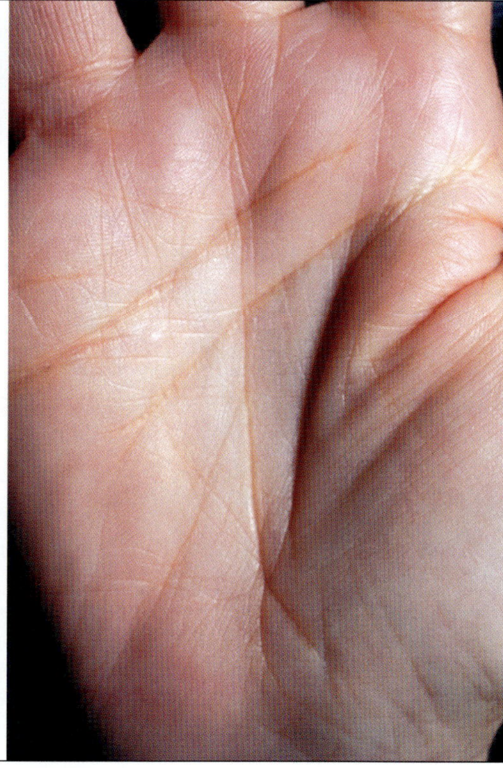

3.19 Orange discoloration of the palmar creases in type III. Before xanthomas of the palmar creases (xanthoma striata palmaris) develop, a discrete discoloration of the palmar creases may be seen, as shown here. This can be seen if the palms are examined closely during a physical examination. The discoloration usually precedes the appearance of a similar discoloration of the plantar creases. The discoloration evolves as seen in **3.20**. In the authors' experience, this sign is not as uncommon as it is reported to be. It differs from the diffuse orange colour of the palm in carotenemia and is pathognomonic of the disease.

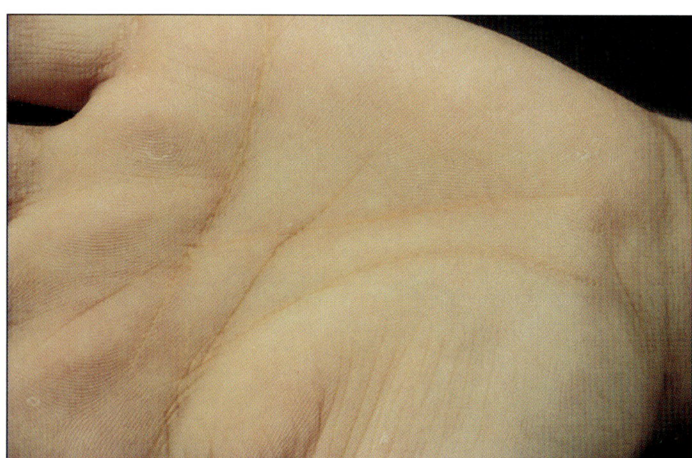

3.20 Orange planar xanthomas of the palmar creases in type III. This figure illustrates a pathognomonic sign of type III that is often missed. It is very discrete and ranges from a yellow-orange pigmentation (**3.19**) to a flat linear xanthoma of orange or yellow-orange colour spilling slightly over the edges of the crease, as shown here. Sometimes it looks like shiny pale yellow planar streaks along the crease (**3.21**). Close examination of the palmar creases should be a routine part of the complete clinical examination in all patients.

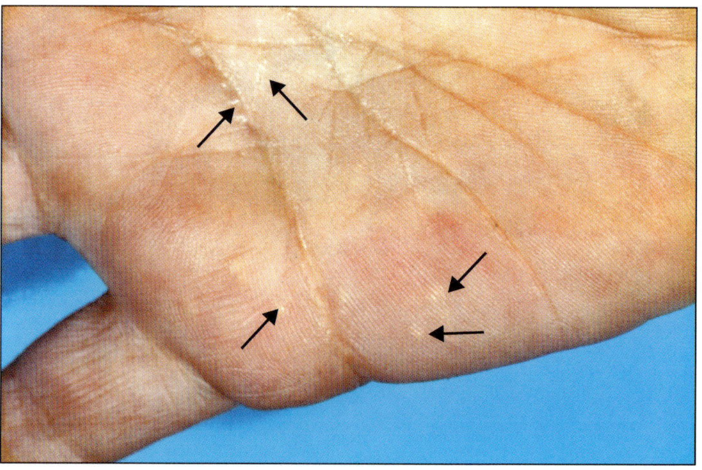

3.21 Whitish-yellow xanthoma striata palmaris and punctate xanthomas. In this patient, a 48-year-old woman with type III dysbetalipoproteinemia, obesity and glucose intolerance, the xanthomas of the palmar creases were discrete and whitish yellow (top arrows). Some had a shiny surface. In addition, she had deep-seated punctate yellowish xanthomas on the cubital aspect of the hand and on the tip of the fingers (see **3.25**). Her plasma total cholesterol level was 15.2 mmol/l (588 mg/dl) and triglyceride level was 12.4 mmol/l (1100 mg/dl).

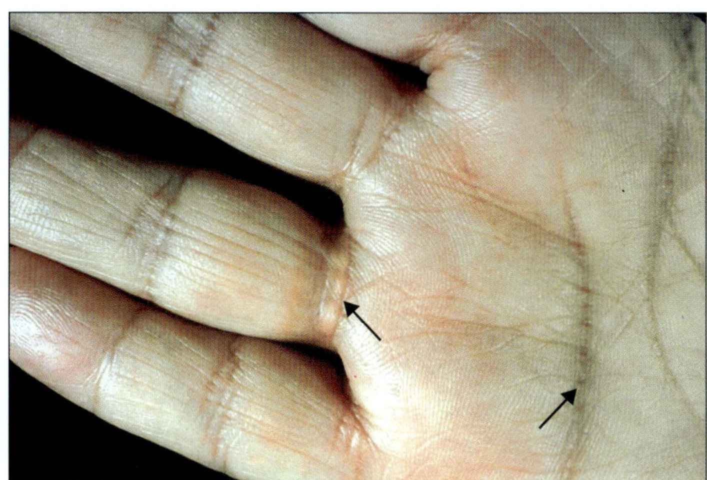 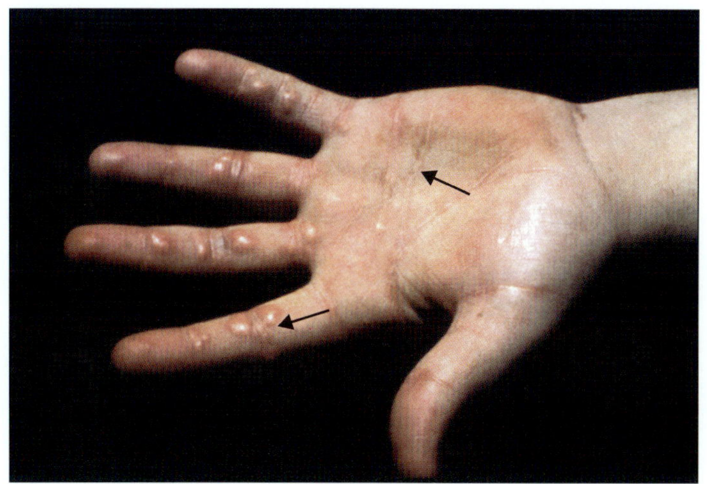

3.22 Planar xanthoma and palmar creases pigmentation in dysbetalipoproteinemia type III. When first seen at the authors' lipid clinic, this 58-year-old woman had a plasma cholesterol of 19.4 mmol/l (750 mg/dl) and triglycerides of 14.6 mmol/l (1290 mg/dl), stable angina, essential hypertension and obesity. She had a brownish pigmentation of the palmar creases (right arrow) that was reminiscent of the discoloration of creases seen in adrenocorticosteroid deficiency (Addison's disease). She also had orange-yellow eruptive xanthomas of the elbows and buttocks. The pathognomonic clue here was the presence of a single planar xanthoma of the left fourth finger that was masked completely by her wedding ring (left arrow). She was treated with clofibrate, her xanthomas resolved, her lipid profile normalized and her angina disappeared within a few months.

3.23 Skin lesions of the hand in a severe case of dysbetalipoproteinemia type III. The skin lesions were very severe in this 22-year-old man with aggressive dysbetalipoproteinemia, obesity and bronchial asthma. His cholesterol was 9.93 mmol/l (384 mg/dl) and his triglycerides 6.21 mmol/l (550 mg/dl) when first seen. He also had tubero-eruptive xanthomas of the elbows. The lesions in the hands were remarkable as the planar xanthomas of the creases were associated with tubero-eruptive xanthomas of the finger creases (left arrow). At times, these lesions in the finger creases split and bled with minor trauma. The xanthoma striata palmaris were well delineated and quite obvious (right arrow). Although the dyslipoproteinemia responded only partially to diet and fibrate therapy, the lesions regressed markedly during treatment.

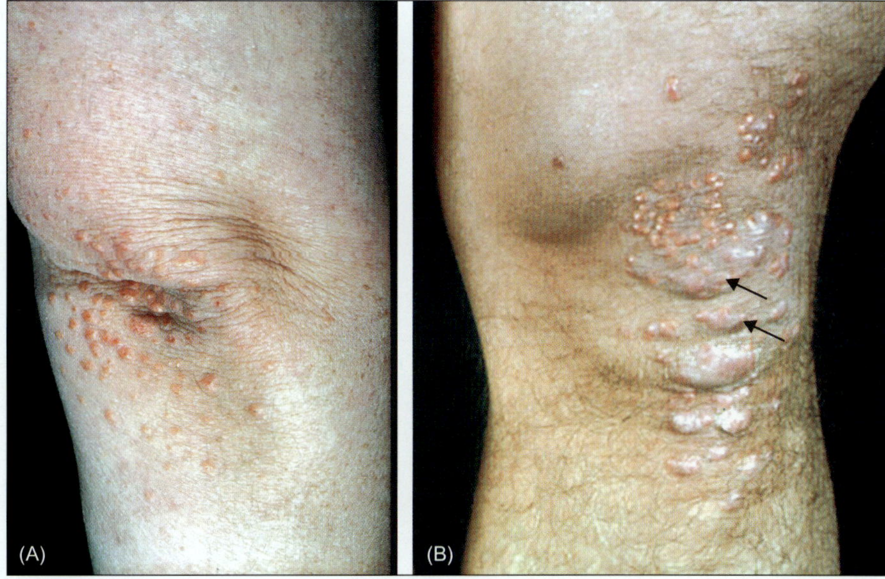

3.24 Eruptive and tubero-eruptive xanthomas of elbow and knee. Eruptive xanthomas tend to be brownish-yellow or orange-yellow in dysbetalipoproteinemia type III. Here are two typical examples. The orange-yellow colour of the eruptive xanthomas stands out in both cases. The image on the left is from the patient described in **3.22**. In this case the xanthomas have a rough texture from surface erosion. The image on the right belongs to a 52-year-old type III patient hospitalized for surgery of a popliteal artery aneurysm in 1976. His plasma cholesterol was 9.6 mmol/l (370 mg/dl), triglycerides 6.43 mmol/l (569 mg/dl). He had orange pigmentation of the palmar creases. The tubero-eruptive xanthomas are typical. As shown here, eruptive xanthomas may at times cluster over a tuberous xanthoma (arrows) or evolve towards a larger tuberous lesion. His xanthomas yielded gradually to clofibrate treatment.

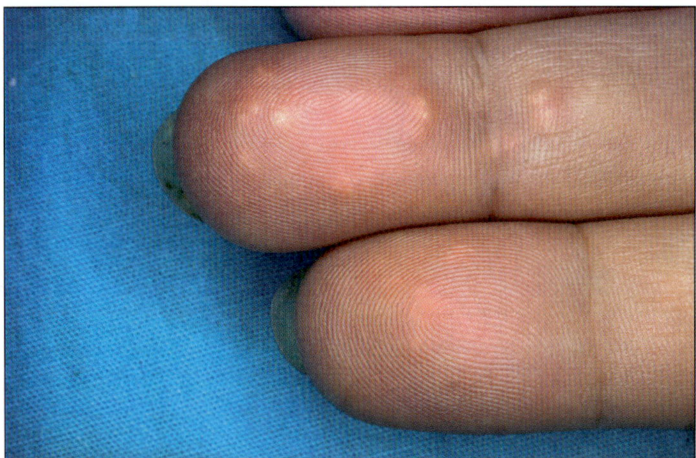

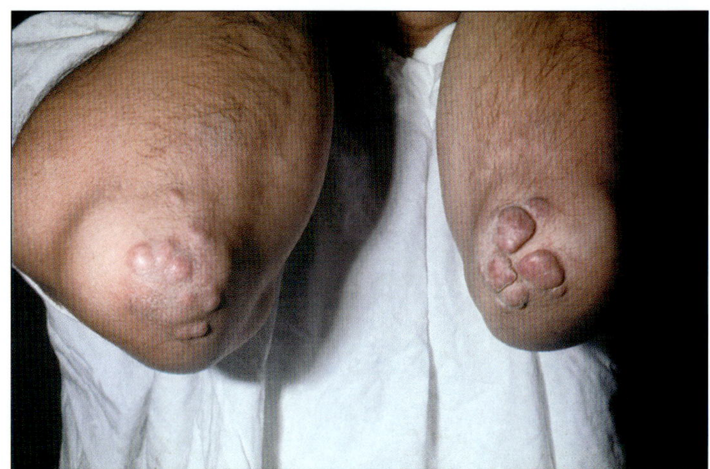

3.25 Punctate eruptive xanthomas of the tip of the fingers in dysbetalipoproteinemia type III. These punctate xanthomas of the tip of the fingers differed from typical eruptive xanthomas in that they seemed more deeply seated in the skin, and not raised as much as the eruptive xanthomas of hyperchylomicronemia, although they tend to appear in clusters as seen here (same patient as in **3.21**).

3.26 Tuberous xanthomas in dysbetalipoproteinemia type III. Tuberous xanthomas are often seen on the elbows and knees in type III. They rarely occur singly and develop in crops as illustrated here in this 40-year-old man, who was under treatment when first seen at the authors' lipid clinic. The xanthomas on the right elbow had started to regress. When clofibrate was briefly discontinued, his cholesterol was 14.22 mmol/l (550 mg/dl) and triglycerides 16.4 mmol/l (1452 mg/dl).

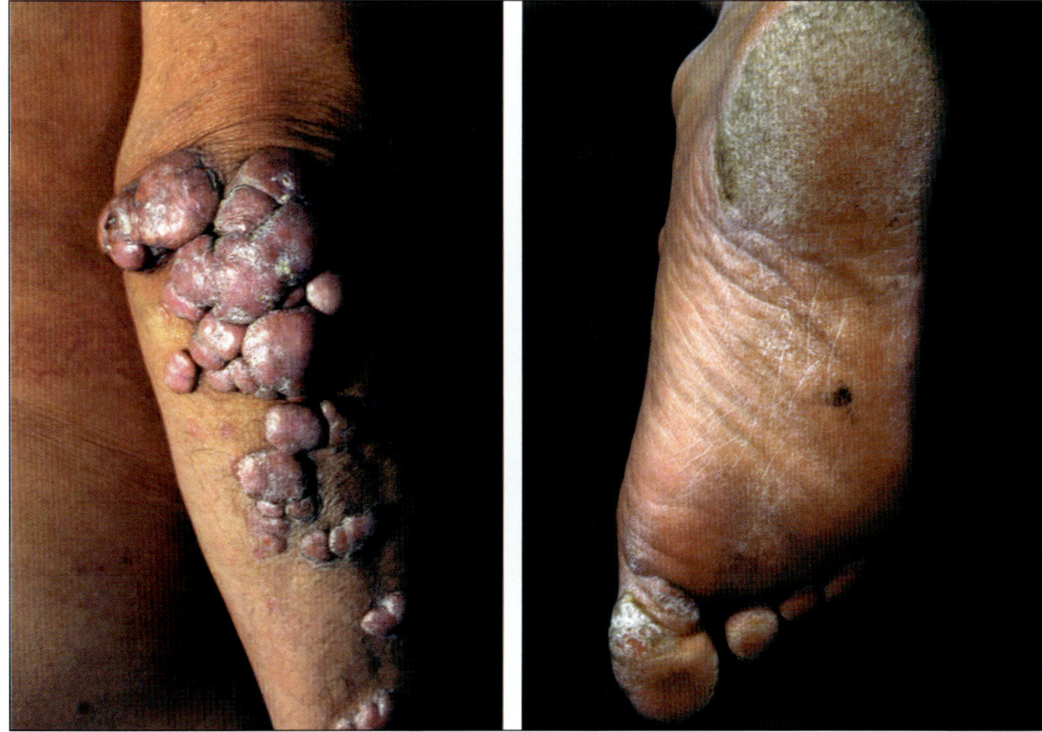

3.27 Extensive tuberous xanthomatosis in dysbetalipoproteinemia type III. If xanthomatous type III is not treated or is poorly treated, the lesions may attain extreme proportions as seen here on the elbow of this 55-year-old patient (presented in more details in **3.29**). Tuberous xanthomas of the ankles and of the soles were also present. Note the lesion under the first toe in the right panel.

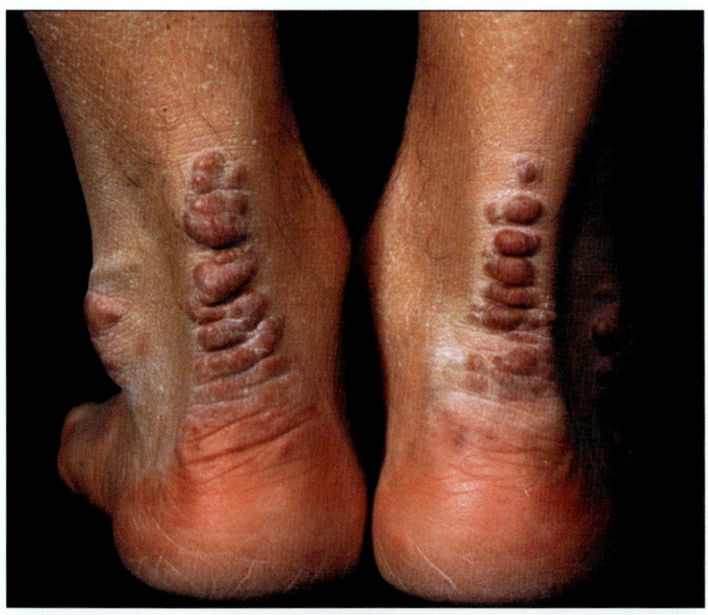

3.28 Tuberous xanthomas of the feet in dysbetalipoproteinemia type III. Occasionally, tuberous xanthomas are seen in the Achilles' tendon and ankle area. They may be accompanied by thickening of the tendon, as in familial hypercholesterolemia. This type III patient was overweight and had coronary artery disease, peripheral arterial disease, multiple arterial aneurysms, and hypothyroidism when first examined at the authors' lipid clinic 32 years ago. He presented with these tuberous lesions, typically arranged in crops. He was 45 years old and his cholesterol was 10.34 mmol/l (400 mg/dl) and triglycerides 11.86 mmol/l (1050 mg/dl).

even tendon xanthomas (essentially Achilles' tendon) may be present. CAD (47%) and/or peripheral arterial atherosclerosis (20%), and less often cerebrovascular disease, may be associated with type III, if untreated. Recently, Hopkins *et al.* (2005) showed that 3.4% of 653 subjects with premature familial CAD have type III dysbetalipoproteinemia and the risk of CAD in type III is five- to ten-fold that of controls depending on the multiple logistic regression model used. These usually develop in middle-aged patients but occasionally may supervene prematurely. An unusual presentation of xanthomas may be associated with the Koebner phenomenon as reported with psoriasis and a variety of other skin diseases. The cutaneous xanthomas develop at sites of trauma or inflammation of normal skin. This is not unique to type III and may occur with severe hypertriglyceridemia. This has been reported, for example, along a scar after accidental laceration, in the hands of a person who had previously suffered severe electric shock while grabbing live wires, and at the site of a bee sting or cat scratch (**3.29**).

Diagnosis of familial dysbetalipoproteinemia (*Table 3.2*) is based on a combination of the presence of the typical xanthomas, high plasma levels of both triglycerides and cholesterol, demonstration of the presence of remnant accumulation with a high plasma VLDL-C/triglyceride ratio, a typical broad beta band on lipoprotein electrophoresis and an E2/2 apoE phenotype or genotype (tests that are not always readily available unfortunately). The Friedewald equation (**3.30**) to measure LDL-C may not be used when triglycerides are 4.52 mmol/l (400 mg/dl) or greater but is particularly unreliable in type III leading to overestimation of LDL-C by approximately 40% (**3.30–3.32**). Exclusion of other causes of remnant accumulation associated with a type III phenotype or a secondary cause is mandatory (see section on other causes of remnant excess below). It is useful to look for the 'second hit' to reveal conditions such as obesity, another hyperlipidemia gene defect, inconspicuous hypothyroidism, or pregnancy-associated overproduction of triglycerides or cholesterol. The most common mistake is failure to detect the tell-tale typical lesions which may be very discrete especially in the palmar creases: orange or brownish discoloration and thin planar xanthomas. A planar xanthoma may be hidden under a ring for instance (**3.22**). These lesions will be revealed only by close and careful inspection. The remarkably good response to drug therapy is another helpful diagnostic component (**3.32** and see **3.34** later). It is to be noted that, even when the hyperlipoproteinemia is normalized, remnants may still be present in plasma as illustrated in **3.32**.

Differential diagnosis must be made with familial hypercholesterolemia when tendon xanthomas are present (remnant accumulation is unusual), severe hypertriglyceridemia with eruptive xanthomas (familial hyperchylomicronemia, mixed hypertriglyceridemia especially in diabetic patients), primary biliary cirrhosis which may harbour similar planar lesions (liver dysfunction, different clinical features, high bilirubin levels) and other rare causes of remnant accumulation copying the type III phenotype such as hepatic lipase deficiency, pseudo-type III, apoE deficiency, and dominant type III secondary to apoE2 mutations (see below) as well as secondary causes. In rare instances, combination of an E2/2 genotype with a mutation of the LDL receptor gene may result in a peculiar phenotype displaying features of both inherited lipid disorders. These individuals have palmar as well as tendon xanthomas, higher total cholesterol than in type III, but triglycerides and LDL-C intermediate between FH and type III (**3.33**), and a VLDL-C/triglyceride

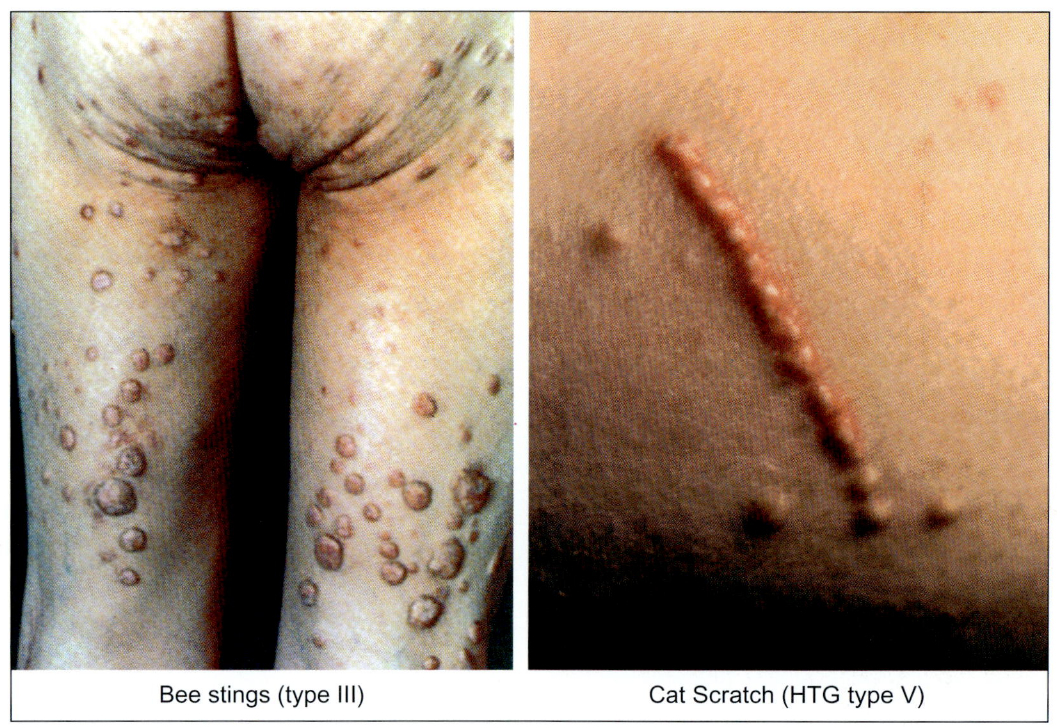

| Bee stings (type III) | Cat Scratch (HTG type V) |

3.29 Eruptive xanthomas at site of injury (Koebner phenomenon). The Koebner phenomenon (koebnerization) relates to the appearance of lesions at the site of skin injury. The cutaneous xanthomas develop at sites of trauma or inflamed normal skin. A 55-year-old farmer (left panel), whose hyperlipidemia had been treated with a lipid-lowering diet alone since its discovery at age 22, was stung by a swarm of bees at the age of 25. This was followed by a severe allergic reaction. Four months after this event, a constellation of brownish raised xanthomas of various sizes appeared rapidly at the site of each bee sting on the buttocks and the thighs. The picture shown here was taken when he first attended the authors' lipid clinic, where the diagnosis of type III was made. His cholesterol was 7.87 mmol/l and triglycerides 3.74 mmol/l (304 and 331 mg/dl). The zipper-like lesion in the right panel appeared at the site of a cat scratch within a week in a 39-year-old woman with severe endogenous hypertriglyceridemia – triglycerides 51.6 mmol/l (4556 mg/dl) and cholesterol 13.52 mmol/l (523 mg/dl) – associated with type 2 diabetes and obesity. She had lipemia retinalis and widespread eruptive xanthomas on the thighs, knees and arms. The xanthomas regressed with diet and fibrate therapy. These two cases were reported previously (Roederer G *et al.* [1988]. Eruptive and tubero-eruptive xanthomas of the skin arising on sites of prior injury: two case reports. *JAMA*, **260**: 1282–1283. Erratum in: *JAMA* [1989]. **261**: 1280).

ratio >0.7 (>0.30 for mg/dl calculation). A LDLR mutation should be suspected in a type III patient with a LDL-C level above 3.0 mmol/l and a family history of premature CAD (Carmena *et al.* 2000).

A lipid-lowering diet is very useful and a fibrate is the drug of choice in the treatment of type III. Striking regression of even the most severe xanthomas can be observed (**3.34**). Statins are also effective and useful for patients intolerant to fibrates.

Other inherited causes of remnant excess
Apolipoprotein E deficiency

ApoE is a ligand for receptors involved in plasma lipoprotein homeostasis, including LDL receptor-related protein (LRP), VLDL receptor (VLDLR), and LDL receptor (LDLR). It is a multifunctional protein and its importance has been well established in mice by inactivation of the apoE gene. Indeed the *apoE* knockout mouse, with no circulating apoE, has become a valuable animal model for the study of atherosclerosis. ApoE deficiency occurs spontaneously in humans and is associated with the type III phenotype and its typical clinical findings including tubero-eruptive xanthomas and premature atherosclerosis. Only a few cases of this condition have been reported, the first in 1981 by Brewer Jr. and colleagues at the NIH in Bethesda. Five kindreds with apoE deficiency have been reported. Different mutations of the apoE gene, such as an acceptor splice site mutation in intron 3, or a point mutation ($Trp_{210} \rightarrow$ Stop) which encodes the truncated apoE3$_{WASHINGTON}$, may cause this disease. The pattern of inheritance seems to be reces-

Table 3.2 Useful elements for diagnosis of classic type III dysbetalipoproteinemia

Clinical	• Pigmentation of palmar creases • Xanthoma striata palmaris • Tubero-eruptive xanthomas • Eruptive xanthomas • Tuberous xanthomas • Atherosclerosis >50 (men), >60 (women)
Family	• CAD, PAD or CVD >50 (men) >60 (women) • Apparent recessive inheritance
Biochemistry	• High TC, high TG, low LDL-C • VLDL-C/TG high • Broad β-band • Floating β-lipoprotein or β-VLDL • ApoE E2/2 phenotype or genotype
Exclusion	• Type III features in the absence of the E2/2 phenotype or genotype

CAD, coronary artery disease; PAD, peripheral arterial disease; CVD, cardiovascular disease; TC, total cholesterol; TG, triglycerides; VLDL, very-low-density lipoproteins.

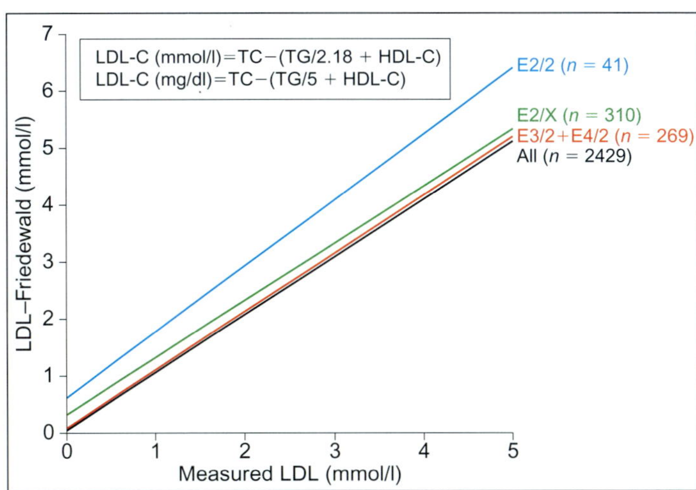

3.30 The Friedewald equation used to measure low-density lipoprotein-cholesterol (LDL-C) is unreliable in dysbetalipoproteinemia type III. The Friedewald equation (box at the top) has been used for many years to derive values for LDL-C when the concentration of plasma total cholesterol (TC), triglycerides (TG) and HDL-C is known from direct measurement. TG divided by a constant provides an estimate of VLDL-C. The equation is not applicable by definition when triglycerides are ≥ 4.52 mmol/l (400 mg/dl). Some modifications have been suggested to improve the original equation, but in practice it reflects LDL-C measured by the gold standard method (see **3.12**) relatively well. As seen here, the presence of the E2/2 phenotype is responsible for an overestimation of LDL-C of about 40% in this study (blue line). The few E2/2 subjects (n = 41), when included among patients expressing at least one ε2 allele (E2/X, X representing all the other alleles, ε2, ε3 and ε4, n = 310) pushed the regression line upward with a slight overestimation (green line), which was virtually normalized when they are excluded (E3/2 + E4/2, n = 269) (red line). This study was undertaken in collaboration with Daniel Bouthillier on 2429 untreated patients seen between 1987 and 1996 at the author's lipid clinic with TG ≤ 4.5 mmol/l. Separation by sex had little effect on these relationships.

sive as only the homozygotes have the clinical manifestations and the biochemical features of type III. However, one case of severe type III has been reported in a patient with an E1/0 (0 standing for 'E null') phenotype. The E1 was ascribed to a $Gly_{127} \rightarrow Asp$ mutation, reported several times before and also known as $ApoE1_{BETHESDA}$ (see next section on ApoE mutations, dominant type III and lipoprotein glomerulopathy and **3.40** later). The null allele was due to a base deletion in codon 31 causing a frameshift and a premature stop at codon 60, with no fragment of apoE detected in plasma. Kinetic studies in apoE deficiency have shown a markedly impaired catabolism of VLDL, chylomicrons and their remnants because of a lack of direct removal and lipolysis of small VLDL and IDL, an increased rate of LDL-apoB catabolism secondary to upregulation of the LDL receptor and reduced VLDL-apoB production. Interestingly, large VLDL devoid of apoE were cleared normally and a portion of circulating lipoprotein(a) (Lp(a)) was more buoyant (lesser density) than normal Lp(a), and

had a delayed catabolism in these subjects, but were cleared twice as rapidly as normal Lp(a) in normal subjects (**3.35** and **3.36**). This demonstrates how human apoE deficiency can be used as a tool to study lipoprotein metabolism.

The following features may help in separating this condition from classic familial dysbetalipoproteinemia which has an identical clinical phenotype: plasma cholesterol is relatively higher than plasma triglycerides (mg/dl), plasma apoE is low (about half of normal or less in marked contrast to classical type III), and an apoE2 is not observed on isoelectric focusing of circulating VLDL. Specialist laboratories may help establish the diagnosis by demonstrating the causal mutation.

Standard Friedewald equation (mmol/l) LDL-C = TC−(TG/2.18 + HDL-C) Where TG/2.18 = VLDL-C	
If phenotype is:	2.18 should be replaced by:
E2/2	1.18
E3/2	1.83
E4/2	1.84
E4/4	2.20
E3/3	2.21
E4/3	2.26

3.31 Modification of the Friedewald equation to correct for variation imparted by the apolipoprotein E (apoE) phenotype. In the study mentioned in **3.30** a regression analysis for each of the six apoE phenotypes allowed derivation of correction constants to calculate an accurate very-low-density lipoprotein (VLDL)-C value. These are given here for values calculated in mmol/l using a modification of the Friedewald equation. In practice, in the absence of the knowledge of the apoE phenotype one may use 2.18 which provides sufficient accuracy, except for dysbetalipoproteinemia type III subjects for whom triglycerides (TG) should be divided by 1.18. The mean overestimation in per cent was ≤1.5% for E3/3, E4/4 and E4/3 but was 38.5 ± 25.5% for E2/2, 7.1 ± 9.7% for E4/2 and 4.8 ± 10.4% for E3/2. Without correction, the overestimation of the standard Friedewald equation was 2.5 ± 8.9% for the entire group.

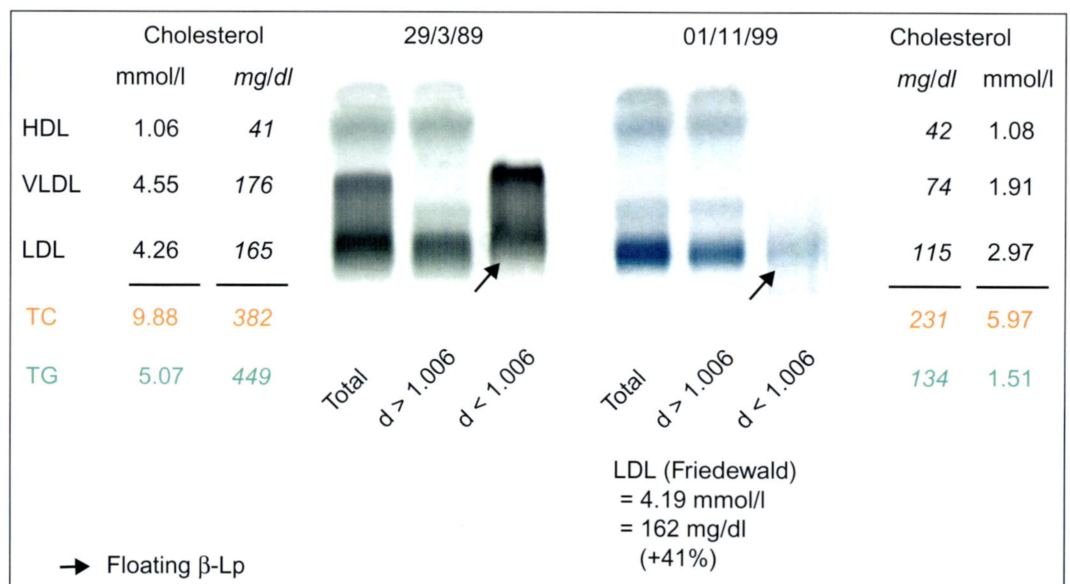

3.32 Persistence of a floating β-lipoprotein after correction of the hyperlipidemia in dysbetalipoproteinemia type III and unreliability of the Friedewald equation for measuring low-density lipoprotein-cholesterol (LDL-C). After 9 years of treatment with fenofibrate, the floating β-very-low-density lipoproteins (VLDL) observed on agarose gel electrophoresis of separated lipoprotein fractions (**3.12**) persisted in this patient even after full correction of the hyperlipidemia (arrows). She therefore remains dyslipoproteinemic with presence of remnants in her plasma. The hyperlipoproteinemia was first noted at 59 years of age when a diagnosis of hypothyroidism was made and treatment started. The diagnosis of type III dysbetalipoproteinemia was made at the age of 64 and the presence of the E2/2 phenotype noted. She had none of the clinical manifestations of type III. On both occasions, her VLDL-C/triglyceride (TG) ratio was >0.7 (0.89 before and 1.24 after treatment) when calculated in mmol/l, or >0.3 (0.39 before and 0.54 after treatment) when calculated in mg/dl. The figures for cholesterol in the major lipoprotein fractions as well as total cholesterol (TC) and triglycerides (TG) are given for samples taken 9 years apart. The calculation of the Friedewald equation on the 1999 specimen without correction is given (bottom right) showing a 40% overestimation (4.19 instead of 2.97 when measured). Calculation using the correction factor given in **3.31** above gives a value of 2.98.

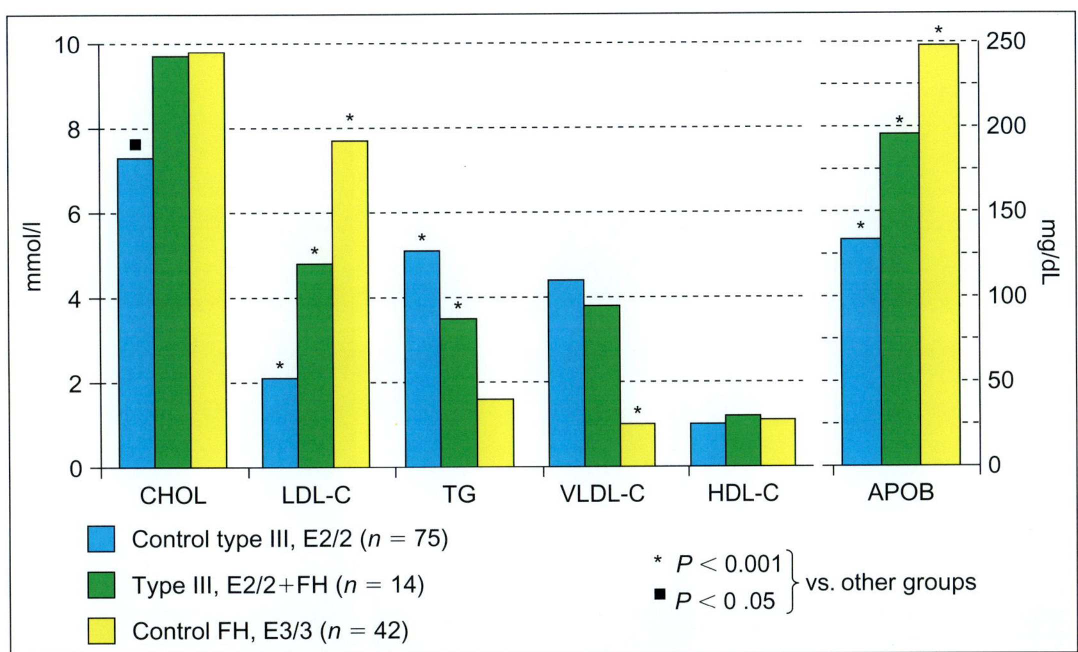

3.33 Lipid profile in dysbetalipoproteinemia type III, type III + familial hypercholesterolemia (FH) and FH. If both type III and familial hypercholesterolemia (FH) are expressed in the same subject, low-density lipoprotein-cholesterol (LDL-C) and total plasma apolipoprotein B (apoB) are intermediate between those of pure type III and pure FH as seen here. Even clinically, the phenotype may be intermediate with features of type III and FH. The high-density lipoprotein (HDL) levels do not differ in the three groups while very-low-density lipoprotein-cholesterol (VLDL)-C is increased in the combined disorders. There was a trend for coronary artery disease to be higher in FH and for carotid artery disease to be higher in the combination. This figure represents pooled data of males and females from a study carried out in the authors' laboratory and lipid clinic (Carmena R *et al.* [2000]. Coexisting dysbetalipoproteinemia and familial hypercholesterolemia. Clinical and laboratory observations. *Atherosclerosis*, **148**: 113–124).

Apolipoprotein E mutations, dominant type III and lipoprotein glomerulopathy

Several mutations of apoE are associated with a *co-dominant transmission of type III* in contrast to the more common 'recessive' type III hyperlipoproteinemia associated with the E2/2 phenotype. Mutations involving the helical regions of the apoE molecule (residues 130–150, helix 4) are especially likely to be associated with type III hyperlipoproteinemia in a dominant fashion. The apoE2 (Lys$_{146}$→Gln) variant is a good example (**3.37**). Heterozygous carriers of this variant have elevated levels of plasma triglycerides, cholesterol and apoE. Expression of this mutant apoE2 in mice causes a specific inhibition of VLDL-triglyceride lipolysis and a 7 to 50-fold increase in triglycerides depending on the level of expression. These mutations may change the charge of apoE so that delipidated VLDL apoE does not necessarily migrate as apoE2. This is the case for ApoE1$_{HAMMERSMITH}$ (Lys$_{146}$→Asn; Arg$_{147}$→Trp), due to a dinucleotide substitution, which is associated with early manifestation of dominant type III hyperlipoproteinemia. The same applies to apoE1$_{HARRISBURG}$, Lys$_{146}$→Glu and apoE*3$_{LEIDEN}$ (7 amino

acids insert). The diagnosis in these variants is based on the dominant pattern of inheritance and demonstration of the apoE mutant in specialist laboratories.

Lipoprotein glomerulopathy is a rare kidney disease associated with the clinical and biochemical type III phenotype. It has been mainly observed in Asians, especially Japanese and Chinese, but a few cases have been reported in Caucasians (France, Poland and USA). It is characterized by the presence of lipid or lipoprotein droplets in dilated mesangial glomeruli (**3.38**). The latter are filled with stratified lipoprotein-laden thrombi but no fibrinogen, complement or immunoglobulin. This leads to proteinuria, progressive decline in renal function, glomerulosclerosis and nephrotic syndrome with eventual renal failure. It is mostly associated with an abnormal apoE2 (apoE2$_{SENDAI}$, apoE2$_{MAEBACHI}$, apoE1$_{TOKYO}$ and others, see **3.37**). Recurrence has been observed after renal transplantation so that the cause is extra-renal. Furthermore, the disease is reproduced when apoE2$_{SENDAI}$ is transfected into an apoE$^{-/-}$ mouse. The diagnosis is based on the occurrence of progressive kidney disease associated with the dysbetalipoproteinemia phenotype, high plasma levels of

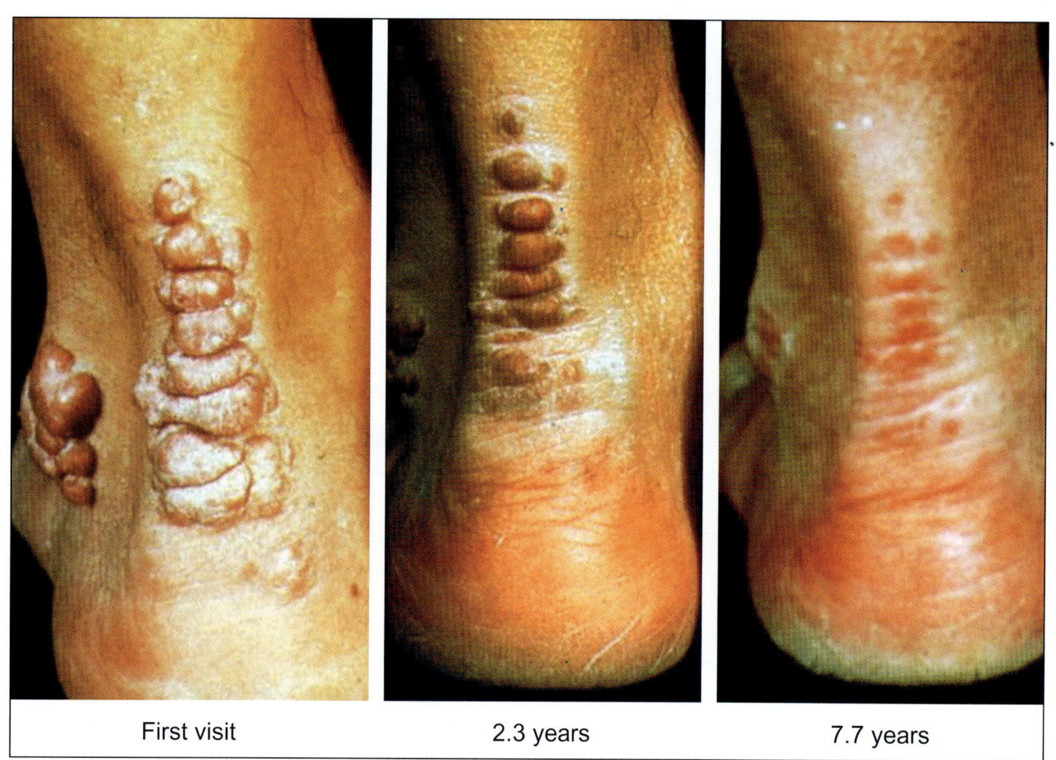

3.34 Regression of severe tuberous xanthomas with fibrate treatment. One of the characteristics of dysbetalipoproteinemia type III is its responsiveness to treatment. Even well-established florid tuberous xanthomas may regress over time. This patient (described above in **3.28**) responded at first to clofibrate and dietary management but an escape from the lipid lowering effect took place over time despite the addition of niacin and dextro-thyroxine. When fenofibrate became available, this patient began to respond again to treatment and his dyslipoproteinemia could be resolved. In spite of the escape to treatment the xanthomas regressed almost completely over 7.7 years of follow-up.

apoE and demonstration of an abnormal apoE. The renal biopsy is pathognomonic (**3.38**). It will reveal the strikingly dilated glomerular capillaries and the presence of lipoprotein-laden obstructive thrombi. Treatment with a fibrate or probucol in combination has been shown to induce regression of renal lesions (**3.38**).

It is to be noted that not all *'natural' APOE mutations* (OMIM No. 107741) (http://www.ncbi.nlm.nih.gov/entrez/dispomim.cgi?id=107741, see 'allelic variants') result in the type III phenotype – some may be associated with normolipidemia, hypertriglyceridemia, hypercholesterolemia or both. When the mutation alters the charge of the protein, its migration is changed. Adding a basic amino acid with a positive charge (Arg, Lys or His) will displace the molecule towards the cathode (and basic pH) whereas removing a positive charge or adding an acidic negatively charged amino acid (Asp or Glu) will move the apoE in the other direction (anode, acidic pH) on isoelectric focusing gels (IEF), see **3.15**, and **3.39** and **3.40**. ApoE1 (2 positive charges less than E3) or apoE5 (2 more positive charges) and apoE7

(4 more positive charges than E3) will be readily identified by their unusual place on the gel. However, other mutations may add a charge to E3 and move it to the E4 position or remove a charge from E3 and move it to the apoE2 position. Separation on IEF gels does not allow the identification of such mutations directly. Combining phenotyping (**3.15**) with genotyping (**3.16**) may give a clue as they may show a discrepancy between the genotype and the phenotype. In the case of the apoE1$_{HAMMERSMITH}$ mutation, Lys$_{146}$→Asn–Arg$_{147}$→Trp for instance, the IEF phenotype is E3/1 whereas the *HhaI* genotype is E3/E3. Modification by cysteamine adds a charge unit for each cysteine present in the molecule, thus E2 that has two Cys moves to the E4 position, and E3 with one Cys moves to the E4 position (**3.40**). This helps to determine which parent molecule is modified by a mutation. Finally, the change in charge may be slightly less then expected when the substituted amino acid is histidine as is the case for the apoE3′$_{MONTREAL}$ (**3.41**). This is because His has a slightly lower pKa than Arg and the mutant E3′ does not display a full charge difference as E3 does. The natural apoE

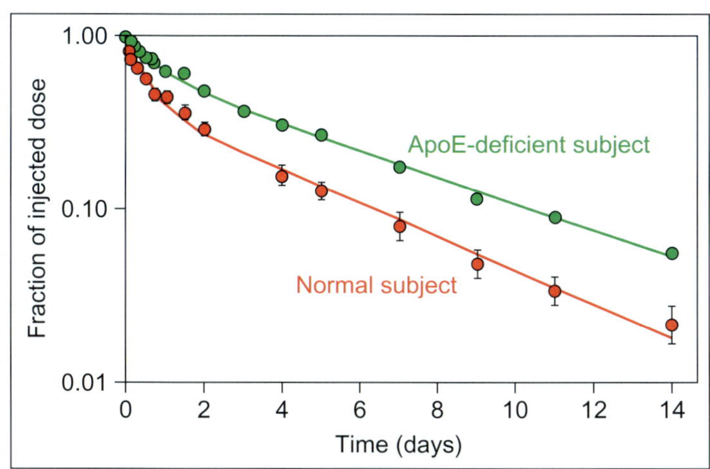

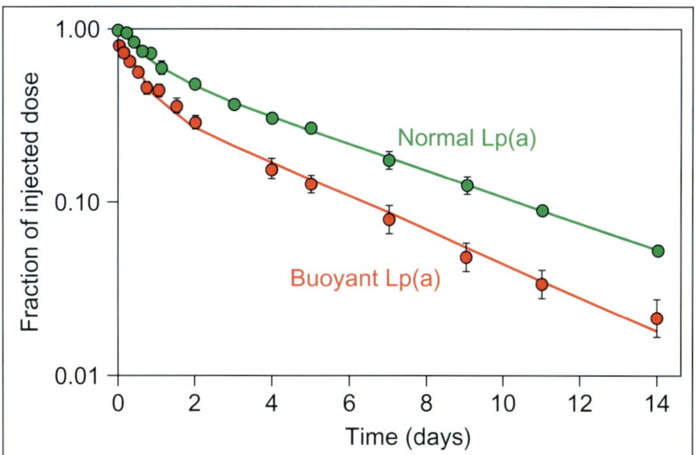

3.35 Delayed metabolism of labelled buoyant lipoprotein (Lp) (a) from an apoE-deficient patient infused in this patient and in control subjects. ApoE-deficient patients provide a unique model to study plasma lipoprotein kinetics in clinical research. Ikewaki and co-workers thoroughly studied lipoprotein kinetics in an apoE-deficient patient using stable isotope methodology with ^{13}C-phenylalanine and a multi-compartmental analysis. Their findings are described in the text, and they also noted that there were two species of Lp(a) in this patient: normal Lp(a) and a more buoyant species. The latter contained apoB-48, apoAIV and apoCs and floated in the very-low-density lipoprotein (VLDL) and intermediate-density lipoprotein (IDL) density range. The Lp(a) kinetic study illustrated here was carried out with ^{125}I-labelled buoyant Lp(a) from an apoE-deficient patient. When infused, ^{125}I-buoyant Lp(a) was catabolized at a slower rate in the patient than in control subjects. This was ascribed to apoE-free buoyant Lp(a) of the patient acquiring apoE in the plasma of the normal subjects, which accelerated its catabolism. This demonstrates that apoE can modulate Lp(a) metabolism *in vivo*. Data from the control subjects are given as the mean ± SE. Redrawn from Ikewaki K *et al.* (2004). Abnormal *in vivo* metabolism of apoB-containing lipoproteins in human apoE deficiency. *J Lipid Res*, **45**: 1302–1311.

3.36 Buoyant Lp(a) from an apolipoprotein E (apoE)-deficient patient are cleared more rapidly than normal Lp(a) from the same patient in control subjects. In the second part of their study on Lp(a), Ikewaki *et al.* determined the rate of disappearance of ^{125}I-buoyant Lp(a) and ^{131}I-normal Lp(a) isolated from the apoE-deficient patient, and infused in the plasma of control subjects. The buoyant Lp(a) was cleared in the normal subjects at twice the rate of the normal Lp(a). Ikewaki *et al.* provided information indicating that buoyant Lp(a) is a precursor of normal Lp(a) and because normal Lp(a) from the patient is catabolized at the same rate as normal Lp(a) from a control subject, they surmised that once mature Lp(a) has been formed, the subsequent metabolism of Lp(a) is apoE independent. Data are given as the mean ± SE. Redrawn from Ikewaki K *et al.* (2004). Abnormal *in vivo* metabolism of apoB-containing lipoproteins in human apoE deficiency. *J Lipid Res*, **45**: 1302–1311.

mutations are given in **3.37**. The colour code indicates whether the mutation is associated with type III, dominant type III, lipoprotein glomerulopathy, non-type III lipid changes or normolipidemia. Response to diet and drugs depends on the mutation. If diet therapy is insufficient, starting with a fibrate in subjects with type III and isolated hypertriglyceridemia is the rule, or a statin if high LDL-C predominates. Patients with the apoE3′$_{\text{MONTREAL}}$ have been shown to be highly responsive to dietary management (**3.42**).

Hepatic lipase deficiency

Hepatic lipase deficiency is a rare hereditary recessive disease which may reproduce many of the biochemical character-

istics of type III, since hepatic lipase (HL) plays a role in the catabolism of chylomicron and VLDL remnants.

HL, also called hepatic triglyceride lipase, is a lipolytic enzyme with both triglyceride and phospholipid hydrolase activities. It therefore modulates the triglyceride and phospholipid content of all plasma lipoproteins (remodelling) and has a key role in determining their metabolic fate. It hydrolyses large LDL into smaller denser potentially more atherogenic particles (see **2.12**). Importantly, it contributes to the conversion of IDL into LDL and enhances β-VLDL clearance by bridging the lipoprotein to their cell surface receptor and heparan sulphate proteoglycan in a manner similar to the action of lipoprotein lipase (see **2.2**). The *in vitro* uptake of chylomicrons and β-VLDL is enhanced by hepatic lipase (**3.43**). HL is also involved in reverse cholesterol transport (i.e. return of cholesterol to the liver for excretion) (**3.44**). It decreases plasma HDL, especially HDL particles rich in apoAI and apoAII.

Mature human HL is a 476-amino acid glycoprotein (499 including the signal peptide) coded by a gene of nine

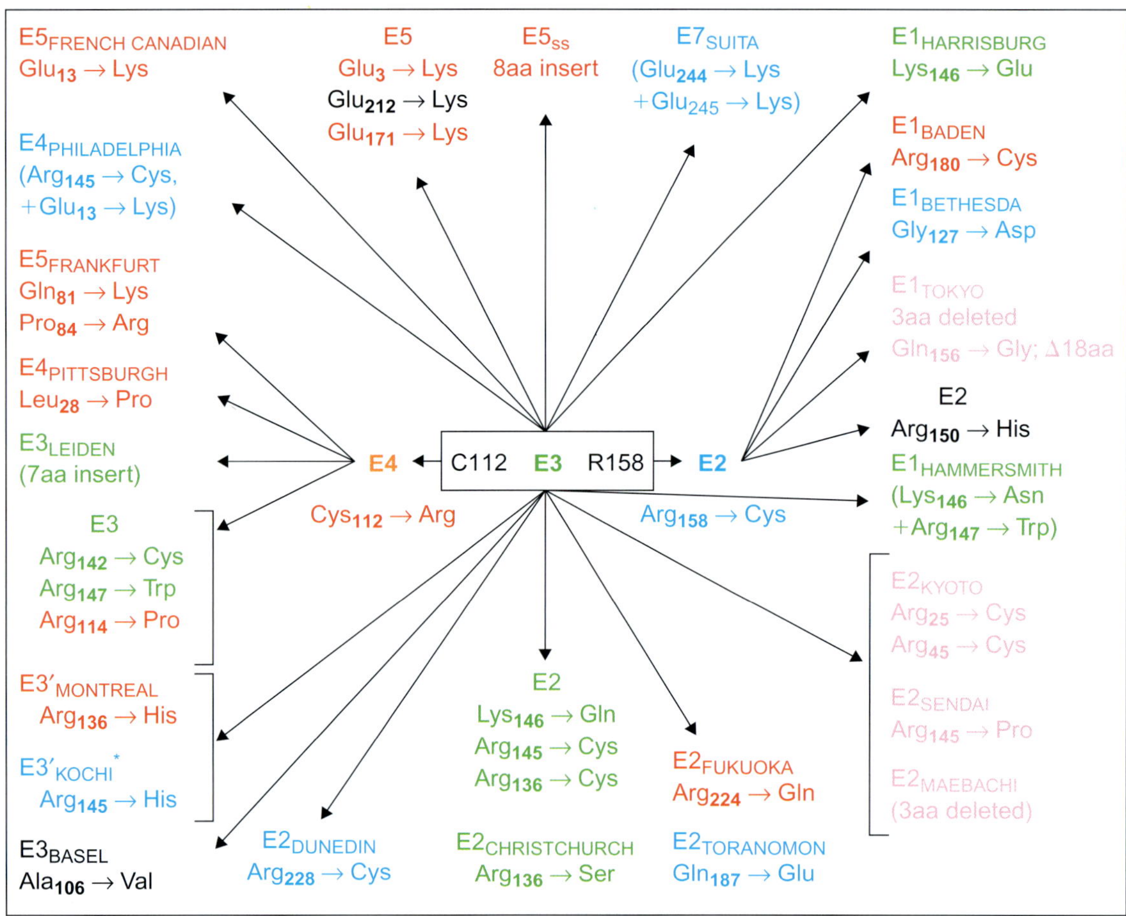

3.37 Natural apolipoprotein E (apoE) mutations. This diagram illustrates most of the APOE gene mutations associated with the dysbetalipoproteinemia type III phenotype (blue), dominant type III (green), lipoprotein glomerulopathy (pink), changes in plasma lipids but not type III (red) and little or no effect on plasma lipids (black). When the mutation has a name the amino acid (aa) change is expressed just under it. If there is more than one line of text under such mutations they express other variants. Amino acid changes in parentheses indicate that two mutations are accounting for the isoelectric focusing (IEF) phenotype (i.e. E4PHILADELPHIA). Note that apo E4PITTSBURGH is also called apo E4FREIBURG. The boxes are to remind the reader about the distinction between E3 Cys112 and Arg158, (C112 and R158), E4 that has an Arg112 and E2 that has a Cys158. 'Δ18 aa' refers to the deletion of 18 amino acids. The arrows indicate the original isoform that mutates to yield the IEF protein isoform migration observed. Note that Glu and Asp (acidic amino acids) have a negative charge, so that when they are lost the molecule gains a charge (moves one charge unit towards the cathode). The basic amino acids Arg, Lys and His add a positive charge when introduced. In the case of E5 Glu3→Lys for example, E3 loses a negative charge (Glu) and acquires a positive charge (Lys) therefore moving two charge units towards the cathode into an E5 position. The difference in charge between Arg and His may account for the presence of a doublet on IEF gels when the normal and the mutated isoforms are present. This is seen with apoE3'MONTREAL and APOE3KOCHI (Suehiro T *et al.* [1990]. *Jpn J Med*, **29**: 587); this explains why we have called it E3'KOCHI in this figure (*). Interestingly, this mutation was associated with some of the characteristics of type III but the very-low-density lipoproteins (VLDL)-C/triglyceride ratio was normal. The E5 and E7 mutations are more commonly reported in Asia but have also been found in Turkey, Ethiopia, Italy, the USA and at the authors' lipid clinic in Canada. Another French-Canadian E5 mutation identified at the authors' lipid clinic is the E5 Glu19 →Lys (unpublished data). This diagram is an update and modification of a previous figure in Davignon J (1993). ApoE polymorphism and atherosclerosis. In: Born G, Schwartz CJ, eds. *New Horizons in Coronary Heart Disease,* Current Science Ltd, London; from an idea of Rall SC Jr *et al.* presented at an international meeting in 1990.

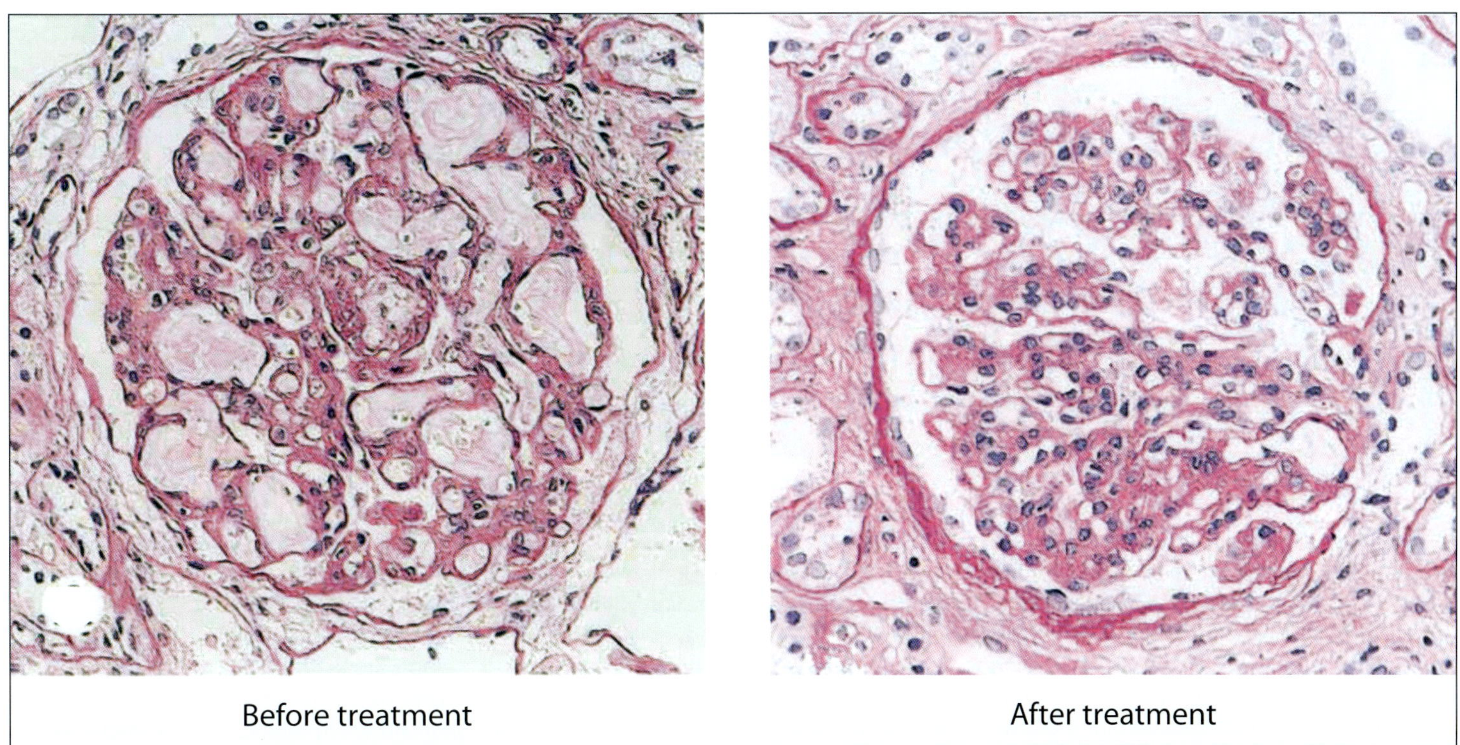

3.38 Resolution of lipoprotein glomerulopathy lesions using lipid-lowering treatment. Renal biopsy is used to confirm the diagnosis of lipoprotein glomerulopathy. Light microscopy of glomerulus before treatment (periodic acid–Schiff stain; original magnification × 200; left panel) shows the typical balloon-like dilatations of the capillaries which are filled with lipoprotein thrombi. The glomeruli are enlarged and exhibit moderate mesangial cell proliferation and a moderately increased mesangial matrix. The second biopsy specimen from this 36-year-old woman with nephrotic syndrome (right panel) was obtained 11 months after initiation of intensive lipid-lowering therapy with fenofibrate (300 mg), niceritrol (750 mg), ethyl-icosapentate (1800 mg), and probucol (500 mg) daily. Lipoprotein thrombi are no longer visible. The quantity of mesangial cells and matrix has increased; a manifestation of glomerular healing. Similar improvements have also been reported with bezafibrate therapy. Reproduced with permission from Ieiri N *et al.* (2003). Resolution of typical lipoprotein glomerulopathy by intensive lipid-lowering therapy. *Am J Kidney Dis*, **41**: 244–249.

exons and eight introns spanning 60 kb on chromosome 15q21 and referred to as *LIPC*. Its promoter contains insulin-responsive elements. Mutations of *LIPC* in humans may cause suboptimal activity of hepatic lipase or result in an inactive enzyme. The first family with HL deficiency was reported in Ontario, Canada, by Breckenridge and colleagues in 1982. Three brothers in this family had complete HL deficiency that was eventually ascribed to a compound heterozygosity for the $Thr_{383} \rightarrow Met$ and $Ser_{267} \rightarrow Phe$ mutations as neither are sufficient alone to produce complete HL deficiency. In patients heterozygous for $Thr_{383} \rightarrow Met$, hepatic lipase is expressed with 40% residual enzyme activity. The $Leu_{334} \rightarrow Phe$ mutation results in the production of a hepatic lipase protein that is secreted but has only 30% of the activity of wild-type hepatic lipase. The $Arg_{186} \rightarrow His$ mutation leads to a protein that is not secreted. Two homozygotes have been reported in Seattle by Brunzell and

colleagues. One was homozygous for an intron 1 acceptor splice site mutation (Seattle-1) and the other for a deletion of exon 1 and promoter (Seattle-3). Neither had the presence of HL protein in the circulation. Simple heterozygotes are usually normolipidemic unless other factors intervene. Partial HL deficiency can be picked-up by measuring post-heparin plasma hepatic lipase activity and by detecting the enrichment of LDL and HDL in triglycerides, which occurs even in normolipidemic individuals. Mutations of *LIPC* that associate with HL deficiency and polymorphisms of the promoter region are given in **3.45**. Polymorphisms of the promoter region of *LIPC* have been associated with changes in HDL levels, insulin resistance, atherosclerosis and even atherosclerosis progression in women on hormone replacement therapy (HRT). Their reported effect on HL activity varies from none to 20–30% variation. There is also evidence that the amount of HL activity increases with

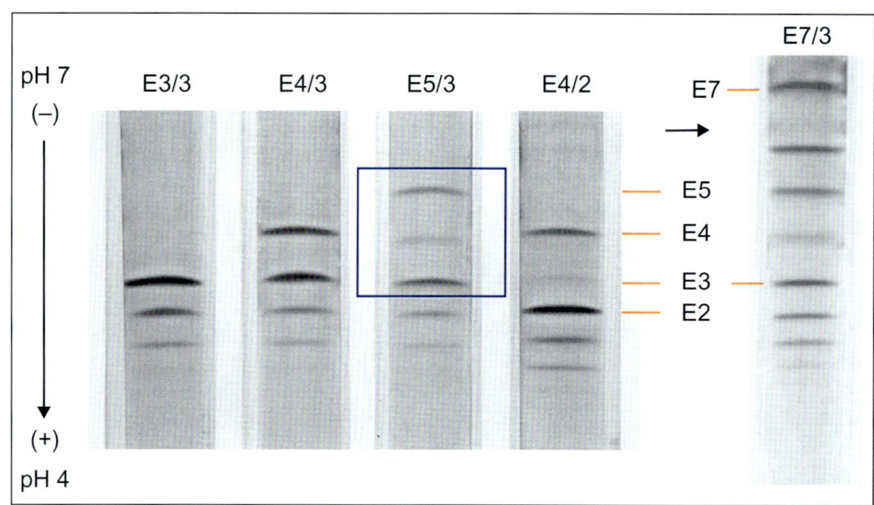

3.39 Demonstration of apolipoprotein E5 (apoE5) and apoE7 mutations on IEF gel of delipidated very-low-density lipoproteins (VLDL). The unusual position of the E5 band on IEF gels makes this mutation readily detectable by IEF. This is the French-Canadian mutation $Glu_{13} \rightarrow Lys$ reported by the authors' research group in collaboration with Humphries' group in London in 1991. The triglycerides were two-fold higher in the affected than in the non-affected individuals. Note that E5 is accompanied by a faster band of sialylated apoE5 as occurs with all isoforms. Only the part of the gels where apoE isoforms separate is shown. Gels from subjects expressing the E3/3, E4/3 and E4/2 phenotypes are used for comparison with the E5/2 phenotype. Yamamura and co-workers first reported such variants in Japan in 1984, whereas Ordovas and colleagues were the first to report an E5 mutation in Caucasians in 1987. The IEF gel on the right shows an E7/3 phenotype for comparison from a patient seen at the authors' lipid clinic. The ambiguity of the numerous bands seen was resolved using the same strategy. The arrow indicates where serum amyloid A (SAA) migrates on these gels (a common contaminant sometimes mistaken for apoE4). ApoE7 has been found to be associated with normolipidemia as well as moderate hyperlipidemia or severe hypercholesterolemia with tendon xanthomas and premature coronary artery disease. These variants were first reported by Japanese investigators.

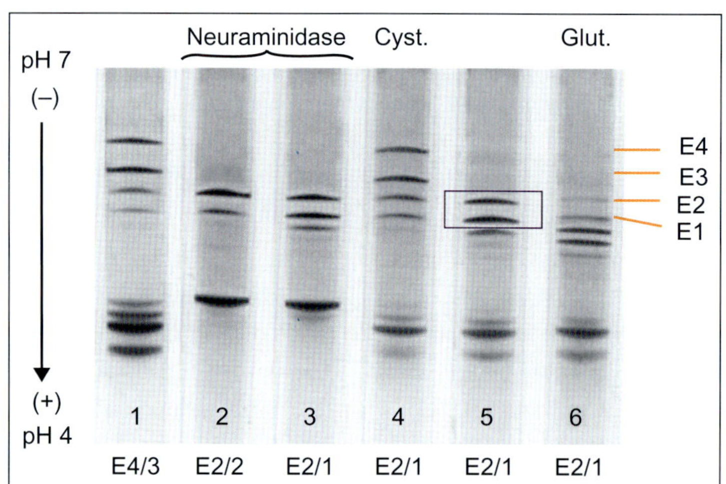

3.40 Resolving the ambiguity of an E2/E1 phenotype using IEF and neuraminidase, cysteamine or glutathione. The identity of an ApoE1 occurring with an apoE2 isoform can be confirmed using simple tools and IEF. The standard IEF gel of the presumed E2/1 subject is in gel 5 (box). An E4/3 phenotype was run simultaneously for comparison (gel 1). Delipidated very-low-density lipoproteins (VLDL) from a normal E2/2 individual and from the E2/1 subject were treated with neuraminidase to ensure that the E1 band is not monosialylated E2 as observed in the E2/2 gel (gel 2). For the E2/2 phenotype, the lower band is less intense but not for the E2/1 sample, supporting the notion that it is an E2 band. Note how neuraminidase affects the sialylated apoC proteins in the lower part of the tubes. Cysteamine (Cyst) treatment moved both apoE2 and apo E1 by two positive charge units indicating that the parent isoform of E1 could be E2 (gel 4). A similar result was demonstrated by treating the sample with glutathione (Glut), which introduces a negative charge with each Cys, confirming that E2 and E1 each have 2 Cys residues (gel 6). This apo E1 could be apoE1$_{BETHESDA}$ (**3.37**) or another unknown mutation. The gene was not sequenced in this patient, who was seen at the authors' lipid clinic to further characterize the variant.

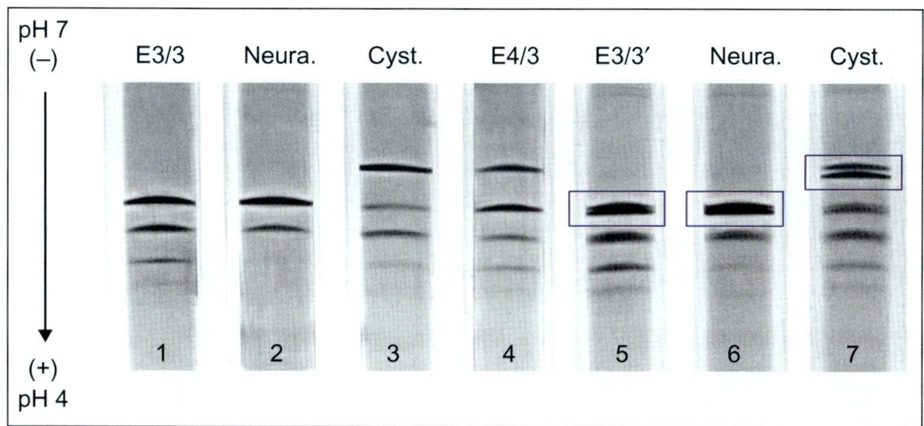

3.41 Effect of cysteamine and neuraminidase on apolipoprotein E (apoE) isoform migration on IEF gels and demonstration of the E3′ mutation: Cysteamine (β-mercaptoethylamine) introduces an amino group on Cys residues through disulphide bond formation and increases the net charge of the protein by one unit for each Cys present. It is therefore helpful in determining whether the apoE has one (E3), two (E2) or no cysteine (E4). This is illustrated here: in the third IEF gel, cysteamine treatment (Cyst) of the E3/3 isoform brings the isoform one positive charge towards the cathode, occupying the site where E4 normally migrates (as in the E4/3 gel next to it, gel 4). Neuraminidase (sialydase) which splits off sialyl (or neuraminic acid) residues, helps determine whether the protein band seen is a sialylated apoE.

In the second IEF tube E3 is treated with neuraminidase (Neura), the tri- and the di-sialylated apoE3 bands disappear, whereas the monosialylated band is less intense and the unsialylated E3 band becomes more accentuated. The last three tubes show the E3′ mutation migrating as a doublet with normal apoE3; even the sialylated derivatives migrate as doublets and become less intense when treated with neuraminidase. The lower band (the more acidic one) is apoE3′, the Arg$_{136}$→His mutation identified in the authors' laboratory (ApoE3′$_{MONTREAL}$). Both apoE3 species move up (cathodic) by one positive charge unit when treated with cysteamine because they both have only one Cys residue (gel 7 on the right). Cysteamine is used as a drug for the treatment of cystinosis and is an inhibitor of somatostatin. These images show the apoE region of the original gels reproduced in Minnich A *et al.* (1995). Identification and characterization of a novel apolipoprotein E variant, apolipoprotein E3′ (Arg$_{136}$→His): association with mild dyslipidemia and double pre-β very low density lipoproteins. *J Lipid Res*, **36**: 57–66.

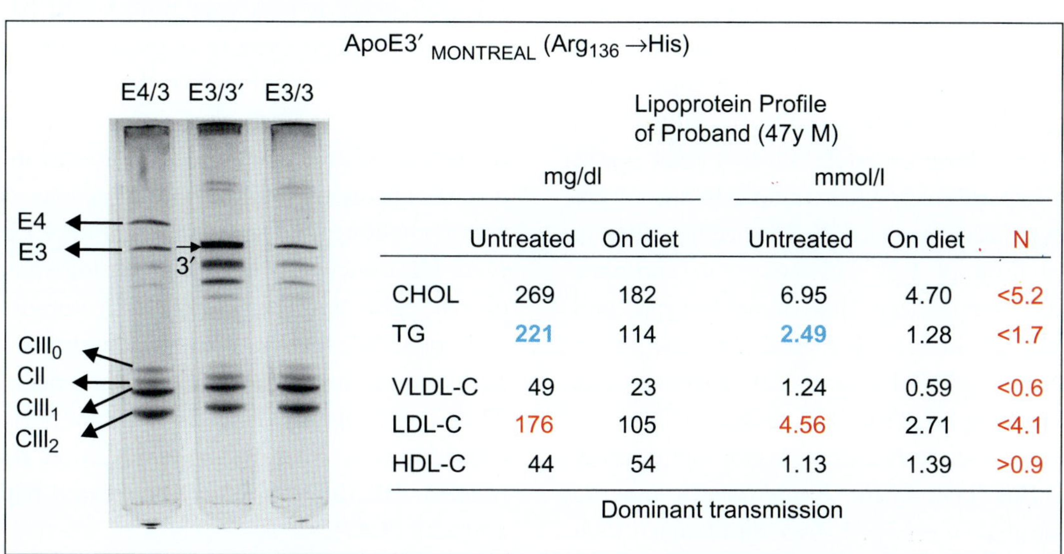

Lipoprotein Profile of Proband (47y M)

	mg/dl		mmol/l		
	Untreated	On diet	Untreated	On diet	N
CHOL	269	182	6.95	4.70	<5.2
TG	221	114	2.49	1.28	<1.7
VLDL-C	49	23	1.24	0.59	<0.6
LDL-C	176	105	4.56	2.71	<4.1
HDL-C	44	54	1.13	1.39	>0.9

Dominant transmission

3.42 Response to diet of a patient with apoE3′$_{MONTREAL}$. The treatment of dyslipidemia associated with uncommon apoE mutations should be guided by the phenotype. The telltale IEF apoE phenotype is shown in the left panel between an E4/3 and an E3/3 phenotype for comparison. This 47-year-old man, carrier of the apoE3′$_{MONTREAL}$ mutation, had a mild combined hyperlipidemia phenotype, peripheral atherosclerosis and a family history of premature coronary artery disease. His plasma lipid abnormalities were corrected within 3 months on a low animal fat and low cholesterol diet restricted in simple carbohydrates. Lipids and lipoproteins before and after treatment are shown on the left in mg/dl and in mmol/l on the right. See Minnich A *et al.* (1995). Identification and characterization of a novel apolipoprotein E variant, apolipoprotein E3′ (Arg$_{136}$→His): association with mild dyslipidemia and double pre-β very low density lipoproteins. *J Lipid Res*, **36**: 57–66.

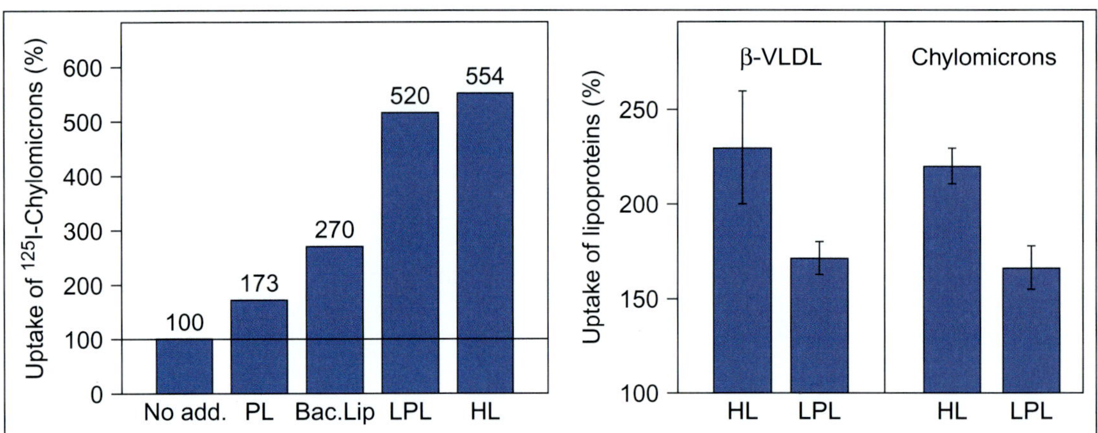

3.43 Uptake of labelled chylomicrons and β-very-low-density lipoproteins (β-VLDL) by hepatocytes is enhanced by lipoprotein lipase (LPL) and hepatic lipase (HL). This classical experiment performed by Krapp in Beisiegel's laboratory demonstrates the facilitating role of hepatic lipase in favouring remnant uptake by liver cell receptors. In the left panel, the uptake of ^{125}I-labelled human chylomicrons by human hepatoma cells Hep3b (1 μg/ml, 37 °C, 90 min) is enhanced by LPL and hepatic lipase (0.1 μg/ml) but not by phospholipids (PL) or bacterial lipase (Bac.Lip). In the absence of chylomicrons, the uptake is 16 ng/mg cell protein and this is expressed as 100%. In the right panel, labelled chylomicrons and β-VLDL uptakes are enhanced by LPL and hepatic lipase purified from post-heparin plasma in similar experimental conditions. Here the final concentration of LPL was 0.2 μg/ml and that of hepatic lipase, 0.1 μg/ml. The authors further showed that the LDL receptor-related protein (LRP) probably mediated the uptake as the effect was the same in normal and LDLR null fibroblasts. They also demonstrated that expression of proteoglycans was essential for the effect to take place because in Chinese hamster ovarian (CHO) cells deficient in proteoglycans the effect did not occur as in normal CHO cells. This kind of interaction is illustrated in **2.2**. Redrawn with permission from Krapp A, Ahle S, Kersting S, Hua Y, Kneser K, Nielsen M, Gliemann J, Beisiegel U (1996). Hepatic lipase mediates the uptake of chylomicrons and β-VLDL into cells via the LDL receptor-related protein (LRP). *J Lipid Res*, **37**: 926–936.

increases in visceral obesity, possibly as an anti-atherogenic defence mechanism.

Absence of HL leads to hypertriglyceridemia which is usually mild but may be severe, a consistent increase in β-VLDL (electrophoresis) or IDL (ultracentrifugation), and a usually modest elevation in HDL that may reach, however, levels of hyperalphalipoproteinemia in the severe phenotype. All lipoproteins are enriched in triglycerides (a consistent manifestation of HL deficiency). In complete HL deficiency, LDL are enlarged and more buoyant and plasma apoB levels are increased several-fold due to an increase in the number of VLDL and IDL particles. The phenotype is less striking in partial HL deficiency because even a small amount of active HL protein may significantly affect VLDL and IDL catabolism. Sometimes it may be confused with familial combined hyperlipidemia (high plasma cholesterol, triglycerides and apoB). Premature atherosclerosis is part of this disease. Eight out of ten patients over 35 years of age developed CAD in their forties and early fifties. The atherogenic potential of this condition is illustrated by the fact that β-VLDL from a patient with HL deficiency are taken up more avidly by macrophages *in vitro* than β-VLDL from a patient with type III (**3.46**). Eruptive

xanthomas and pancreatitis have been reported. Human HL deficiency is very rare but should be suspected when the type III phenotype is atypical: absence of the expected E2/2 phenotype, normal or increased HDL-C, or high apoB levels. It is likely that a single gene mutation leading to partial HL deficiency may be found in or contribute to a dyslipoproteinemia; this situation may constitute a diagnostic challenge. Diagnosis is established in partial or complete HL deficiency by demonstrating an absent or reduced post-heparin lipolytic activity with impaired or absent HL activity or HL mass *in vitro* and demonstrating one or more *LIPC* mutation by sequencing in specialist laboratories. There are probably more cases where partial HL deficiency contributes to the dyslipoproteinemia than suspected at present. HL deficiency may be treated with a statin and/or a fibrate (**3.47**).

Pseudo-type III hyperlipoproteinemia

Pseudo-type III hyperlipoproteinemia (PT-III) is another condition of unknown etiology where patients may exhibit the type III phenotype in the presence of virtually any apoE isoform combination. It has been reported in one large French-Canadian family in the province of Quebec

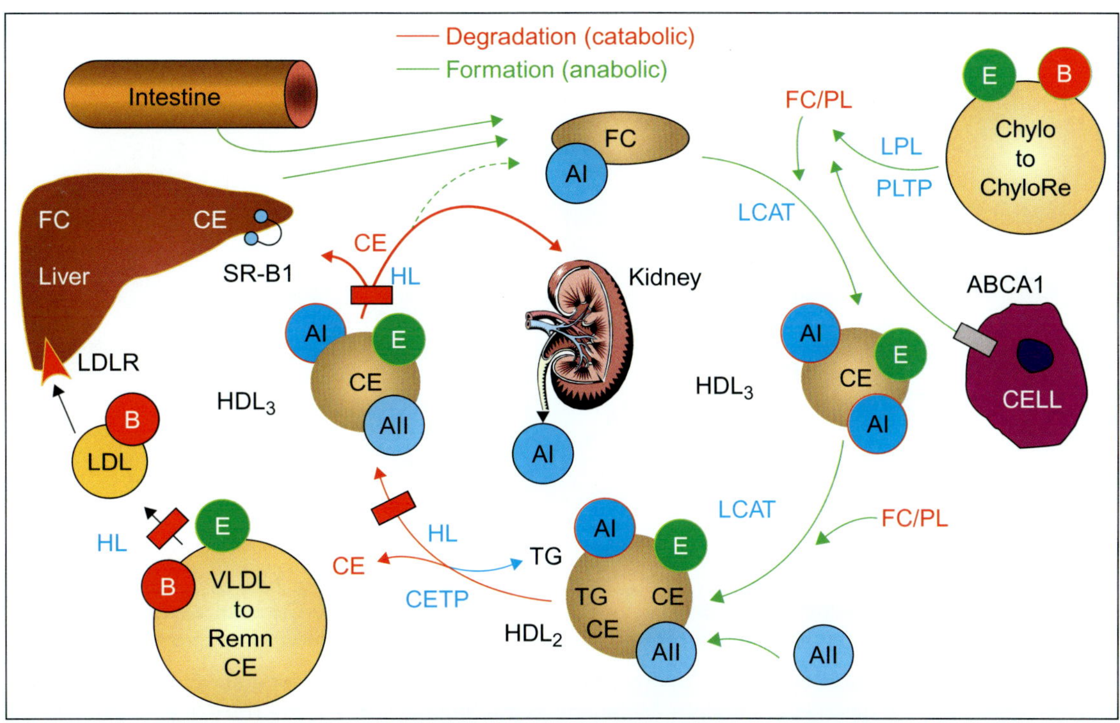

3.44 Role of hepatic lipase (HL) in high-density lipoprotein (HDL) metabolism and hepatic lipase deficiency. This 'circular' pathway of HDL metabolism is based on a model in which HDL is formed via an anabolic pathway (green arrows) involving ATP-binding cassette A1 (ABCA1) and phospholipid transfer protein (PLTP) before entering a catabolic cascade (red arrows). It starts with nascent apoAI discoidal particles (top of circle) originating from the liver, the intestine or the surface of chylomicrons during their catabolism in the circulation (Chylo to ChyloRe). This is followed by their maturation to large apoAI-only HDL$_3$ particles. Cholesteryl esters (CE), phospholipids (PL) and apolipoprotein E (apoE) are acquired in the circulation. The lecithin: cholesterol acyl transferase (LCAT) reaction allows the transformation of free cholesterol (FC) from cells (surface membranes or via ABCA1) to CE for uptake by the HDL particle. The mature HDL$_2$ formed acquires apoAII therefore becoming a preferred substrate for human hepatic lipase. ApoAII is a hydrophobic protein synthesized in the liver and is readily incorporated in the circulation into apoAI-containing spherical HDL particles. It is then directed down the catabolic pathway, where lipids are removed by hydrolysis of PL and triglycerides (TG) and particles get progressively smaller (HDL$_3$) until the apoAI is either cleared through the kidneys or returns into the anabolic pathway (dashed arrow).

Cholesteryl ester transfer protein (CETP) allows transfer of CE to apoB-containing particles in exchange for triglycerides (blue arrow). Acquisition of TG by HDL increases their clearance although it may reduce their interaction with cell surface receptors. For clarity, all of the TG flux is not shown (see **2.12**). This pathway allows for the transfer of FC from the periphery to the plasma compartment for removal by the liver as part of the process of reverse cholesterol transport. CE-loaded HDL$_2$ particles deliver CE to the liver via the scavenger receptor B type 1 (SR-B1) and also indirectly through the apoB-containing particles (very-low-density lipoproteins [VLDL] to LDL cascade, lower left). This leads to formation of small dense TG-poor HDL and LDL. In hepatic lipase deficiency (red bars) these processes are markedly perturbed leading to enrichment of HDL and apoB-containing particles in TG and PL. Large HDL particles are present with an increase in HDL particles containing apoAI and apo AII. The fractional catabolic rate of apoAI is impaired but the levels of preβ-migrating apoAI are normal, therefore cellular cholesterol efflux is not altered. Plasma concentration of β-VLDL, total cholesterol and TG are increased. There is usually a modest elevation in HDL-C. Modification of a diagram from Deeb SS *et al.* (2003). Hepatic lipase and dyslipidemia: interactions among genetic variants, obesity, gender, and diet. *J Lipid Res*, **44**: 1279–1286.

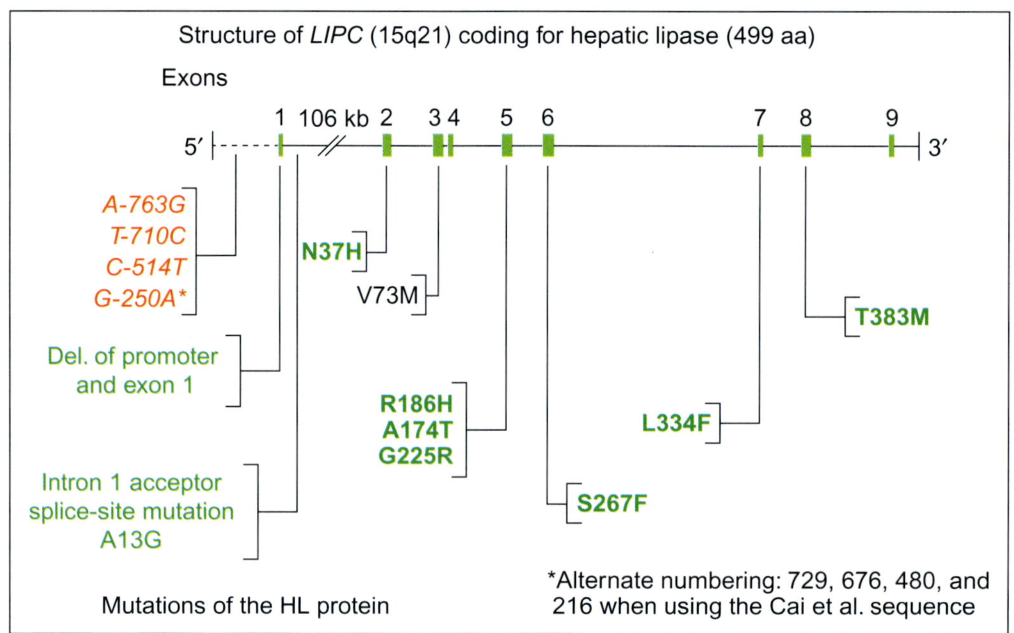

3.45 Hepatic lipase (HL) gene *LIPC* mutations and polymorphisms. In this diagram, the gene structure is given at the top and the mutations in the hepatic lipase protein given in the bottom. Mutations of the hepatic lipase gene (*LIPC*) are rare, and they have been found in all exons except exon 9. They do not all cause complete hepatic lipase deficiency with a severe phenotype. Homozygotes reported for an intron 1 acceptor splice site mutation (Seattle-1) or for a deletion of exon 1 and promoter (Seattle-3) have no circulating hepatic lipase protein. A severe phenotype also occurs in compound heterozygotes such as S267F (exon 6) + T383M (exon 8) reported in an Ontario family in Canada or A174T (exon 5) + T383M (exon 8) in a French-Canadian family in Quebec, as well as L334F (exon 7) combined either with R186H (exon 5) or T383M (exon 8) in Finnish patients. Although the V73M mutation of exon 5 (in black text) was not associated with dyslipoproteinemia in one study, another report has indicated an increased frequency in four Dutch pedigrees with familial combined hyperlipidemia, although it did not segregate with this trait. The G225R mutation is from Seattle. Regarding the common hepatic lipase promoter single nucleotide polymorphisms (SNPs) shown on the upper left in red italics, some confusion exists because of differences in nomenclature.

The sequences of both Cai SJ *et al.* ([1989]. *Biochemistry*, **28**: 2966) and Ameis D *et al.* ([1990]. *J Biol Chem*, **265**: 6552) are used in the current literature (red text). These polymorphisms may or may not affect the expression of hepatic lipase but when there is an influence, lower hepatic lipase activity is linked to higher high-density lipoprotein (HDL)-C. Some of the polymorphisms have also been associated with changes in plasma low-density lipoprotein (LDL) triglyceride levels, insulin resistance, atherosclerosis and obesity. For instance, the T allele of the *C-514T* (C-480T) genotype has been associated with reduced progression of atherosclerosis severity score of the carotids and the abdominal aorta compared with controls in a small prospective study of post-menopausal women (Fan *et al.* [2005]. *J Clin Endocrinol Metab*, **90**: 3786–3792). The T allele was also found to improve insulin sensitivity in young healthy men consuming monounsaturated fatty acids (MUFA) or carbohydrates instead of saturated fatty acids in their diet (Gòmez *et al.* [2005]. *J Mol Endocrinol*, **34**: 331–338). In contrast, the improvement of insulin sensitivity in response to regular exercise was better in the carriers of the CC genotype than in the TT carriers in the HERITAGE family study (Teran-Garcia M *et al.* [2005]. *Diabetes*, **54**: 2251–2255). Furthermore, two studies indicate that another promoter polymorphism, the *G-250A* (G-216A) substitution, is associated with diabetes, the AA genotype favouring a higher conversion from insulin resistance to type 2 diabetes even in young healthy men (2.35-fold higher risk versus GG) (see Zacharova J *et al.* [2005]. *J Intern Med*, **257**: 185–193). Several of these issues remain controversial due to the inherent complexity of such effects. Many gene–environment (i.e. diet, exercise) and gene–gene (i.e. apoE, apoCIII, LPL, CETP) interactions can modulate the presumed functional significance of these polymorphisms. For instance the *LIPC* promoter polymorphism *C-514T* (C-480T) interacts with apoE polymorphism so that carriers of the T allele who have an apoE ε4 allele have an increased proportion of small dense LDL in their plasma relative to CC combined with the other apoE alleles (Skoglund-Andersson C *et al.* [2003]. *Atherosclerosis*, **167**: 311–317). Also the genetic and environmental contexts vary from population to population.

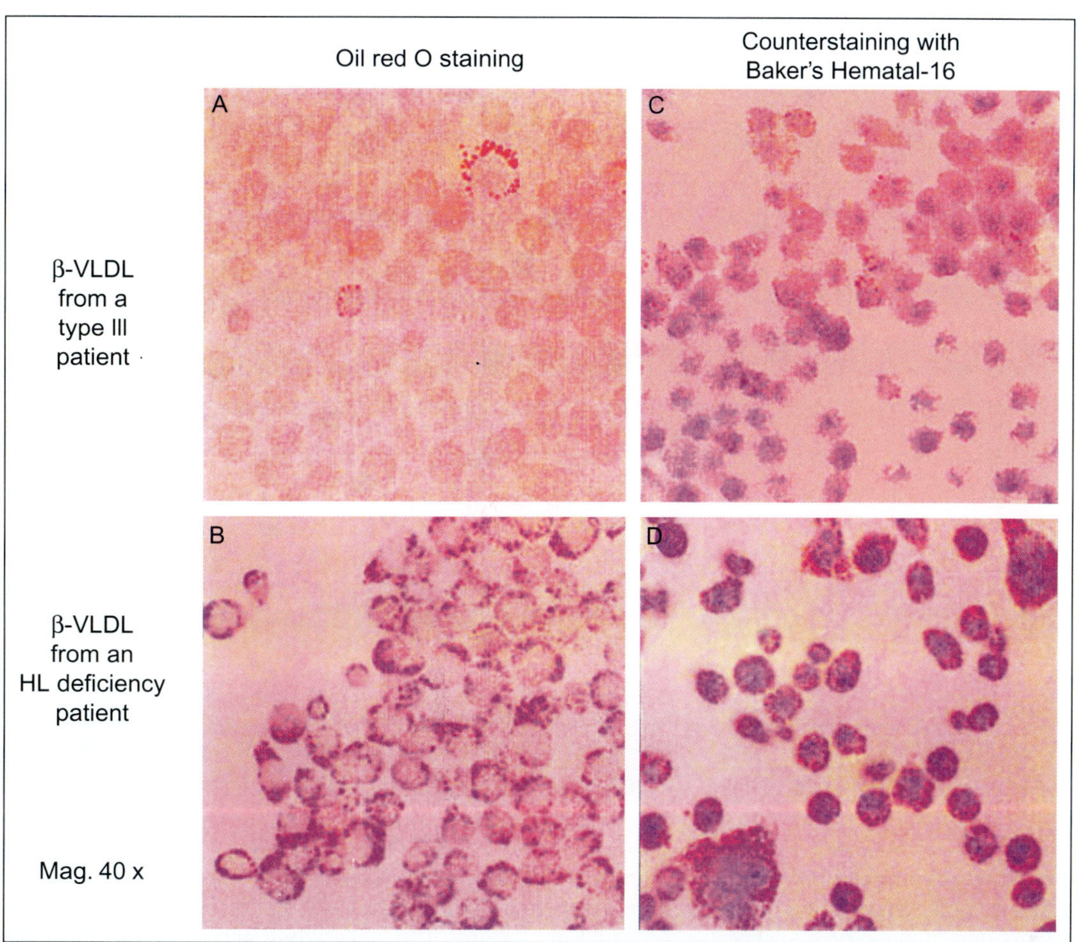

3.46 Uptake of β-very-low-density lipoproteins (β-VLDL) by macrophages in dysbetalipoproteinemia type III versus hepatic lipase deficiency. There is a greater uptake by J774 macrophages of β-migrating VLDL (*Sf* 20 to 400) obtained from a subject with hepatic lipase (HL) deficiency (B, D) than from a type III dysbetalipoproteinemia patient (A, C). These light microscopic images (magnification ×40) were obtained after incubating J774A.1 mouse macrophages for 24 hours with the β-VLDL fraction (50 μg of cholesterol per ml of media) isolated by pevikon block electrophoresis. J774 cells are macrophages that do not secrete apolipoprotein E (apoE). The patient with type III (A and C) had the apoE2/2 phenotype. The patient with hepatic lipase deficiency (B, D) was a compound heterozygote: S267F/T383M (patient B2 of the original Ontario family). The cells were stained with oil red O to identify neutral lipid deposition. Cells in C and D were counterstained with Baker's Hematal-16. Magnification was ×40. Exposure to β-VLDL from a patient with hepatic lipase deficiency increased cholesteryl ester content of macrophages 13-fold compared with 1.5-fold or less with type III β-VLDL. This uptake was found to be mediated by apoE. This figure corresponds to data from the work reported by Huff M *et al.* (1993). VLDL in hepatic lipase deficiency induces ApoE-mediated cholesterol ester accumulation in macrophages. *Arterioscler Thromb*, **13**: 1282–1290. The photomicrographs are courtesy of Murray Huff, Robarts Institute, London, Ontario.

(**3.48**). Affected individuals may exhibit tubero-eruptive xanthomas, arcus corneae, insulin resistance, diabetes, obesity or clinical manifestations of atherosclerosis. Plasma levels of total cholesterol, triglycerides, VLDL-C and apoE are increased. Contrary to classic type III, VLDL-apoB concentration is typically elevated and a double pre-β band (slow-migrating pre-β) is observed when the VLDL fraction is separated by agarose gel electrophoresis, consistent with the presence of TRL remnants. The VLDL-C/TG ratio is usually high as in type III. Discrete lipoprotein particles LpCIII:B and LpB:E (measured by a double antibody enzyme-linked immunosorbent assay [ELISA]) and β-VLDL are not increased as in type III. After an oral fat load, plasma triglyceride concentration and VLDL-apoB are markedly elevated (**3.49**). Post-heparin plasma lipolytic activity is not impaired, with normal HL and LPL activity. The HL gene sequence is normal. Plasma VLDL of PT-III are taken up more avidly by macrophages than VLDL from type III patients or controls. VLDL of PT-III compete efficiently with LDL for uptake

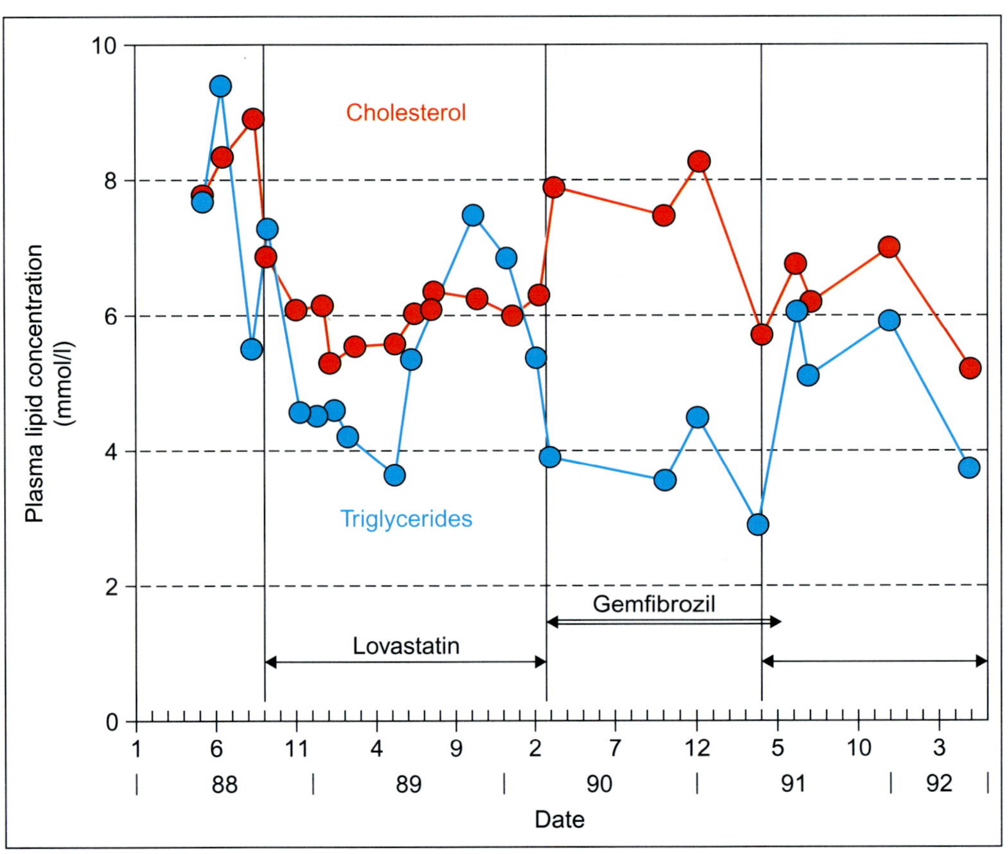

3.47 Drug treatment of hepatic lipase deficiency. The response of plasma cholesterol and triglycerides to lovastatin, gemfibrozil and, for a short period, a combination of the two, is illustrated here in a patient from the Ontario original family with complete hepatic lipase deficiency (compound heterozygote for $Thr_{383} \rightarrow Met$ and $Ser_{267} \rightarrow Phe$). This patient had angina and multiple coronary vessels disease requiring angioplasty at the age of 53 years. At 58 years he had a myocardial infarction despite treatment with lovastatin. Lovastatin (40 mg/day) effectively reduced plasma cholesterol (65%), triglycerides (TG) (62%), low-density lipoprotein-cholesterol (LDL-C) (68%), VLDL-C (56%), apolipoprotein B (apoB) (25%) as well as β-VLDL and the C/TG ratio. When lovastatin was replaced by gemfibrozil (1200 mg/day), the triglycerides fell and cholesterol rose. During follow-up, this patient was eventually given atorvastatin 20 mg daily (Hegele R *et al.* [1999]. *Atherosclerosis*, **143**: 219–222. It substituted for all other previous lipid-lowering agents including combination therapy with simvastatin and fenofibrate, and completely normalized the lipoprotein profile. The patient was also diabetic and was treated with insulin. Redrawn from Hegele R *et al.* (1993). Hepatic lipase deficiency: Clinical, biochemical, and molecular genetic characteristics. *Arterioscler Thromb*, **13**: 720–728.

and degradation by fibroblasts in contrast to VLDL from an individual affected with type III. There is no evidence so far that this condition is due to an apoE receptor defect (LRP, LDLR and the lipolysis-stimulated receptor). The etiology remains unknown. The diagnosis is based on the differences listed in *Table 3.3*. The dyslipoproteinemia is responsive to a diet low in animal fat, cholesterol and simple sugars and to fibrate therapy.

Other dyslipidemic conditions associated with apolipoprotein E

Mild hypertriglyceridemia has been reported in cases of '*sea-blue histiocytosis*' in the presence of the inherited domi-nant apoE mutation ΔLeu_{149} (i.e. deletion of a leucine at position 149, a 3 bp deletion) in the receptor-binding region of apoE. This syndrome is characterized by splenomegaly, thrombocytopenia and the presence of histiocytes in the bone marrow smear that have cytoplasmic granules display-ing a sea-blue colour with the usual hematological stains (**3.50**). This syndrome (OMIM No. 269600) is rare and may develop in lipid storage disorders such as cholesteryl ester storage disease, Niemann–Pick and Gaucher's dis-ease, and in severe hypertriglyceridemia (>11.36 mmol/l or 1000 mg/dl), lecithin: cholesterol acyl transferase (LCAT) deficiency and Tangier disease. The cause of the primary syndrome and the reason for the blue colour are not known

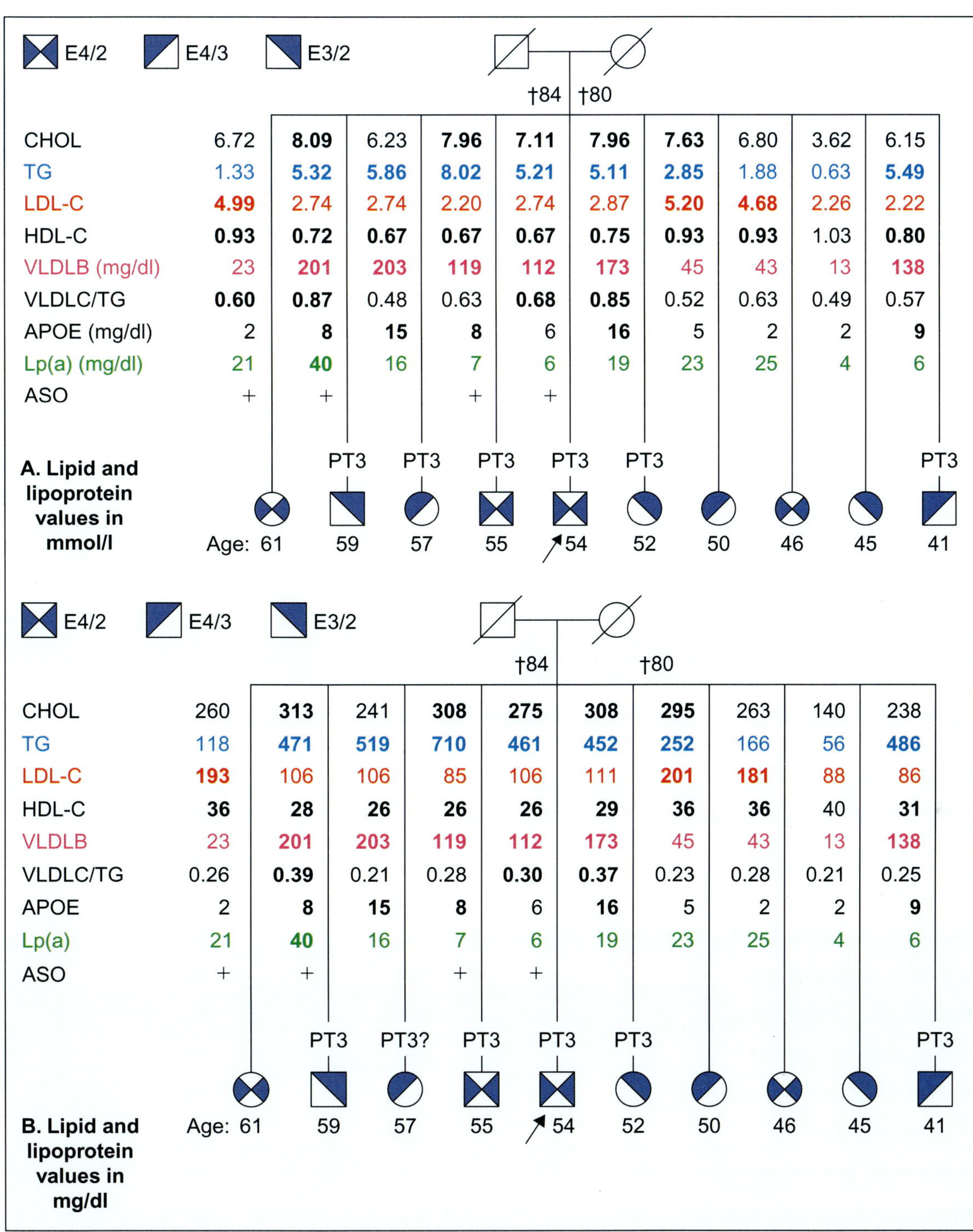

A. Lipid and lipoprotein values in mmol/l

CHOL	6.72	**8.09**	6.23	**7.96**	**7.11**	**7.96**	**7.63**	6.80	3.62	6.15
TG	1.33	**5.32**	**5.86**	**8.02**	**5.21**	**5.11**	**2.85**	1.88	0.63	**5.49**
LDL-C	**4.99**	2.74	2.74	2.20	2.74	2.87	**5.20**	**4.68**	2.26	2.22
HDL-C	**0.93**	**0.72**	**0.67**	**0.67**	**0.67**	**0.75**	**0.93**	**0.93**	1.03	**0.80**
VLDLB (mg/dl)	23	**201**	**203**	**119**	**112**	**173**	45	43	13	**138**
VLDLC/TG	**0.60**	**0.87**	0.48	0.63	**0.68**	**0.85**	0.52	0.63	0.49	0.57
APOE (mg/dl)	2	**8**	**15**	**8**	6	**16**	5	2	2	**9**
Lp(a) (mg/dl)	21	**40**	16	7	6	19	23	25	4	6
ASO	+	+			+	+				
PT3		PT3	PT3	PT3	PT3	PT3				PT3
Age:	61	59	57	55	54	52	50	46	45	41

B. Lipid and lipoprotein values in mg/dl

CHOL	260	**313**	241	**308**	**275**	**308**	**295**	263	140	238
TG	118	**471**	**519**	**710**	**461**	**452**	**252**	166	56	**486**
LDL-C	**193**	106	106	85	106	111	**201**	**181**	88	86
HDL-C	**36**	**28**	**26**	**26**	**26**	**29**	**36**	**36**	40	**31**
VLDLB	23	**201**	**203**	**119**	**112**	**173**	45	43	13	**138**
VLDLC/TG	0.26	**0.39**	0.21	0.28	**0.30**	**0.37**	0.23	0.28	0.21	0.25
APOE	2	**8**	**15**	**8**	6	**16**	5	2	2	**9**
Lp(a)	21	**40**	16	7	6	19	23	25	4	6
ASO	+	+			+	+				
PT3		PT3	PT3?	PT3	PT3	PT3				PT3
Age:	61	59	57	55	54	52	50	46	45	41

3.48 Pseudo-type III hyperlipoproteinemia in a family. In this figure of the 'M Family' the lipid and lipoprotein values are reported separately in mmol/l (A) and in mg/dl (B); the readings when these were measured were in mg/dl. In both figures, very-low-density lipoproteins (VLDL) apolipoprotein B (VLDLB), apolipoprotein E (apoE) and Lp(a) are given in mg/dl. The arrow indicates the proband. The numbers in bold indicate abnormal plasma levels. 'ASO' stands for the presence of atherosclerotic vascular disease; PT3 for the typical phenotype of pseudo-type III, the question mark (PT3?) the absence of a high VLDL-C/triglyceride ratio (VLDL-C/TG), which varied but often hovered above 0.70 (mmol/l) or 0.30 (mg/dl). Typically, triglycerides are elevated, high-density lipoprotein cholesterol (HDL-C) is low but VLDLB is markedly elevated. The striking feature here, besides high VLDLB, is a clinical and biochemical phenotype resembling type III dysbetalipoproteinemia in the presence of the apoE phenotypes E4/2, E4/3 and E3/2, not the E2/2 phenotype. This is part of a figure taken from Davignon J *et al.* In: Stein O, Eisenberg S, Stein Y, eds. *Atherosclerosis IX*, R & L Creative Comm., Tel Aviv, 1992: 199–203).

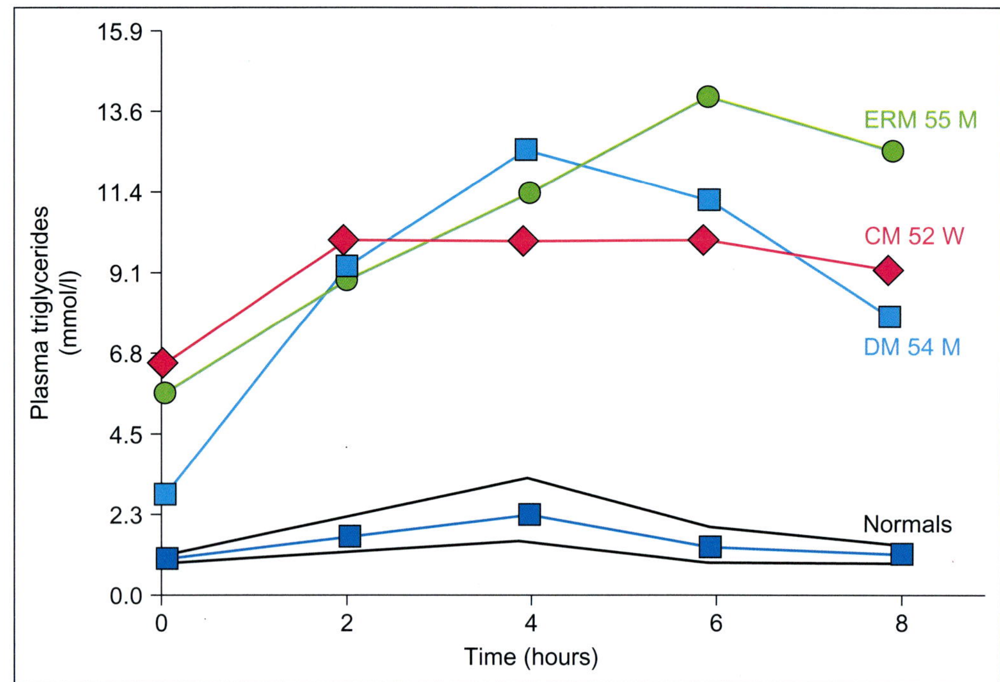

3.49 Elevation of plasma triglycerides after a fat load in patients with pseudo-type III. At time 0, the subjects, two men (M) and one woman (W) between 52 and 55 years of age with pseudo-type III, drank 350 ml/2.5 m² of body surface area of sweetened heavy cream. The response of plasma triglycerides (mean ± SD) in six normal subjects is given for comparison. The marked increase in plasma triglycerides for the different baseline levels is remarkable. This is also rather usual in type III dysbetalipoproteinemia and other forms of hypertriglyceridemia. Redrawn from Davignon J *et al.* (1991). A phenocopy of type III dysbetalipoproteinemia occurring in a candidate family for a putative Apo E receptor defect. *Ann Med*, **23**: 161–167.

Table 3.3 Similarities and differences between type III and pseudo-type III		
Phenotype	**Type III**	**Pseudo-type III**
Tubero-eruptive xanthomas ±	Yes	Yes
Atherosclerosis or obesity ±	Yes	Yes
Glucose intolerance ±	Yes	Yes
High plasma cholesterol, triglycerides and apoE	Yes	Yes
Low LDL-C and HDL-C	Yes	Yes
High VLDL-C/triglyceride	Yes	Yes
Marked fat intolerance	Yes	Yes
Responsiveness to fibrate	Yes	Yes
E2/2 phenotype	Usual	Rare
Any APOE phenotype	No	Yes
High LpE:B and LpCIII:B	Yes	No
β-VLDL	Yes	No
Slow pre-β	Rare	Yes
High VLDL-apoB	No	Yes
Low VLDL-C/VLDLB	No	Yes

LDL-C, low-density lipoprotein-cholesterol; VLDL, very-low-density lipoproteins.
Derived from Davignon J *et al.* (1991). A phenocopy of type III dysbetalipoproteinemia occurring in a candidate family for a putative Apo E receptor defect. *Ann Med*, **23**: 161–167.

although glycosphingolipids and ceroids have been identified in these cells. In the original report, splenectomy was followed by a worsening of the hypertriglyceridemia and the presence in plasma of β-VLDL which prompted the apoE genotyping (E3/3) and sequencing of exon 4 of *APOE*. The β-VLDL formed are taken up readily by macrophages to form foam cells rich in cholesteryl ester. The abnormal apoE has an impaired ability to be taken up by the normal clearance pathway. These effects could account for the foam cell-loaded enlarged spleen and explain the worsening of the hyperlipidemia after splenectomy. An important insight into the apoE structure–function relationship was thus derived from the study of an unusual case. In a family described more recently the phenotype was more severe because of the presence of an ε2 allele. Fibrate or statin therapy was found to be effective in reducing the lipoprotein abnormality.

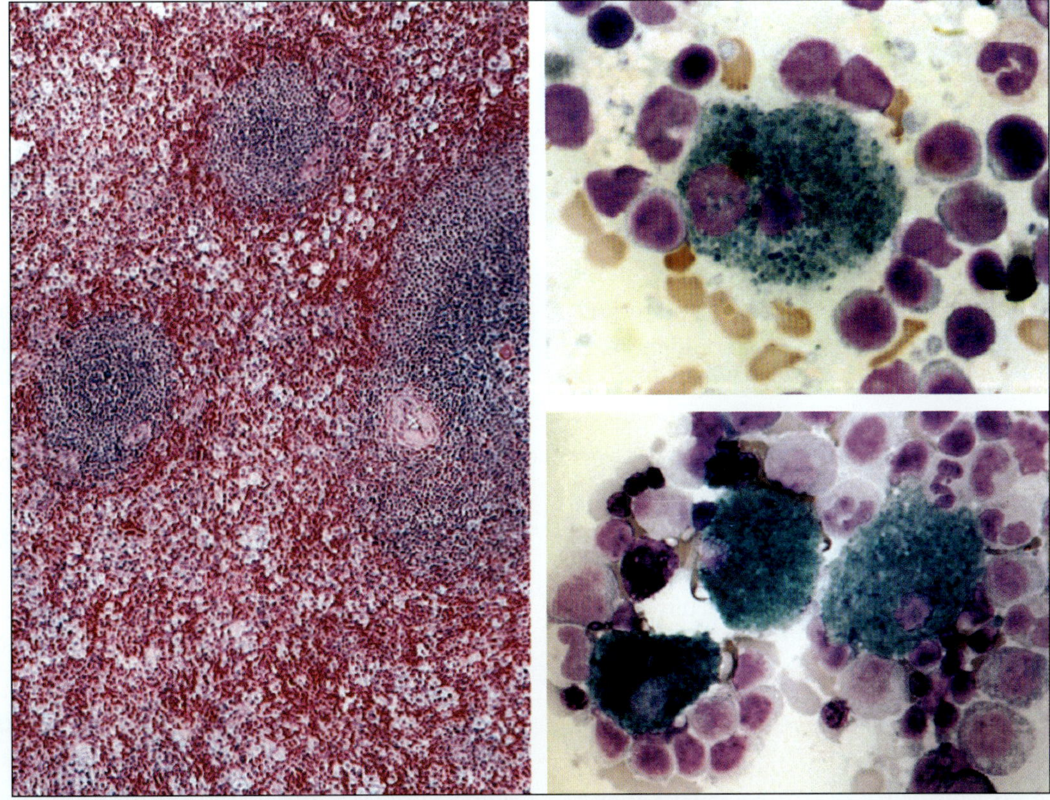

3.50 Histopathological features of the sea-blue histiocytosis syndrome. The panel on the left is a photomicrograph (magnification ×85) of the spleen, stained with hematoxylin and eosin and showing expansion of the red pulp by foamy histiocytes, in a 29-year-old 'healthy' subject with a combination of splenomegaly, reduced platelet count, the sea-blue histiocyte syndrome and the apoE ΔLeu149 mutation. He also had fatty infiltration of the liver, and his plasma cholesterol was 2.32 mmol/l, triglycerides 2.09 mmol/l and high-density lipoprotein-cholesterol (HDL-C) 0.54 mmol/l (90, 184 and 21 mg/dl, respectively) before splenectomy. One year after splenectomy the plasma cholesterol increased to 5.17 mmol/l (200 mg/dl) and triglycerides to 7.27 mmol/l (643 mg/dl). HDL-C was 0.49 mmol/l (19 mg/dl) and the presence of β-VLDL was noted. After 30 days of treatment with a low-fat diet and 1200 mg/day of gemfibrozil, the triglyceride levels fell to 2.31 mmol/l (204 mg/dl) and HLD-C increased to 0.85 mmol/l (33 mg/dl). Total cholesterol was 6.56 mmol/l (254 mg/dl). Reproduced with permission from Nguyen TT *et al.* (2000). *J Clin Endocrinol Metab*, **85**: 4354–4358. The two panels on the right illustrate the phagocytic sea-blue histiocytes typical of the sea-blue histiocytosis syndrome from a bone marrow biopsy specimen taken from a 52-year-old Laotian woman with a follicular lymphocytic non-Hodgkin lymphoma. These cells are characterized by a single eccentric nucleus and cytoplasm containing large blue lysosomal granules on Giemsa stain. Besides the conditions listed in the text, the sea-blue histiocyte syndrome has been reported in total parenteral nutrition, chronic granulomatous disease, Takayasu's arteritis, and hepatic porphyria. It has also been associated with hematological conditions such as idiopathic thrombocytopenic purpura, chronic granulocytic leukemia, lymphoma, mycosis fungoides, primary myelofibrosis, and myelodysplastic syndromes. This is reproduced with permission from Oo TH *et al.* (2002). Unusual presentations of lymphoma: Case 1. Sea-blue histiocytes in non-Hodgkin's lymphoma. *J Clin Oncol*, **20**:1942–1943.

Further reading

Familial combined hyperlipidemia (FCH)

Aguilar-Salinas CA, Barrett PHR, Pulai J, Zhu XL, Schonfeld G (1997). A familial combined hyperlipidemic kindred with impaired apolipoprotein B catabolism – Kinetics of apolipoprotein B during placebo and pravastatin therapy. *Arterioscler Thromb Vasc Biol*, **17**: 72–82

Aguilar Salinas CA, Zamora M, Gomez-Diaz RA, Mehta R, Gomez Perez FJ, Rull JA (2004). Familial combined hyperlipidemia: controversial aspects of its diagnosis and pathogenesis. *Semin Vasc Med*, **4**: 203–209.

Cianflone KM, Maslowska MH, Sniderman AD (1990). Impaired response of fibroblasts from patients with hyperapobetalipoproteinemia to acylation-stimulating protein. *J Clin Invest*, **85**: 722–730

Davignon J, Genest J, Jr (1998). Genetics of lipoprotein disorders. *Endocrinol Metab Clin North Am*, **2**: 521–550.

Eichenbaum-Voline S, Olivier M, Jones EL, Naoumova RP, Jones B, Gau B, Patel HN, Seed M, Betteridge DJ, Galton DJ, Rubin EM, Scott J, Shoulders CC, Pennacchio LA (2004). Linkage and association between distinct variants of the *APOA1/C3/A4/A5* gene cluster and familial combined hyperlipidemia. *Arterioscler Thromb Vasc Biol*, **24**: 167–174.

Georgieva M, Ten Cate H, Keulen ETP, Van Oerle R, Govers-Riemslag JWP, Hamulyák K, Van der Kallen CJH, Van Greevenbroek MMJ, De Bruin TWA (2004). Prothrombotic markers in familial combined hyperlipidemia evidence of endothelial cell activation and relation to metabolic syndrome. *Atherosclerosis*, **175**: 345–351.

Hopkins PN, Heiss G, Ellison RC, Province MA, Pankow JS, Eckfeldt JH, Hunt SC (2003). Coronary artery disease risk in familial combined – Hyperlipidemia and familial hypertriglyceridemia – A case-control comparison from the National Heart, Lung, Blood Institute Family Heart Study. *Circulation*, **108**: 519–523.

Maitra A, Hirany SV, Jialal I (1997). Comparison of two assays for measuring LDL cholesterol. *Clin Chem*, **43**: 1040–1047.

Meijssen S, Cabezas MC, Twickler TB, Jansen H, Erkelens DW (2000). In vivo evidence of defective postprandial and postabsorptive free fatty acid metabolism in familial combined hyperlipidemia. *J Lipid Res*, **41**: 1096–1102.

Nauck M, Warnick GR, Rifai N (2002). Methods for measurement of LDL-cholesterol: A critical assessment of direct measurement by homogeneous assays versus calculation. *Clin Chem*, **48**: 236–254.

Pajukanta P, Lilja HE, Sinsheimer JS, Cantor RM, Lusis AJ, Gentile M, Duan XQJ, Soro-Paavonen A, Naukkarinen J, Saarela J, Laakso M, Ehnholm C, Taskinen MR, Peltonen L (2004). Familial combined hyperlipidemia is associated with upstream transcription factor 1 (*USF1*). *Nat Genet*, **36**: 371–376.

Reynisdottir S, Eriksson M, Angelin B, Arner P (1995). Impaired actiration of adipocyte lipdysis in familial combined hyperlipidemia. *J Clin Invest*, **95**: 2161–2169.

Shoulders CC, Jones EL, Naoumova RP (2004). Genetics of familial combined hyperlipidemia and risk of coronary heart disease. *Hum Mol Genet*, **13**: R149–R160.

Vakkilainen J, Jauhiainen M, Ylitalo K, Nuotio IO, Viikari JSA, Ehnholm C, Taskinen MR (2002). LDL particle size in familial combined hyperlipidemia: effects of serum lipids, lipoprotein-modifying enzymes, and lipid transfer protein. *J Lipid Res*, **43**: 598–603

Van der Vleuten GM, Van Tits LJ, Den Heijer M, Lemmers H, Stalenhoef AF, De Graaf J (2005). Decreased adiponectin levels in familial combined hyperlipidemia patients contribute to the atherogenic lipid profile. *J Lipid Res*, **46**: 2398–2404.

Veerkamp MJ, De Graaf J, Hendriks JCM, Demacker PNM, Stalenhoef AFH (2004). Nomogram to diagnose familial combined hyperlipidemia on the basis of results of a 5-year follow-up study. *Circulation*, **109**: 2980–2985.

Familial dysbetalipoproteinemia and remnant excess
Classical dysbetalipoproteinemia type III

Carmena R, Roy M, Roederer G, Minnich A, Davignon J (2000). Coexisting dysbetalipoproteinemia and familial hypercholesterolemia – Clinical and laboratory observations. *Atherosclerosis*, **148**: 113–124.

Havel RJ (1982). Familial dysbetalipoproteinemia. New aspects of pathogenesis and treatment. *Med Clin North Am*, **66**: 441–454.

Hopkins PN, Wu LL, Hunt SC, Brinton EA (2005). Plasma triglycerides and type III hyperlipidemia are independently associated with premature familial coronary artery disease. *J Am Coll Cardiol*, **45**: 1003–1012.

Mahley RW, Huang YD, Rall SC Jr (1999). Pathogenesis of type III hyperlipoproteinemia (dysbetalipoproteinemia):

questions, quandaries, and paradoxes. *J Lipid Res*, **40**: 1933–1949.

Mahley RW, Rall SC Jr (2001). Type III hyperlipoproteinemia (dysbetalipoproteinemia): the role of apolipoprotein E in normal and abnormal lipoprotein metabolism. In: Scriver CR, Beaudet AL, Sly WS, Valle D (eds) *The Metabolic and Molecular Bases of Inherited Disease*. McGraw-Hill, New York, pp. 2835–2862.

Smelt AH, De Beer F (2004). Apolipoprotein E and familial dysbetalipoproteinemia: clinical, biochemical, and genetic aspects. *Semin Vasc Med*, **4**: 249–257.

Other inherited causes of remnant excess

Apolipoprotein E deficiency

Feussner G, Funke H, Weng W, Assmann G, Lackner KJ, Ziegler R (1992). Severe type III hyperlipoproteinemia associated with unusual apolipoprotein E1 phenotype and e1/'null' genotype. *Eur J Clin Invest*, **22**: 599–608.

Ghiselli G, Schaefer EJ, Gascon P, Brewer HB Jr (1981). Type III hyperlipoproteinemia associated with plasma apolipoprotein E deficiency. *Science*, **214**: 1239–1241.

Ikewaki K, Cain W, Thomas F, Shamburek R, Zech LA, Usher D, Brewer HB Jr, Rader DJ (2004). Abnormal in vivo metabolism of apoB-containing lipoproteins in human apoE deficiency. *J Lipid Res*, **45**: 1302–1311.

Schaefer EJ, Gregg RE, Ghiselli G, Forte TM, Ordovas JM, Zech LA, Brewer HB Jr (1986). Familial apolipoprotein E deficiency. *J Clin Invest*, **78**: 1206–1219.

Apolipoprotein E mutations, dominant type III and lipoprotein glomerulopathy

De Beer F, Van Dijk KW, Jong MC, Van Vark LC, Van der Zee A, Hofker MH, Fallaux FJ, Hoeben RC, Smelt AHM, Havekes LM (2000). Apolipoprotein E2 (Lys146-->Gln) causes hypertriglyceridemia due to an apolipoprotein E variant-specific inhibition of lipolysis of very low density lipoproteins-triglycerides. *Arterioscler Thromb Vasc Biol*, **20**: 1800–1806.

De Knijff P, Van den Maagdenberg AMJM, Stalenhoef AFH, Leuven JAG, Demacker PNM, Kuyt LP, Frants RR, Havekes LM (1991). Familial dysbetalipoproteinemia associated with apolipoprotein E3-Leiden in an extended multigeneration pedigree. *J Clin Invest*, **88**: 643–655.

Greenow K, Pearce NJ, Ramji DP (2005). The key role of apolipoprotein E in atherosclerosis. *J Mol Med*, **83**: 329–342.

Ieiri N, Hotta O, Taguma Y (2003). Resolution of typical lipoprotein glomerulopathy by intensive lipid-lowering therapy. *Am J Kidney Dis*, **41**: 244–249.

Meyrier A, Dairou F, Callard P, Mougenot B (1995). Lipoprotein glomerulopathy: first case in a white European. *Nephrol Dial Transplant*, **10**: 546–549.

Rall SC Jr, Mahley RW (1992). The role of apolipoprotein E genetic variants in lipoprotein disorders. *J Intern Med*, **231**: 653–659.

Rall SC Jr, Innerarity TL, Weisgraber KH, Wardell MR, Mahley RW (1990). The type of mutation in apolipoprotein E determines whether type III hyperlipoproteinemia is expressed as a dominant or recessive trait. In: Descovich GC, Gaddi A, Magri GL, Lenzi S (eds) *Atherosclerosis and Cardiovascular Disease; 7th International Meeting*. Kluwer Academic Publishers, Dordrecht, pp. 81–88.

Saito T, Oikawa S, Sato H, Chiba J (1997). Lipoprotein glomerulopathy and its pathogenesis. *Contrib Nephrol*, **120**: 30–38.

Hepatic lipase deficiency

Ameis D, Stahnke G, Kobayashi J, McLean J, Lee G, Buscher M, Schotz MC, Will H (1990). Isolation and characterization of the human hepatic lipase gene. *J Biol Chem*, **265**: 6552–6555.

Breckenridge WC, Little JA, Alaupovic P, Wang CS, Kuksis A, Kakis G, Lindgren F, Gardiner G (1982). Lipoprotein abnormalities associated with a familial deficiency of hepatic lipase. *Atherosclerosis*, **45**: 161–179.

Cai SJ, Wong DM, Chen SH, Chan L (1989). Structure of the human hepatic triglyceride lipase gene. *Biochemistry*, **28**: 8966–8971.

Deeb SS, Zambon A, Carr MC, Ayyobi AF, Brunzell JD (2003). Hepatic lipase and dyslipidemia: interactions among genetic variants, obesity, gender, and diet. *J Lipid Res*, **44**: 1279–1286.

Fan YM, Dastidar P, Jokela H, Punnonen R, Lehtimäki T (2005). Review: hepatic lipase C-480T genotype-dependent benefit from long-term hormone replacement therapy for atherosclerosis progression in postmenopausal women. *J Clin Endocrinol Metab*, **90**: 3786–3792.

Gómez P, Pérez-Jiménez F, Marín C, Moreno JA, Gómez MJ, Bellido C, Pérez-Martínez P, Fuentes F, Paniagua JA, López-Miranda J (2005). The -514 C/T polymorphism in the hepatic lipase gene promoter is associated with insulin sensitivity in a healthy young population. *J Mol Endocrinol*, **34**: 331–338.

Hegele RA, Little JA, Vezina C, Maguire GF, Tu L, Wolever TS, Jenkins DJA, Connelly PW (1993). Hepatic lipase deficiency: clinical, biochemical, and molecular genetic characteristics. *Arterioscler Thromb*, **13**: 720–728.

Hime NJ, Drew KJ, Wee K, Barter PJ, Rye KA (2006). Formation of high density lipoproteins containing both apolipoprotein A-I and A-II in the rabbit. *J Lipid Res*, **47**: 115–122.

Huff MW, Sawyez CG, Connelly PW, Maguire F, Little JA, Hegele RA (1993). β-VLDL in hepatic lipase deficiency induces ApoE-mediated cholesterol ester accumulation in macrophages. *Arterioscler Thromb*, **13**: 1282–1290.

Ruel IL, Couture P, Cohn JS, Lamarche B (2005). Plasma metabolism of apoB-containing lipoproteins in patients with hepatic lipase deficiency. *Atherosclerosis*, **180**: 355–366.

Skoglund-Andersson C, Ehrenborg E, Fisher RM, Olivecrona G, Hamsten A, Karpe F (2003). Influence of common variants in the CETP, LPL, HL and APO E genes on LDL heterogeneity in healthy, middle-aged men. *Atherosclerosis*, **167**: 311–317.

Teran-Garcia M, Santoro N, Rankinen T, Bergeron J, Rice T, Leon AS, Rao DC, Skinner JS, Bergman RN, Després JP, Bouchard C (2005). Hepatic lipase gene variant -514C> T is associated with lipoprotein and insulin sensitivity response to regular exercise – The HERITAGE Family Study. *Diabetes*, **54**: 2251–2255.

Tilly-Kiesi M, Schaefer EJ, Knudsen P, Welty FK, Dolnikowski GG, Taskinen MR, Lichtenstein AH (2004). Lipoprotein metabolism in subjects with hepatic lipase deficiency. *Metabolism*, **53**: 520–525.

Van't Hooft FM, Lundahl B, Ragogna F, Karpe F, Olivecrona G, Hamsten A (2000). Functional characterization of 4 polymorphisms in promoter region of hepatic lipase gene. *Arterioscler Thromb Vasc Biol*, **20**: 1335–1339.

Zacharova J, Todorova BR, Chiasson JL, Laakso M, Study Grp STOP-NIDDM (2005). The G-250A substitution in the promoter region of the hepatic lipase gene is associated with the conversion from impaired glucose tolerance to type 2 diabetes: the STOP-NIDDM trial. *J Intern Med*, **257**: 185–193.

Pseudo-type III hyperlipoproteinemia

Davignon J, Dallongeville J, Roederer G, Roy M, Fruchart JC, Kessling AM, Bouthillier D, Lussier-Cacan S (1991). A phenocopy of type III dysbetalipoproteinemia occurring in a candidate family for a putative Apo E receptor defect. *Ann Med*, **23**: 161–167.

Giroux LM, Cohn JS, LaMarre J, Davignon J (1997). Pseudo type III dyslipoproteinemia is associated with normal fibroblast lipoprotein receptor activity. *Atherosclerosis*, **132**: 85–94.

Other dyslipidemic conditions associated with apolipoprotein E

Faivre L, Saugier-Veber P, Pais de Barros JP, Verges B, Couret B, Lorcerie B, Thauvin C, Charbonnier F, Huet F, Gambert P, Frebourg T, Duvillard L (2005). Variable expressivity of the clinical and biochemical phenotype associated with the apolipoprotein E p.Leu149del mutation. *Eur J Hum Genet*, **13**: 1186–1191.

Nguyen TT, Kruckeberg KE, O'Brien JF, Ji ZS, Karnes PS, Crotty TB, Hay ID, Mahley RW, O'Brien T (2000). Familial splenomegaly: Macrophage hypercatabolism of lipoproteins associated with apolipoprotein E mutation [apolipoprotein E (Δ149 Leu)]. *J Clin Endocrinol Metab*, **85**: 4354–4358.

Inherited Dyslipoproteinemias of Various Etiologies

Familial lipoprotein(a) hyperlipoproteinemia

High levels of lipoprotein(a) (Lp(a)) aggregate or segregate in families and may be associated with atherosclerotic vascular disease. In Turkey, a country with a low average low-density lipoprotein-cholesterol (LDL-C) level, familial Lp(a) hyperlipoproteinemia has been reported as one of the most common familial lipoprotein disorder leading to premature myocardial infarction.

Lp(a) or lipoprotein(a) was first described in 1963 by Berg at the University of Oslo. This peculiar lipoprotein has a 'recent' evolutionary history as it is present only in humans, Old World primates and hedgehogs. Essentially, it consists of a typical LDL particle linked by a disulphide bridge to apolipoprotein(a). The latter is a large glycoprotein with no amphipathic helices (lipid-binding sites), which is linked to apolipoprotein B (apoB)-100 by a single disulphide bond in the C-terminal regions of both proteins, close to the LDL receptor binding site of apoB (**4.1**). In the early years of lipoprotein identification, Lp(a) could be demonstrated in plasma using a combination of lipoprotein electrophoresis and preparative ultracentrifugation. It was recovered in the bottom d = 1.006 g/ml ultracentrifugal fraction with high-density lipoproteins (HDL) and was given the name 'sinking preβ-lipoprotein' (**4.2**). In 1987, McLean and colleagues found that both the apo(a) and the plasminogen genes had coding sequences for so-called kringle domains, K I to K V for plasminogen and K IV and K V for apo(a) (**4.3**). The hedgehog apo(a) has K III repeats. The structure of a typical kringle is shown in **4.4**.

The apolipoprotein(a) gene (*LPA*, OMIM No. 152200) maps to chromosome 6q26–27 and is heterogeneous because of the number of sequence repeats (3 to >40) that encode the K IV type 2 domains. The inheritance pattern is complicated by the fact that the apo(a) size polymorphism is controlled by a large number of co-dominant alleles (>35) that vary widely in expressivity (**4.5**). The frequency distribution of kringle IV type 2 repeats and of Lp(a) plasma concentration differs widely across populations (**4.6**). The encoded apo(a) protein thus can have a molecular weight ranging from 300 kDa to 800 kDa. There is a general inverse relationship, with inter-individual variation, between the size of apo(a) and the plasma concentration of Lp(a), and this is believed to be 90% genetically determined. Most individuals are heterozygous for apo(a) size, therefore the plasma concentration of Lp(a) results from the relative contribution of each isoform. It has been observed that black people have two- to three-fold higher levels of Lp(a) than white people or Asians, even when adjusted for apo(a) size. However, an increased risk for coronary heart disease (CHD) associated with higher Lp(a) levels in African-Americans has not been documented. Interestingly, mutations of the apo(a) gene (**4.7**) resulting in no circulating apo(a) (Lp(a) deficiency) are associated with an apparently normal phenotype.

Very little is known about Lp(a) metabolism. However, it has been established that the rate of Lp(a) synthesis in the liver determines its plasma concentration. Lp(a) is assembled extracellularly by a two-step mechanism involving a conformational change and its catabolism is not affected by LDL receptor activity. Studies in an apoE-deficient subject and controls (see **3.35** and **3.36**) have revealed that a buoyant form of Lp(a) associated with very-low-density lipoproteins (VLDL) and intermediate-density lipoproteins (IDL) may be a precursor of mature Lp(a) which does not need apoE to be cleared from plasma. Recent stable isotope studies indicate that in the fed state some apo(a) may dissociate from apoB and reassociate with another newly secreted apoB particle.

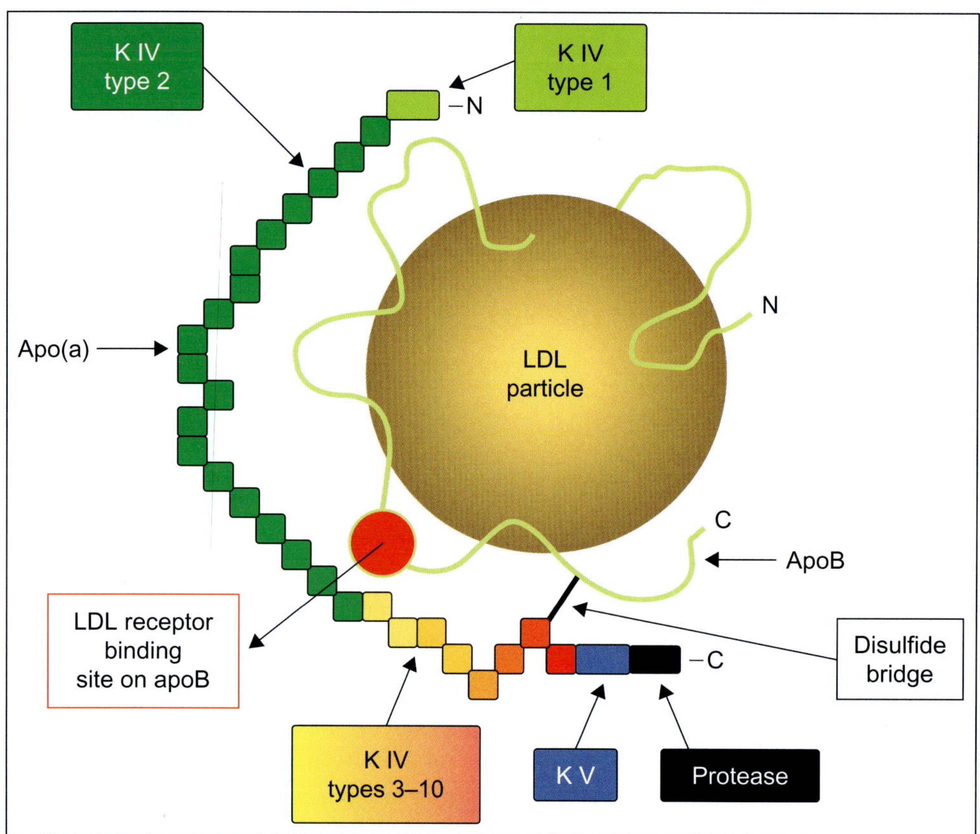

4.1 Model structure of lipoprotein(a) (Lp(a)). The first component of Lp(a) is similar to a low-density lipoprotein (LDL) particle consisting of a lipid core of cholesteryl esters and triglycerides surrounded by a surface layer of phospholipid and free cholesterol. Its single molecule of surface apolipoprotein B (apoB represented by a green-yellow line), is linked to its second component, apolipoprotein(a) through a single disulphide bond (black line). The putative LDL receptor binding domain of apoB is shown as a red circle. The apo(a) moiety consists of a single copy of kringle (K) IV type 1 (light green), kringle IV types 3–10 (yellow to orange), kringle V (blue), and a protease domain analogous to plasminogen (black). In addition, it contains multiple copies (3–>40) of kringle IV type 2 (green) which are responsible for the size polymorphism of Lp(a). Kringles contain 80–85 amino acids for a molecular weight of about 10 kDa and so the molecular weight of apo(a) may range from 300 kDa to 800 kDa, depending on the number of kringle IV type 2 that are repeated. Note that apo(a) location is such that it might interfere in the interaction between apoB and its receptor. This diagram is redrawn and slightly modified from Berglund L, Ramakrishnan R (2004). Lipoprotein(a) An elusive cardiovascular risk factor. *Arterioscler Thromb Vasc Biol*, **24**: 2219–2226.

Peptide fragments of apo(a) have been found in the urine. Lp(a) is an acute phase reactant and increases markedly in plasma in response to the inflammatory cytokine interleukin (IL)-6. Beside the implication in athero-thrombogenesis, the physiological function of apo(a) is not fully understood. Some of the structure–function relationships that have been established are described in **4.7**.

Many clinical studies, carried out mostly in white populations, have found significant correlations between the plasma level of Lp(a), and the risk for a variety of vascular diseases including coronary artery disease (CAD), peripheral vascular disease, vein graft stenosis after coronary artery bypass surgery, stroke, dementia and deep vein thrombosis.

Plasma Lp(a) is elevated in patients with abdominal aortic aneurysm, systemic sclerosis, hypothyroidism, Behçet's syndrome (a multisystem inflammatory disease with skin and mucosal lesions involving eyes, mouth and genitals, complicated by arthritis, thrombophlebitis and vascular events), gangrenous diabetic foot lesions, hemodialysis or end-stage renal disease. In the latter, Lp(a) is independently associated with cardiovascular events. A recent meta-analysis of 27 prospective studies cumulating in 5436 deaths from CAD or non-fatal myocardial infarction over a mean follow-up of 10 years yielded a significant 70% increase of cardiovascular risk for individuals in the top third of baseline plasma Lp(a) compared with those in the bottom third (**4.8**).

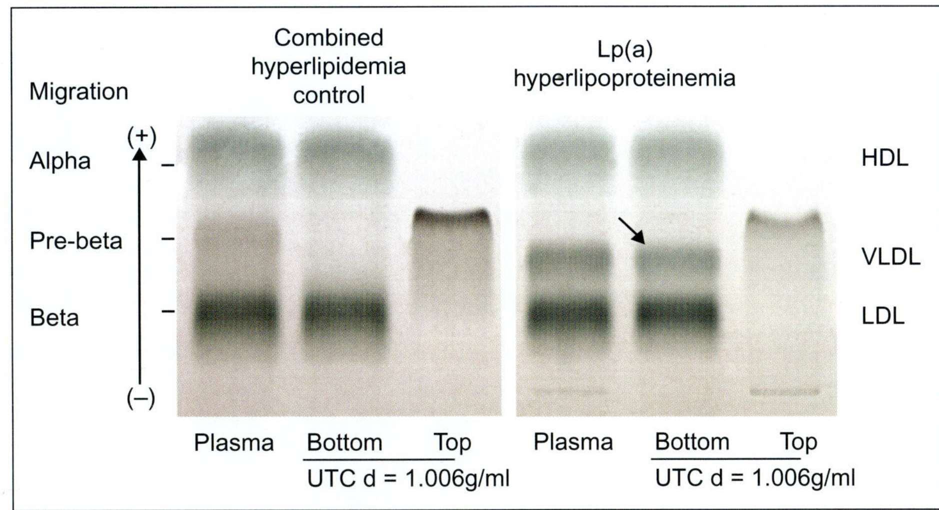

4.2 Demonstration of Lp(a) as a 'sinking preβ-lipoprotein'. Using a combination of ultracentrifugation of plasma at density d = 1.006 g/ml and agarose gel electrophoresis as described in **2.17**, one can demonstrate that Lp(a) shows preβ migration, but sinks to the bottom of the ultracentrifugation (UTC) tube (right panel, arrow), hence its previous name of 'sinking preβ lipoprotein'. The lipoprotein profile was as follows: cholesterol 6.93 mmol/l, low-density lipoprotein-cholesterol (LDL-C) 5.17 mmol/l, triglycerides 0.89 mmol/l, and HDL-C 1.11 mmol/l (268 mg/dl, 200 mg/dl, 79 mg/dl and 43 mg/dl, respectively); the Lp(a) was 100 mg/dl. The left panel shows a control with combined hyperlipidemia (high LDL and very-low-density lipoproteins [VLDL]). The preβ lipoprotein seen in total plasma floats in the top fraction and is not seen in the bottom fraction. This technique was popular before commercial kits became available for the measurement of Lp(a). It is important to know because when analysing whole plasma by lipoprotein electrophoresis the band of Lp(a) may be mistaken for an excess of VLDL.

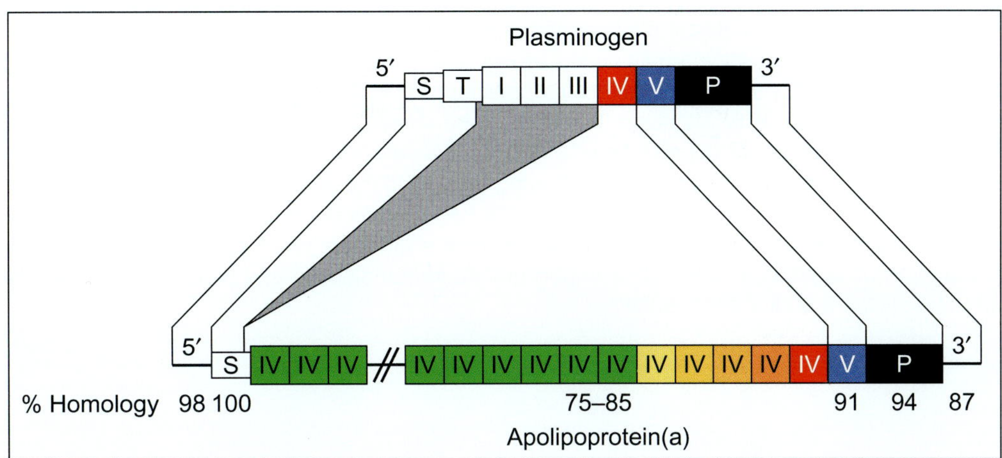

4.3 Homology between plasminogen and apo(a) genes. Discovery of the homology between the apo(a) gene and the plasminogen gene was a breakthrough that provided new insight into the role of Lp(a) in athero-thrombogenesis. Both plasminogen (*PLG*) and apo(a) (*LPA*) genes are member of the same gene superfamily and both are localized on chromosome 6. Both genes have nucleotide sequences coding for different kringle domains, a signal sequence (S) allowing secretion and a protease domain (black rectangle). Whereas plasminogen is a plasma serine protease zymogen, apo(a) has an inactive protease domain. Both genes share a sequence coding for a kringle (K) V (blue) and a kringle IV (in red in both genes to illustrate the marked similarities between K IV of PLG and K IV type 10 of apo(a) which is closest to K V). *LPA* does not share the 'tail region' (T) and kringles I, II and III of *PLG*. The other major difference is in the diversity of the kringle domain sequences for *PLG* and the numerous (and variable) repetitions of the sequences coding for a kringle IV domain in *LPA*. Also, kringles of apo(a) are glycosylated but kringles of plasminogen are not. Connecting lines indicate regions of homology with shading in grey to represent domains that are lacking in apo(a). The percentage of identity of plasminogen and apo(a) cDNA sequences for the following domains is shown at the bottom: 98% for the 5′-untranslated region, 100% for the signal sequence, 75–85% for kringle IV, 91% for kringle V, 94% for the protease sequence, and 87% for the 3′-untranslated region. This high degree of homology has raised the possibility that the apo(a) gene originated via duplication and remodelling of the plasminogen gene. It is thought that they evolved from a common precursor about 40 million years ago when Old and New World monkeys diverged. Redrawn from McLean JW *et al.* (1987). cDNA sequence of human apolipoprotein(a) is homologous to plasminogen. *Nature*, **330**: 132–137.

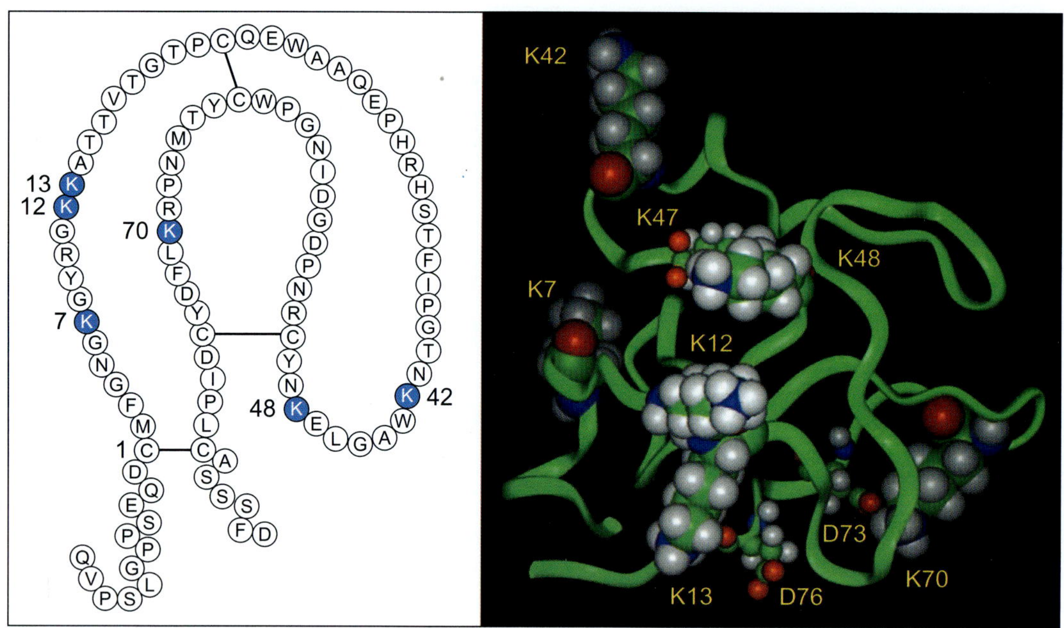

4.4 Amino acid sequence and spatial model of kringle V. Kringle V immediately proximal to the protease domain is important in apo(a) because it is the site for covalent binding of oxidized phospholipids and is pro-inflammatory, both consistent with an atherogenic potential. The amino acid sequence and the loop structure of the kringle domain stabilized by intrachain disulphide bonds are given in the left panel. This three-loop structure resembles the Danish pastry bearing this name. The numbering begins with Cys (C) in position 1. The six Lys (K) in positions 7, 12, 13, 42, 48, and 70 are shown as blue circles. The amino acid residues preceding Cys-1 and following Cys-80 are portions of the linker regions joining K IV$_{10}$ to Cys-1 and Cys-80 to the protease domain. These kringle structures are also present in plasminogen, prothrombin, tissue plasminogen activator, urokinase, coagulation factors VII, IX, X, XII and protein C. These peptides are members of a protein superfamily acting as regulatory proteases in the fibrinolytic and coagulation systems. Kringles help binding of these peptides to other macromolecules or receptors. In the right panel, the spatial model of K V derived from the crystal structure of human apo(a) K IV$_{10}$ is given. The six Lys are shown by space-filled atoms. Lys-48 and Lys-70 form salt bridges with the carboxyl side chains of Glu-47 (E) and Asp-73 (D), respectively (shown in smaller space-filled atoms). Lys-13 makes hydrogen bonds with the main chain carbonyl of Asp-76. Lys-7 being located in the inner surface groove is excluded from interactions. Lys-12 and Lys-42 protrude from the kringle surface and appear to be free of constraints and may be the likely candidates for covalent linkage to oxidized phospholipids. White = hydrogen; green = carbon; blue = nitrogen; red = oxygen. Reproduced from: Edelstein C *et al.* (2003). Lysine-phosphatidylcholine adducts in kringle V impart unique immunological and potential pro-inflammatory properties to human apolipoprotein(a). *J Biol Chem*, **278**: 52841–52847.

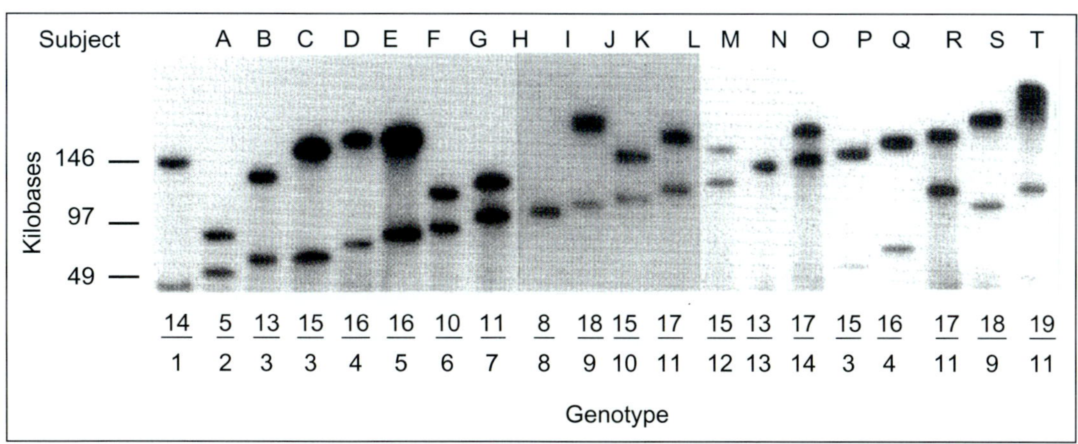

4.5. Multiple alleles and high heterozygosity of the apo(a) gene. Genomic DNA from 102 unrelated Caucasians was obtained from blood mononuclear cells, digested with the restriction enzyme *Kpn*I and separated according to size by pulse-field gel electrophoresis, transferred to a nylon membrane, and the restriction fragments revealed by hybridizing with a ^{32}P-labelled apo(a) kringle IV specific probe. This study, carried out by Lackner and colleagues at Hobbs' laboratory at the University of Texas Southwestern Medical School, revealed the high degree of heterozygosity of the apo(a) gene. In these 102 individuals, 19 different alleles were identified and 94% of these individuals had two different alleles. Lackner also demonstrated that the size of the apo(a) gene correlated directly with the size of the apo(a) protein and inversely with concentration of Lp(a) in plasma. Interestingly, an allele can be associated with similar levels of Lp(a) among members of a given family, but the same allele in another family may be associated with markedly different levels that also remain consistent among family members. This suggests that levels may be determined by interaction with another factor (i.e. a 'second hit'). Although more insight might be obtained regarding the inheritance of Lp(a) in families using this technique and perhaps refine cardiovascular risk predictability as some studies have indicated, it has not received much interest from the standpoint of clinical practice. This is owing to the fact that the technique is labour-intensive, time-consuming, expensive, needs to be done in dedicated laboratories and has not been simplified for the study of large numbers of subjects.

Measurement of the Lp(a) mass is the only approach used at present. Lp(a) may be quantified by a variety of techniques using either antibodies to the kringle IV type 2 domain (unfortunately influenced by size polymorphism), a latex-enhanced immunonephelometric assay using monoclonal anti-Lp(a) (simple, automated), or isolation of intact Lp(a) particles by lectin affinity and measurement of its cholesterol content. This topic was critically reviewed by Lippi and Guidi ([2003]. *Critical Rev Cin Lab Sci*, **40**:1), and these authors raised important practical points: the need to assess confounding factors to avoid undue delays before measurements after sampling; recognition of temperature sensitivity (Lp(a) is sensitive to prolonged storage at room temperature or at 4 °C [oxidation, degradation]; best storage is at −70 °C; repeated freezing and thawing is deleterious); awareness that the method of calibration is difficult because of the 1000-fold variation in plasma levels; and use of a definitive standard is necessary. This figure is reproduced from Lackner C *et al.* (1991). Molecular basis of apolipoprotein(a) isoform size heterogeneity as revealed by pulsed-field gel electrophoresis. *J Clin Invest*, **87**: 2153–2161.

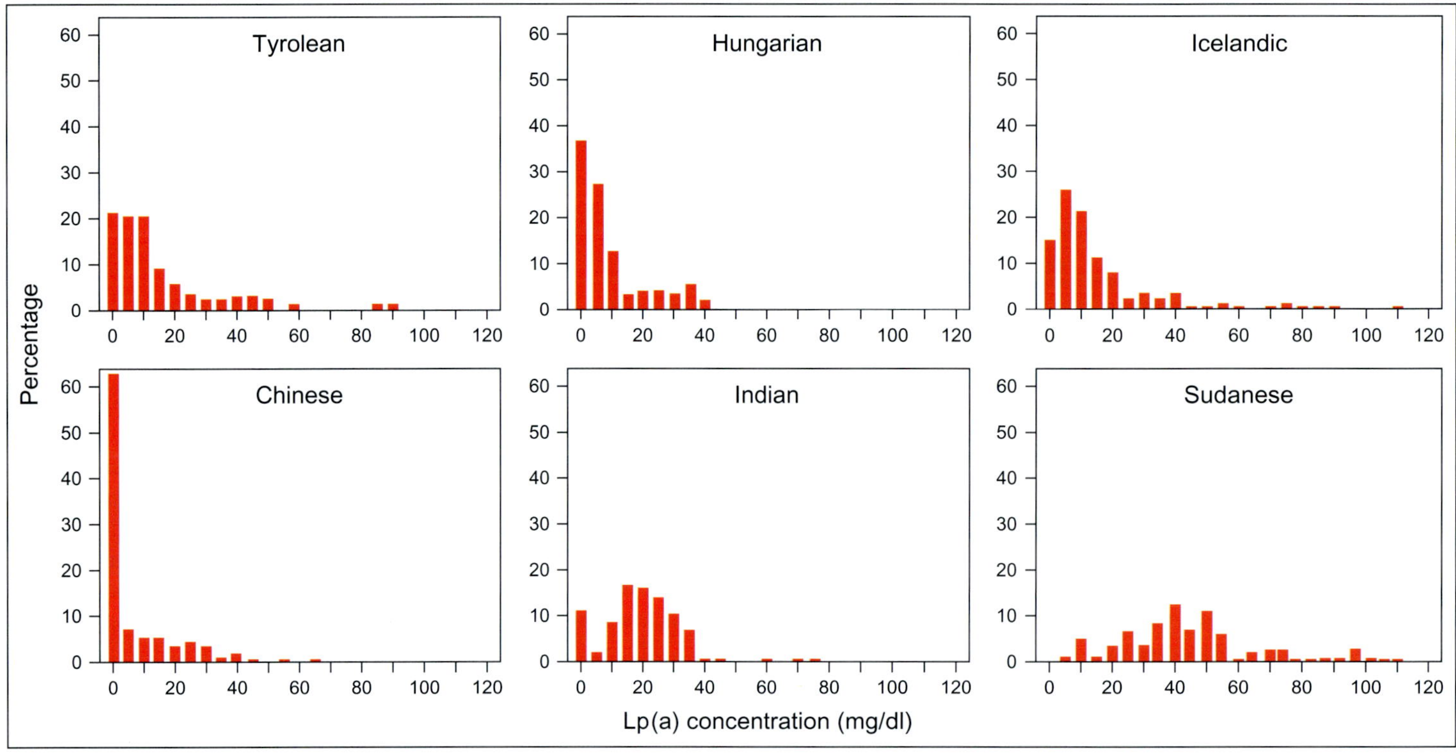

4.6 Frequency distribution of lipoprotein(a) (Lp(a)) plasma levels vary widely across populations. The frequency distribution of Lp(a) plasma concentrations was measured in seven different ethnic groups by Sandholzer C *et al.* in 1991 (six are shown here). The distribution is skewed to the right in most populations warranting log transformation for statistical analysis. However, this distribution varies widely across populations of different ethnic origin; this is particularly striking here when comparing the Chinese and black Sudanese cohorts. In the latter the distribution is nearly Gaussian. The authors also carried out apo(a) phenotyping in these populations. They observed that: there is considerable heterogeneity of Lp(a) polymorphism among populations; differences in apo(a) allele frequencies alone did not explain differences in Lp(a) levels among populations; and in some populations, such as the Sudanese blacks, Lp(a) concentrations are determined by factors that are different from the apo(a) size polymorphism. Redrawn from Sandholzer C *et al.* (1991). Effects of the apolipoprotein(a) size polymorphism on the lipoprotein(a) concentration in 7 ethnic groups. *Hum Genet*, **86**: 607–614.

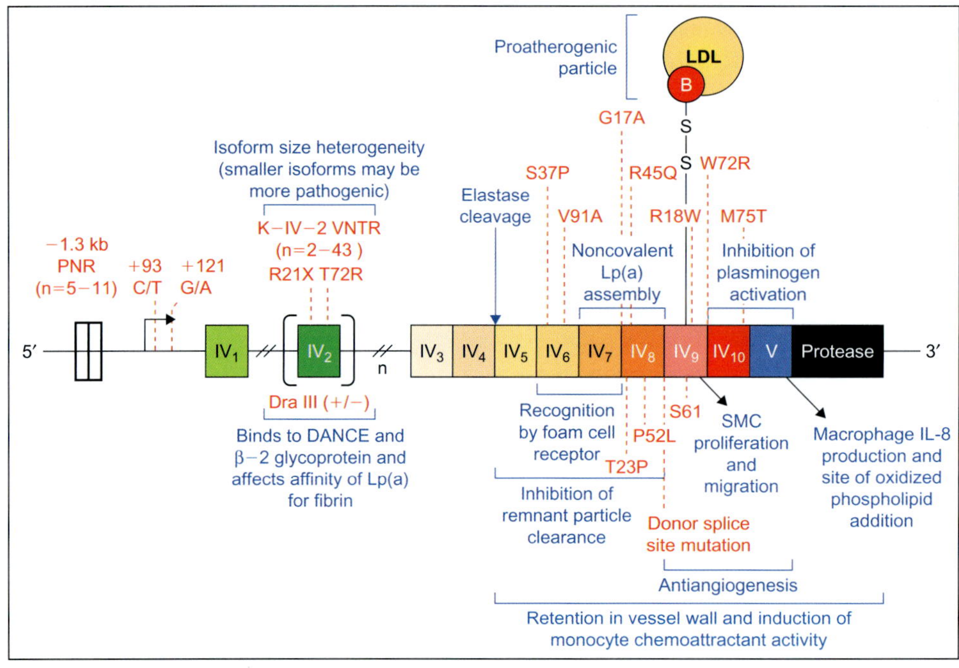

4.7 – *Figure caption opposite.*

4.7 (*Figure bottom of previous page*) **Apo(a) gene mutations and structure–function relationships.** The apo(a) gene size varies between 32 kb and 189 kb and differs by increments of 5.6 kb corresponding to one kringle unit. Each kringle is coded by two exons, and because of the variable number of kringle repeats the total number of exons also varies. This composite and hybrid diagram, which refers to the gene as well as to the protein, is used to display the polymorphic sites and mutations of the apo(a) gene (or protein) in red and the structure–function relationships in blue. The disulphide bond that links kringle (K) IV type 5 of apo(a) to apoB of LDL is indicated as part of the review of the structure–function relationships. On the apo(a) gene in the middle of the diagram the location of the regions coding for the ten different types of kringles from 1 (IV_1) to 10 (IV_{10}) are depicted. The polymorphisms, mutations and sources of variation are given (red text) from the 3′ to the 5′ end of the gene. PNR denotes the penta-nucleotide repeat polymorphism in the promoter, the number ranging from 5 to 11. K IV_2 VNTR denotes the variable number of tandem K IV type 2 repeat polymorphisms responsible for size variation of apo(a) (n = 2–43). *Dra*III refers to a polymorphic site detected using the restriction enzyme *Dra*III present in a subset of K IV type 2 kringle sequences. It occurs with higher frequency in Chinese and is invariably associated with low plasma levels of Lp(a) in Caucasians. The substitution of C by T at position +93 leads to negative regulation in expression of the gene, while a change of G to A at position +121 leads to positive regulation. The T72R mutation of K IV_2 abolishes the lysine binding capabilities of apo(a) and should therefore produce a more benign Lp(a) with less athero-thrombogenic potential. The R21X (Arg_{21}→Ter) in exon 1 of K IV type 2 domain and the donor splice site mutation of the 6 kb intron separating the two exons of K IV type 8 repeat cause Lp(a) deficiency. These subjects appear healthy. There are sequence variants in K IV_6 to K IV_{10} exons whose effects are neutral or undetermined except for a rare mutation W72R in K IV_{10} (Trp_{72}→Arg) affecting the lysine binding of apo(a) which has been observed in some individuals from the black population in the USA. This part of the figure is redrawn and updated from Utermann G (1999). Genetic architecture and evolution of the lipoprotein(a) trait. *Curr Opin Lipidol*, **10**: 133–141.

Specific functions that have been ascribed to discrete functional units of Lp(a) are given in blue on this diagram. These functional domains have been identified on apo(a) using a combination of the expression of recombinant variants of apo(a) and elastase cleavage of apo(a) and Lp(a). Elastase cleaves the protein between K IV_4 and K IV_5 as shown. The atherogenic role is attributed in part to the: (1) isoform size heterogeneity that relates smaller size to higher Lp(a) levels and greater atherogenic potential, (2) presence of a site (K IV_6 and K IV_7) that recognizes a specific receptor on monocyte/macrophages favouring uptake of the pro-atherogenic Lp(a) with its LDL moiety to form foam cells, (3) interference of apo(a) with normal interaction of apoB with the LDL receptor, (4) ability of a region (K IV types 5, 6, 7 and 8) to delay clearance of circulating remnant lipoproteins (overexpression of this fragment in mice fed a high-fat diet enhances atherosclerosis), (5) K IV type 9 that stimulates smooth muscle cell (SMC) migration and proliferation, (6) induction of cytoskeletal rearrangements in the endothelial cells increasing their permeability and resulting in a dysfunctional endothelium, (7) presence of K V that stimulates interleukin (IL)-8 production by macrophages, and allows addition of oxidized phospholipids (the pro-atherogenic oxidized phospholipids are preferentially associated with Lp(a) compared with free LDL) (see **4.4**, K12 and K42). All of the above and the propensity of apo(a) to adhere to arterial wall components such as fibrin, fibrinogen, fibronectin and glycosaminoglycans favour retention of Lp(a) in the arterial wall. The same applies to binding of apo(a) and Lp(a) via the K IV_2 repeats to β2-glycoprotein-1 (also called apoH) and to the extracellular matrix protein DANCE (developmental arteries and neural crest epidermal growth factor [EGF]-like). Regarding the antifibrinolytic and thrombogenic role, the following mechanisms apply: (1) apo(a) interference with the efficient activation of plasminogen to plasmin attributed to the combined effect of K IV_{10} and K V binding to the complex plasminogen, tissue-type plasminogen activator (t-PA) and fibrin, (2) competition of apo(a) for binding of plasminogen to fibrin and fibrinogen via K V and the protease domain, (3) enhancement of plasminogen activator inhibitor (PAI)-1 activity. In addition, the fragment containing K IV_9, K IV_{10} and K V inhibits basic fibroblast growth factor-stimulated venous endothelial cell proliferation and migration and represses neovascularization in chick embryos and tumour growth in nude mice. These observations suggest anti-angiogenic and anti-carcinogenic effects. It has also been speculated that Lp(a) transports cholesterol to sites of injury and wound healing, but as an untoward side effect it may also trigger deposition of cholesterol in growing atherosclerotic plaques. This part of the diagram has been modified slightly from Koschinsky ML, Marcovina S (2004). Structure–function relationships in apolipoprotein(a): insights into lipoprotein(a) assembly and pathogenicity. *Curr Opin Lipidol*, **15**: 167–174, and Koschinsky ML (2005). Lipoprotein(a) and atherosclerosis: new perspectives on the mechanism of action of an enigmatic lipoprotein. *Curr Atheroscler Rep*, **7**: 389–395.

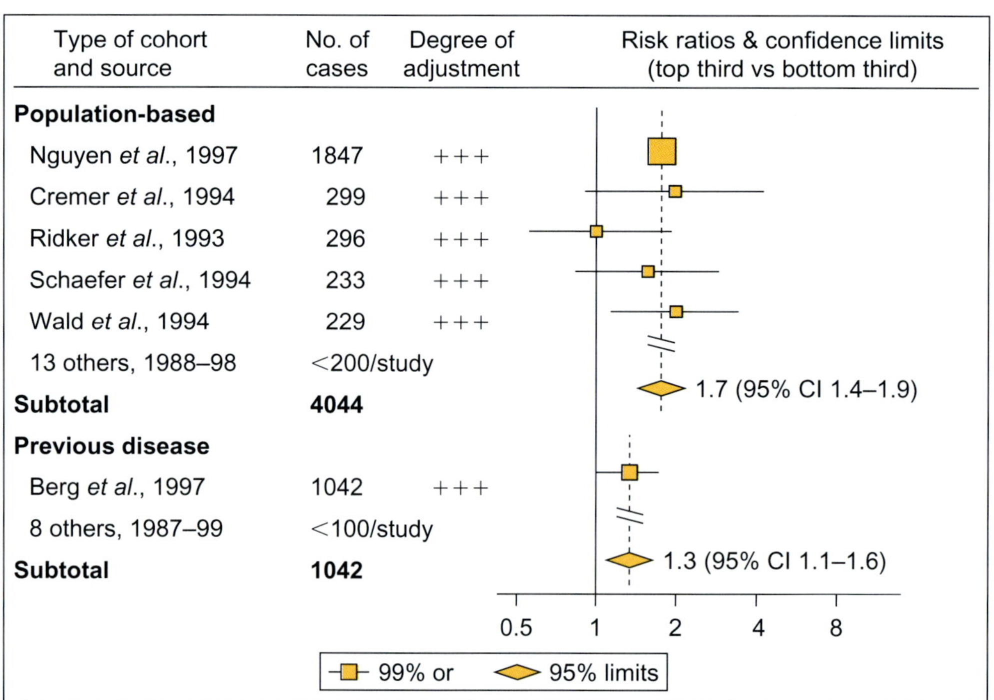

4.8 Meta-analysis of prospective studies on coronary artery disease (CAD) risk impact of lipoprotein(a) (Lp(a)). For many years it was controversial whether Lp(a) is an independent CAD risk factor because both negative and positive studies had been published. This large meta-analysis, along with other recent studies, has resolved the issue. It took into account geographical location of study, size, type of cohort (population-based or selected because of previous disease), mean age, follow-up duration, blood storage temperature and duration. It included 5436 deaths from coronary heart disease or non-fatal myocardial infarctions during a weighted mean follow-up of 10 years in 27 eligible studies. The risk ratios compare top and bottom thirds of baseline measurements. Orange-yellow squares indicate the risk ratio in each study, with the size of the squares proportional to number of cases and horizontal lines representing 99% confidence intervals (CIs). The combined risk ratios and their 95% CI are indicated by orange-yellow diamonds. Degree of adjustment for possible confounders is denoted as follows: +, adjustment for age and sex only; ++, adjustment for the preceding plus smoking; and +++, adjustment for the preceding plus some other classical vascular risk factors. For sake of simplicity, population-based studies including fewer than 200 cases or previous disease studies including fewer than 100 cases are not shown on this partial reproduction of the figure published by Danesh J et al. In the prospective studies not shown (n = 11–191) all but one had a +++ level of adjustment. Comparison of individuals in the top third of baseline plasma Lp(a) measurements with those in the bottom third in each study yielded a combined risk ratio of 1.6 (95% CI 1.4–1.8, $2P$ < 0.00001). Reproduced with permission from Danesh et al. (2000). Lipoprotein(a) and coronary heart disease – meta-analysis of prospective studies. *Circulation*, **102**: 1082–1085.

In the large Prospective Epidemiological Study of Myocardial Infarction (PRIME), subjects with levels of Lp(a) in the highest quartile had more than 1.5 times the risk than subjects in the lowest quartile. Moreover, the risk was a function of LDL-C levels as observed previously. A Lp(a) concentration above 33 mg/dl combined with a LDL-C >163 mg/dl (>4.22 mmol/l) was associated with a 4.5-fold increase in CAD risk compared with a relative risk of 0.82 when combined with an LDL-C <121 mg/dl (<3.13 mmol/l) (**4.9**). Some studies of familial hypercholesterolemia (FH) with or without CAD have shown a higher frequency of high Lp(a) levels in the presence of CAD (**4.10**). The association between Lp(a) and cardiovascular disease and stroke in particular may be stronger in men than in women.

The mechanism whereby Lp(a) may promote cardiovascular disease (CVD) has been ascribed to both its LDL-related structure and its plasminogen-like antifibrinolytic function. Lp(a) (and free apo(a)) is found in the atherosclerotic arterial wall, and kringle IV-type 10 has a dominant role in the binding of apo(a) to fibrin or fibrinogen and components of the extracellular matrix (**4.7**). Lp(a) is also readily oxidizable *in vitro* similar to LDL (**4.11**) and is taken up by monocyte-macrophages, resulting in a potentially atherogenic particle (**4.12**). The expression of tissue plasminogen activator (t-PA) and inhibitor-1 (PAI-1) in the vascular wall is influenced by the presence and concentration of Lp(a), which is retained more avidly than LDL. Small apo(a) size polymorphism has also been found to be associated with CVD in men. The

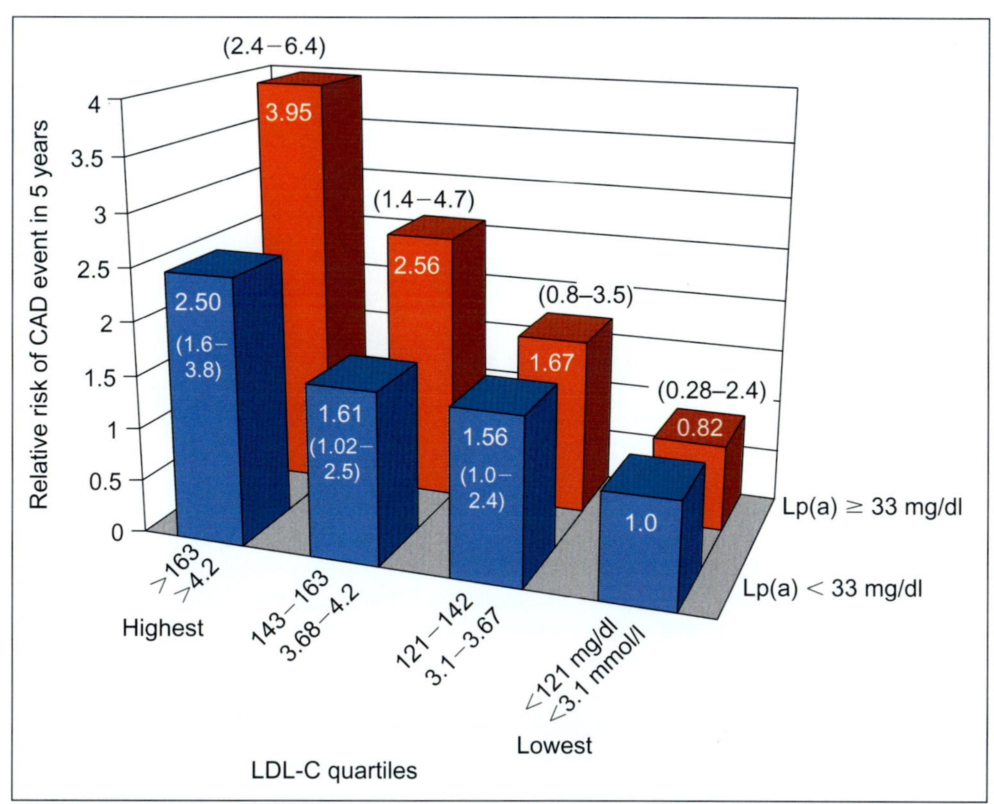

4.9 Lipoprotein(a) (Lp(a)) enhances coronary artery disease (CAD) risk associated with high low-density lipoprotein-cholesterol (LDL-C). Several studies have indicated an interaction between Lp(a) and LDL-C, a notion of prime importance in clinical practice. The PRIME study (Prospective Epidemiological Study of Myocardial Infarction) provided a clear demonstration of this interaction as illustrated here. PRIME included 9133 French and Northern Irish men aged 50–59 at entry, without a history of CAD and not on lipid-lowering drugs. During 5 years of follow-up, 288 subjects experienced at least one CAD event (myocardial infarction, coronary death, angina pectoris). Logistic regression analysis was used to evaluate Lp(a) levels as a predictor of CAD. Lp(a) was a highly significant predictor of CAD events in the entire cohort ($P < 0.0006$) with a relative risk between top and lower quartile of Lp(a) of 1.56 (95% CI 1.10–2.21). As shown on this graph derived from data reported by Luc G *et al.* the relative risk (RR) of a CAD event associated with a Lp(a) level of <33 mg/l increased gradually from the referent value of 1.0 to 2.50 (95% CI 1.6–3.8) from the lowest (<121 mg/dl; <3.1 mmol/l) to the highest (>163 mg/dl; >4.2 mmol/l) quartile of low-density lipoprotein-cholesterol (LDL-C). In contrast, the RR of a CAD event associated with a Lp(a) level ≥33 mg/dl increased more steeply from 0.82 (95% CI 0.28 to 2.4) to 3.95 (95% CI 2.4–6.4) from the lowest to the highest quartile of LDL-C. Therefore, high levels of Lp(a) increase the risk of CAD associated with high LDL-C (upper half of the distribution), conversely high levels of Lp(a) in the absence of elevated LDL-C (lower half of the distribution) do not add to the risk already associated with the LDL-C level. Bar graph drawn from data in Luc G *et al.* (2002). Lipoprotein(a) as a predictor of coronary heart disease: the PRIME Study. *Atherosclerosis*, **163**: 377–384.

kringle V of Lp(a) (**4.4** and **4.7**) covalently binds oxidized phospholipids (especially phosphatidylcholine), which may accumulate into the vessel wall and promote atherosclerosis. Kringle V also stimulates IL-8 production by human macrophages in culture, a pro-inflammatory effect. An association of Lp(a) with coronary calcifications in human atherosclerosis specimens has been reported, consistent with observations in the WHHL transgenic rabbit expressing human apo(a) (**4.13**). Although three studies failed to find an association between coronary calcification and Lp(a), one of them, the Dallas Heart Study, showed that there was a higher prevalence of coronary artery calcium (CAC) measured by electron beam computed tomography (EBCT) among Caucasians with high plasma levels of Lp(a) plus elevated plasma levels of LDL-C (men) or reduced levels of HDL-C (men and women). Finally, in men with CAD and high LDL-C in the Familial Atherosclerosis Treatment Study (FATS), Lp(a) concentration was a major correlate of baseline disease severity, atherosclerosis progression, and event rate over 2.5 years. Moreover, with substantial LDL-C reductions, persistent elevations of Lp(a) were no longer atherogenic or clinically threatening.

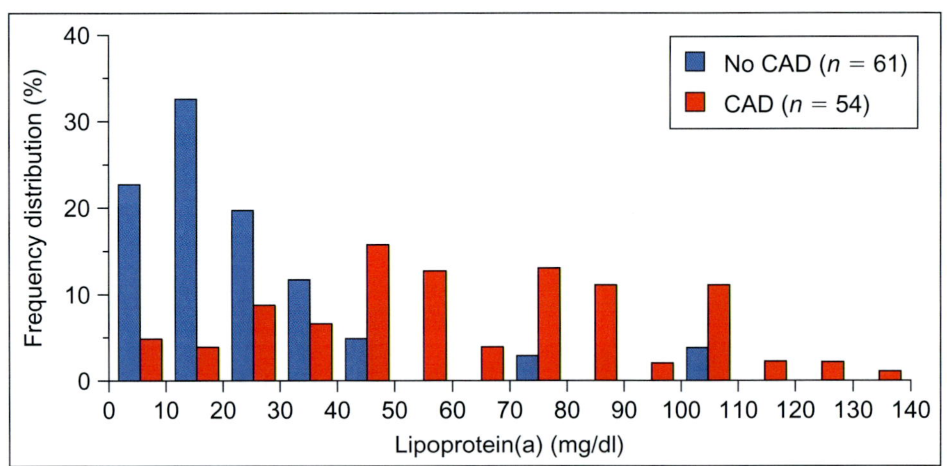

4.10 Higher frequency of elevated lipoprotein(a) (Lp(a)) levels in familial hypercholesterolemia (FH) patients with coronary artery disease (CAD) than in patients without CAD. The frequency distribution of serum Lp(a) concentration in heterozygous FH subjects from a UK lipid clinic without CAD (blue columns) resembles that observed in normal Caucasians (see **4.6**) with only a few individuals having very high levels. In contrast, the frequency distribution in FH subjects with CAD (red columns) is clearly displaced towards higher Lp(a) concentrations. This is reflected in the median Lp(a) levels being 18 mg/dl in the absence of CAD and 57 mg/dl in its presence. This finding has been confirmed in some studies but not in others. This may reflect the differences in ethnicity, age, type of *LDLR* mutation or variation in other associated modulating factors. In practice, the family history and severity of the disease in a proband should guide the need to measure Lp(a) in other family members. Redrawn from Seed M *et al.* (1990). *N Engl J Med*, **322**: 1494–1499.

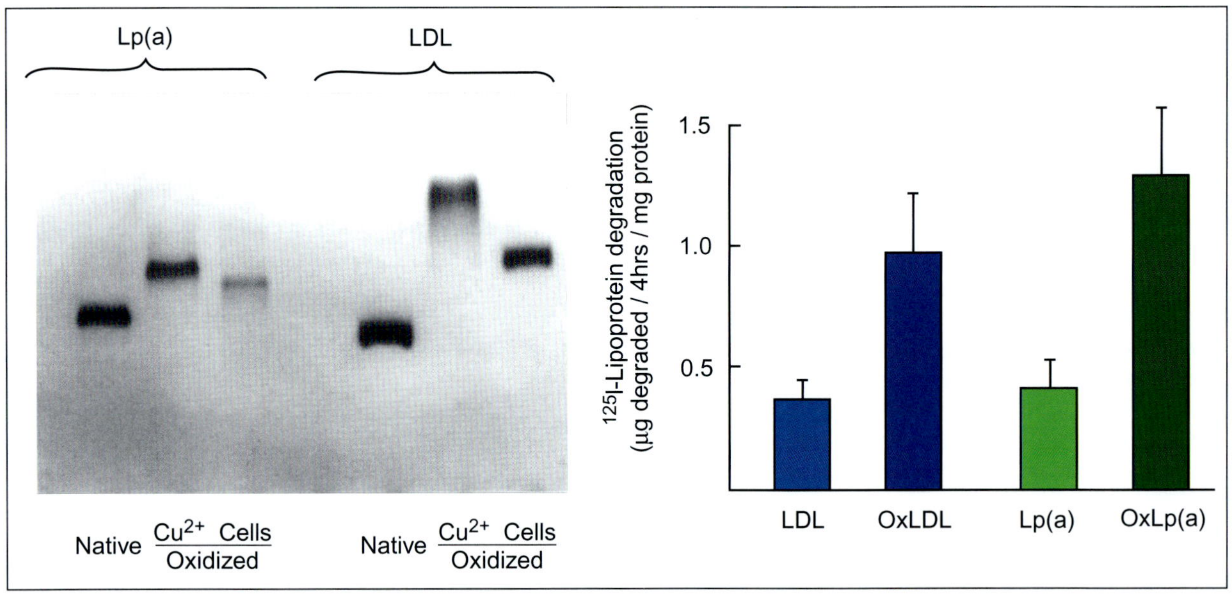

4.11 *In vitro* oxidation and macrophage uptake of native or oxidized lipoprotein(a) (Lp(a)) and low-density lipoproteins (LDL). The left panel illustrates that native LDL and Lp(a) isolated from the same patient with familial combined hyperlipidemia (FCH) and Lp(a) hyperlipoproteinemia can be oxidized *in vitro* when exposed to 10 µM CuCl$_2$ (Cu^{++}) or to human mononuclear cells (Cells), as shown by a faster electrophoretic mobility on agarose gel electrophoresis. This effect, which is completely abolished by the antioxidant probucol, modifies the structure of Lp(a) and enhances its atherogenic properties. Indeed, oxidized Lp(a) (OxLp(a)) as well as oxidized LDL (OxLDL) are taken up readily and degraded by human monocyte macrophages (right panel) to induce accumulation of cholesteryl esters and form foam cells. They have also been isolated from human atheromatous lesions (see **4.12**). When the apo(a) was clipped off from LDL with dithiothreitol the remaining particle was degraded at a lower rate than the whole OxLp(a) indicating a preferential uptake and degradation. Work in the laboratory of Scanu at the University of Chicago has demonstrated that the size of the LDL moiety of Lp(a) may vary as the size of native LDL varies. It is likely that in FCH Lp(a) particles are smaller and denser as LDL are compared to those of a patient with familial hypercholesterolemia. These figures from work carried out in the authors' laboratory are redrawn from Naruszewicz M *et al.* (1992). Oxidative modification of lipoprotein(a) and the effect of beta-carotene. *Metabolism*, **41**: 1215–1224.

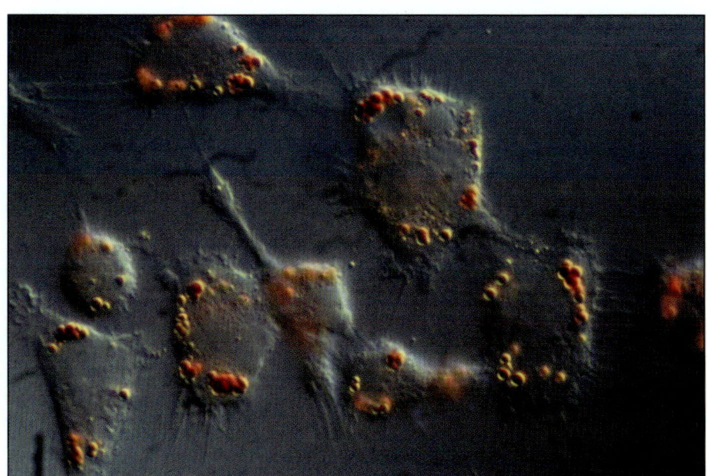

4.12 Macrophage uptake of lipoproteins isolated from human atheroma. In the early 1990s, Hoff at the Cleveland Clinic Research Institute isolated lesion low-density lipoproteins (LDL) and lipoprotein(a) (Lp(a)) from human atherosclerotic plaques obtained at autopsy. They were characterized and their properties evaluated. Lp(a) was present in a form resembling intact but oxidized Lp(a), larger particles representing Lp(a) complexed to itself or to other plaque components and a slightly smaller particle probably representing partially degraded Lp(a). He had similarly isolated and studied lesion LDL. The figure is an interference contrast photomicrograph of mouse peritoneal macrophages in culture exposed to lesion-derived LDL (100 μg/ml) and incubated 48 hours at 37 °C and stained for lipids with Oil red O. Oxidized Lp(a) is similarly taken up by macrophages. The authors are grateful to Henry Hoff for having generously provided this unpublished picture. For further information, see Hoff HF, O'Neil J. (1991). *J Arterioscler Thromb*, **11**: 1209–1222; Hoff HF *et al.* (1993). *J Lipid Res*, **34**: 789–798; and Hoff HF *et al.* (1994). *Chem Phys Lipid*, **67–68**: 271–280.

The current Canadian clinical guidelines (but not all guidelines) include measurement of Lp(a) to quantify the CVD risk. A concentration of 30 mg/dl or more is considered high and an indicator of risk. The overall relationship of Lp(a) with cardiovascular disease and the quantitative contribution of elevated Lp(a) to CAD risk in the presence of high LDL-C are sufficiently well established (see **4.8–4.10**) to warrant this attitude. A link between thromboembolic events and Lp(a) has been clearly demonstrated in several conditions; however, there are some caveats. Accurate standardized methods of measurements are not widely available in clinical chemistry laboratories and assays may be affected by apo(a) size heterogeneity (see **4.5**). Several conditions may spuriously increase plasma Lp(a) levels, a confounding factor (see above). Serum Lp(a) is relatively resistant to lowering by diet, exercise, weight loss or statins. There is no evidence from clinical trials as yet to support a benefit from

lowering Lp(a) levels; such a trial needs to be done but is difficult because nicotinic acid, the most effective agent, has multiple beneficial lipoprotein effects.

The diagnosis of 'familial Lp(a) hyperlipoproteinemia' is made difficult because of the variation in the apo(a) gene, its high heterozygosity and the dependence of the CVD risk on the size polymorphism of apo(a). Also, it does not have a specific clinical profile. Therefore, measurement of Lp(a) is particularly important in people with a moderate CVD risk, a strong family history of premature cardiovascular disease, and elevated LDL levels (especially if associated with low HDL-C), in those who have an unexpectedly severe atherosclerotic phenotype and in subjects from a family in which high Lp(a) segregates with manifestations of atherosclerosis. In these cases an elevated Lp(a) concentration should entail a more vigorous treatment of dyslipidemia and concomitant risk factors. Treatment with nicotinic acid (that may induce Lp(a) lowering up to 40%) and its slow-release derivatives, LDL apheresis, neomycin, and estrogen therapy in postmenopausal women can effectively decrease Lp(a) plasma concentration.

Familial phytosterolemia (*ABCG5-ABCG8* defects)

Familial phytosterolemia (familial sitosterolemia, familial β-sitosterolemia, familial ATP-binding cassette family G type 5 and/or type 8 defect, sterolin deficiency), is an autosomal recessive disease characterized by elevated plasma plant sterols and relatively normal plasma cholesterol concentrations, xanthomatosis and premature CAD. It has raised much interest because study of this disease led to new discoveries that allowed a better understanding of cholesterol transport mechanisms in the liver and the intestine. The term phytosterolemia is preferred to sitosterolemia because all plant sterols are affected, not just sitosterol.

Healthy subjects have very low plasma levels of plant sterols (phytosterols), which are mostly derived from vegetable oils, seeds and nuts, mainly because they are poorly absorbed. Plant sterols also interfere with cholesterol absorption because of their ability to displace cholesterol from intestinal micelles. This led, before the era of fibrates and statins, to the use of a plant sterol emulsion as a cholesterol-lowering agent. The content of phytosterol in a normal diet is in the order of 150–450 mg/day. However, it takes 2 gm/day of this supplement to achieve a mere 10% cholesterol

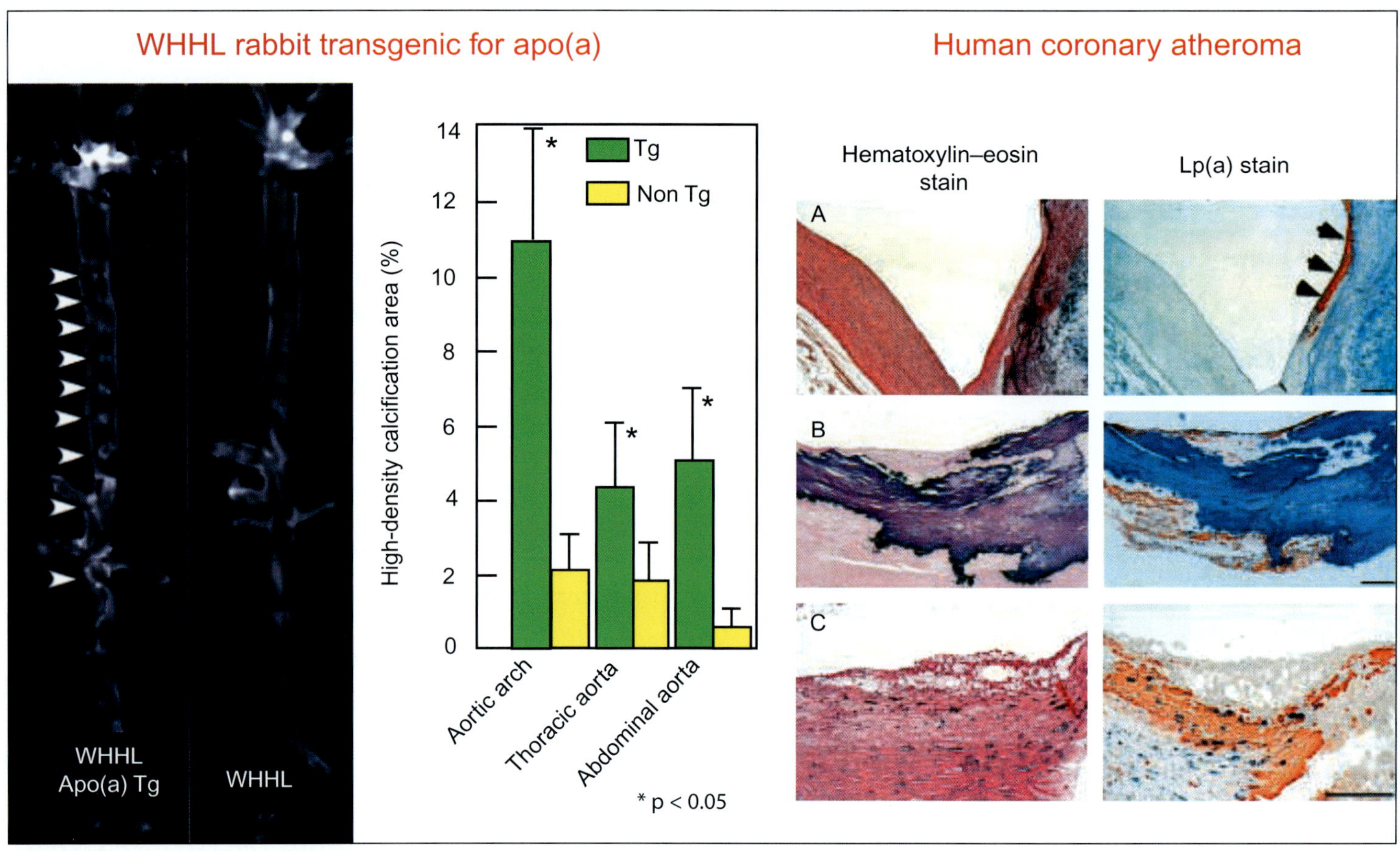

4.13 Lipoprotein(a) (Lp(a)) associates with calcifications in atherosclerotic lesions. The left panels provide a radiographic demonstration of multiple aortic calcification sites in the low-density lipoprotein (LDL) receptor-deficient Watanabe heritable hyperlipidemic rabbit (WHHL) transfected with the human apo(a) transgene (apo(a) Tg) compared with the non-transgenic (non Tg) WHHL. In this model, apo(a) markedly enhanced the spontaneous development of atherosclerotic lesions that resemble complex lesions observed in advanced human disease. The arrowheads point to the calcifications. The high-density areas (calcification) were quantitated on X-ray films by a computerized image analysis system and plotted in the bar graph. Values are expressed as a per cent of each segment of the aorta ($P < 0.05$ vs. the non Tg WHHL rabbits). They were significantly higher in the apo(a) transgenic WHHL in the three aortic segments studied. Immunostaining with antibodies against apo(a) and apoB showed that apo(a) was frequently deposited around the calcified areas and co-localized with apoB.

The authors also found that human Lp(a)-treated rabbit aortic smooth muscle cells (SMC) showed increased alkaline phosphatase activity and enhanced calcium accumulation. In addition, Lp(a) tended to stimulate SMC toward osteoblastic differentiation by inducing Osf2 (osteoblast specific factor-2) mRNA expression. The right panel demonstrates that Lp(a) is intimately associated with areas of calcification in human coronary arteries as observed in the rabbit model. (A) Lp(a) deposition (orange) along the surface of calcified area on the right side (indicated with arrowheads), (B) Lp(a) around ossification, and (C) in this lesion, calcium deposition is sparsely distributed beneath the foam cells and Lp(a) deposition is intermingled with SMC. Scale bars represent 200 μm. Reproduced with permission from Sun H *et al.* (2002). Lipoprotein(a) enhances advanced atherosclerosis and vascular calcification in WHHL transgenic rabbits expressing human apolipoprotein(a). *J Biol Chem*, **277**: 47486–47492.

reduction on average. The need for multiple doses and flatulence were the trade-offs that caused its demise. The structural formula of plant sterols is shown in **4.14**. The major plant sterols are sitosterol (because there are no α forms of plant sterols, this is no longer called β-sitosterol), campesterol and stigmasterol. They follow the same pathway of absorption and enterohepatic recirculation as cholesterol (**4.15**). They are taken up by micelles, enter the enterocytes via a specific transporter, Niemann–Pick C-1 like-1 protein (NPC1L1), and the bulk is rapidly returned to the intestinal lumen via the heterodimeric transporters ABCG5 (*ATP-binding cassette family G type 5*) and ABCG8 (also called sterolin-1 and sterolin-2). The small amount not re-excreted is esterified and transferred into chylomicrons and passes

Sterols

Cholesterol
HO

Avenosterol
HO

Campesterol
HO

β-sitosterol
HO

Stigmasterol
HO

Brassicasterol
HO

Stanols

Campestanol
HO
H

Sitostanol
HO
H

Stigmastanol
HO
H

4.14 Comparison of the structure of plant sterols and stanols with cholesterol. The chemical structure of plant sterols is similar to that of cholesterol. Campesterol and β-sitosterol, the 24-methyl and the 24-ethyl analogues of cholesterol respectively, are the most abundant plant sterols. They occur at low concentrations in human plasma and they represent 95% of dietary phytosterols. Dehydrogenation of the carbon 22–23 bond of sitosterol leads to stigmasterol which is another common phytosterol. The others, brassicasterol, avenasterol, ergosterol, and stigmasterol, and also shellfish sterols, have been identified in plasma in minute amounts. Plant sterols are abundant in the diet and found in considerable amounts in seeds, nuts, fruits and vegetable oils. Daily intake ranges from about 180 mg in the USA to 480 mg in Japan. Saturation of the Δ5 double bond of the three major plant sterols leads to the formation of 5α-derivatives, sitostanol, campestanol and stigmastanol. Although present in the diet in small amounts they are almost totally unabsorbable. As they may effectively compete with cholesterol in the formation of mixed micelles and interfere with cholesterol absorption they have raised interest as cholesterol-lowering agents, and have been introduced in 'functional foods' such as sitostanol margarines.

into the lymph to reach the circulation and the liver to be unesterified and re-excreted into the bile via liver ABCG5-ABCG8 transporter. The normal plasma level of phytosterol averages 0.7 mg/dl and represents less than 1% of the total sterol content of plasma lipoproteins. Excessive absorption of plant sterols may disrupt cholesterol homeostasis. Mice lacking the ABCG5 and ABCG8 half transporters have a 30-fold increase in plasma levels of plant sterols, and low biliary cholesterol concentration. Their plasma and liver cholesterol concentrations are reduced by 50% but rapidly increase with cholesterol feeding. They also display a massive reduction in the adrenal content of cholesterol. The human form of ABCG5-ABCG8 deficiency is familial phytosterolemia.

Familial phytosterolemia (OMIM No. 210250) is a rare autosomal recessive condition with a frequency estimated at 1:1 500 000, which shares the clinical features of familial hypercholesterolemia (FH). Tuberous, planar and tendinous xanthomatosis (**4.16** and **4.17**), developing in childhood, may be moderate or severe enough to determine a clinical phenotype that is indistinguishable from that of homozygous FH. A generalized eruptive xanthomatosis has even been reported in a 6-year-old child. Arthralgia and arthritis (knees and ankle joints), hypersplenism, thrombocytopenia and hemolysis may be present. Plasma cholesterol concentrations may be normal or moderately elevated, but in some children may reach levels found in homozygous

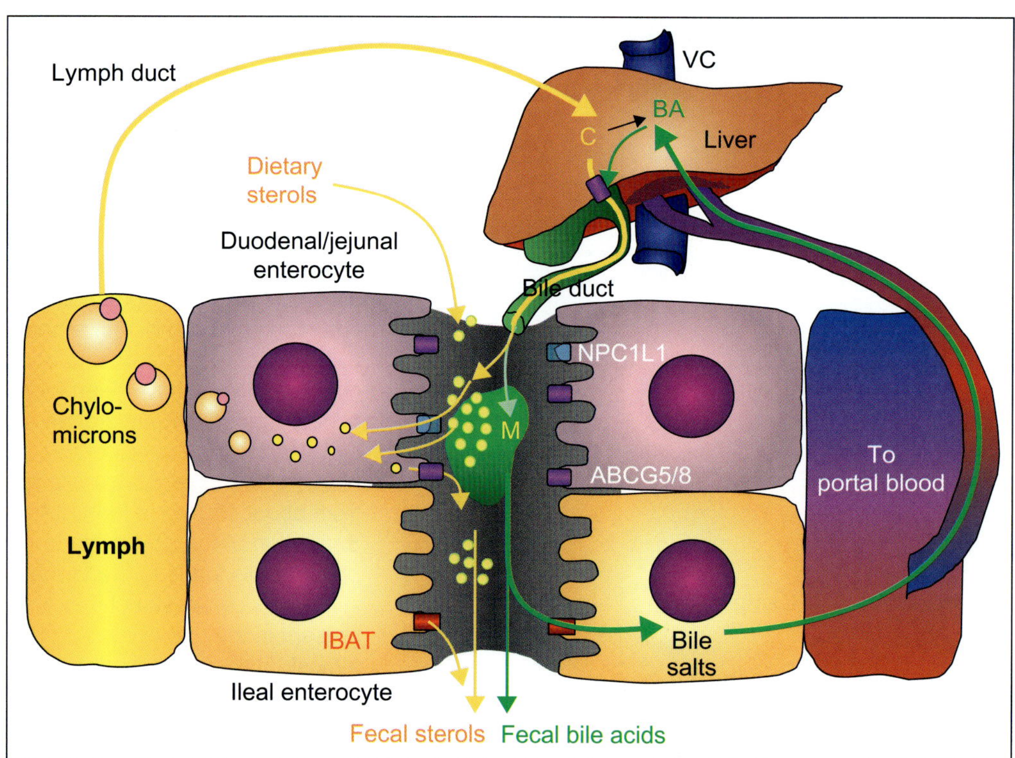

4.15 Sterol absorption and the two enterohepatic recirculations. In this diagram, the yellow path is that of cholesterol and the green path that of bile salts; they each have an enterohepatic recirculation that is key to understanding their respective roles in cholesterol homeostasis of the body. Intestinal cells are in contact with both lymphatics and blood capillaries. The duodenal and jejunal enterocytes (pink) handle lipids and bile acid differently from the ileal enterocytes (orange). Dietary cholesterol (~400 mg/day) and other sterols (~200 mg/day) enter the intestine and mix with free sterols and bile salts coming from the bile (1200 mg/day). The liver synthesizes about 400 mg/day of cholesterol. The unesterified sterols are taken up by enterocytes as part of mixed micelles (M) – formed in the lumen with bile salts, fatty acids, and phospholipids – by diffusion or by membrane transporter molecules such as Niemann–Pick C-1 like protein-1 (NPC1L1). The sterols are esterified in the enterocyte and packaged into chylomicrons for transfer into the lymph, a very active process after a fatty meal. This takes place mostly in the proximal small intestine. The chylomicrons reach the main circulation via the thoracic duct into the left subclavian vein thus eventually reaching the liver through the hepatic artery. Some of the sterols are also re-excreted into the intestine.

Cholesterol absorption varies from 25% to 75%, fluctuates with time and is context dependent. Phytosterol absorption is usually less than 5%. Unabsorbed sterols and neutral sterols are excreted in the feces. About 800 mg of neutral sterols and acidic sterols (from bile salts) are excreted daily in the feces. Bile salts are synthesized from cholesterol in the liver. They enter the intestine in the bile, favouring absorption of cholesterol by their contribution to the formation of mixed micelles. In the intestine, 95% is removed mostly by active transport in the distal third of the small intestine, thanks to the highly effective ileal bile acid transporter (IBAT) also called apical sodium dependent bile acid transporter (ASBT). The remainder ends up in the feces as 'acidic sterols'. Knockout of the IBAT gene (*Slc10a2*) in the mouse abolishes the enterohepatic recycling of bile acids. The reabsorbed bile salts are exported to the liver directly by the portal system to be reutilized in bile formation.

FH (>13 mmol/l; >500 mg/dl) whereas triglycerides are normal. Elevated apoB is another feature of familial phytosterolemia. Premature atherosclerosis is typical and death from CAD has been reported as early as age 13 (**4.18**). The disease is characterized primarily by an increased intestinal absorption (15–16% instead of <5%) and a reduced biliary secretion of plant sterols. This results in plasma levels of sitosterol and campesterol approximately 50-fold higher than normal (14–65 mg/dl vs. 0.3–1.0 mg/dl for β-sitosterol).

Plasma levels of other plant sterols such as stigmasterol, campesterol, sitostanol and campestanol (**4.14**) are also elevated. A high vegetable oil diet may worsen the disease. The plant sterols are carried by LDL and HDL particles and accumulate in tissues but not in the brain (although spinal intradural xanthomatosis has been reported in this condition). The etiology of this disease, which was first reported in 1974 by Bhattacharyya and Connor and by Kwiterovitch and colleagues, was unknown until recently when Hobbs and

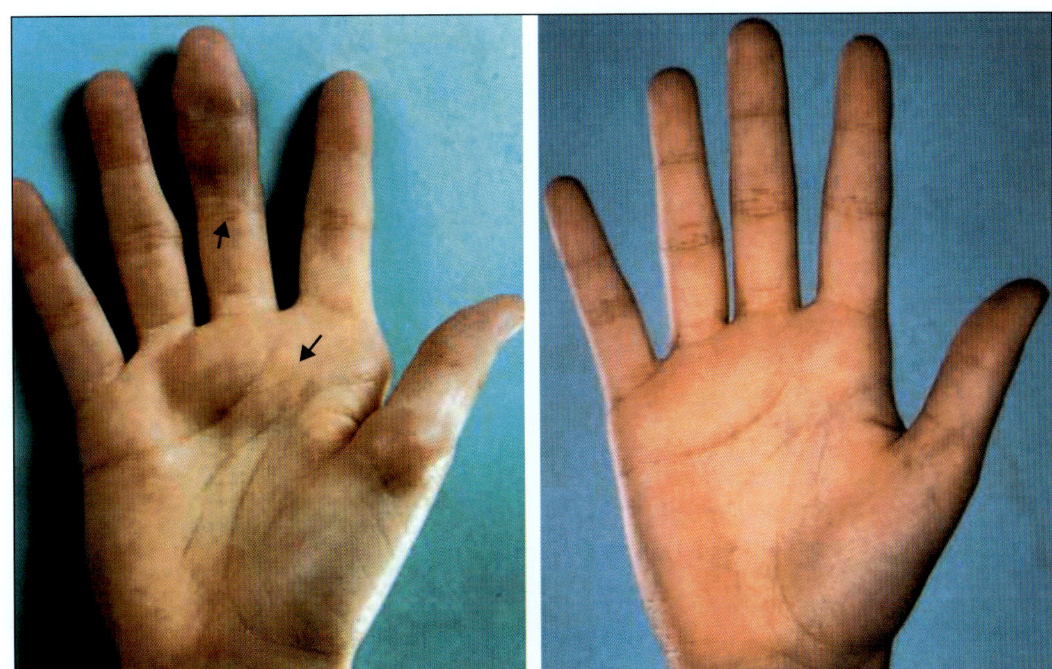

4.16 Tubero-eruptive xanthomas of the palm and finger in familial phytosterolemia before and after treatment. This 17-year-old girl presented with palmar and finger lesions (left), Achilles tendon xanthomas (**4.17**) and only mildly elevated plasma cholesterol levels. She had a family history of vascular disease. Her plasma sitosterol was 950 µmol/l (normal <16 µmol/l) and campesterol 378 µmol/l (normal <24 µmol/l). She was instructed in following a diet low in plant lipids (oil and margarine), nuts, chocolate and seeds and prescribed a bile acid binding resin. Although the patient's plasma levels of plant sterols remained markedly elevated, her tendon xanthomas diminished strikingly, as shown in the photograph taken five years later (right). These palmar xanthomas are reminiscent of some of the planar and tubero-eruptive lesions seen in dysbetalipoproteinemia type III (see **3.23** and **3.25**). The apoE phenotype of this patient was E4/2, there were no β-very-low-density lipoproteins (β-VLDL) and the VLDL-C/triglyceride ratio was low at 0.28 (calculations from mmol/l) confirming absence of remnants and virtually excluding a type III (Anton Stalenhoef, personal communication, 2006). Reproduced with permission from Stalenhoef AF (2003). Image in Medicine. *N Engl J Med*, **349**: 51.

colleagues, at the University of Texas Southwestern Medical Center in Dallas, discovered that it segregated with mutations of the adenosine triphosphate (ATP) binding cassette transporters G5 and G8 (ABCG5, ABCG8) genes (**4.19**). Each gene codes for a 'half transporter' ABCG5 (sterolin-1) and ABCG8 (sterolin-2) that exert their function together in the heterodimeric form (**4.20**) to mediate efflux of dietary sterol in the intestine and protect humans against over-accumulation of sterols.

The metabolic defects associated with familial phytosterolemia include increased sterol absorption encompassing cholesterol and shellfish sterols as well as plant sterols, reduced biliary cholesterol excretion and decreased cholesterol biosynthesis. The defective transporter prevents re-entry of plant sterols (and cholesterol) that had been absorbed via micelles and the NPC1L1 transporter into the intestinal lumen (**4.21**). Plasma apoB levels have been reported to be inherited as an autosomal co-dominant trait in this disease with homozygotes having very high levels and heterozygotes having intermediate levels. However, using phytosterolemia as the marker phenotype, the mode of inheritance is that of an autosomal recessive trait. In heterozygotes, increased sitosterol absorption is compensated by a rapid elimination of plant sterols. About 75–85% of plasma phytosterols and stanols are transported by LDL, and the remainder are transported by HDL.

The genetic defect underlying familial phytosterolemia is a mutation in the genes coding for the transporters ABCG5 or ABCG8. They normally co-operate in the heterodimeric form at the brush border of the intestine to limit intestinal absorption and promote biliary excretion of sterols. These adjacent and oppositely orientated genes are highly expressed in the intestine and in the liver (**4.19**). *ABCG5* was mapped to chromosome 2p21, a region (*STSL*) which had been predicted to contain the familial phytosterolemia gene by Patel and co-workers in 1998. It codes for a 651-amino acid

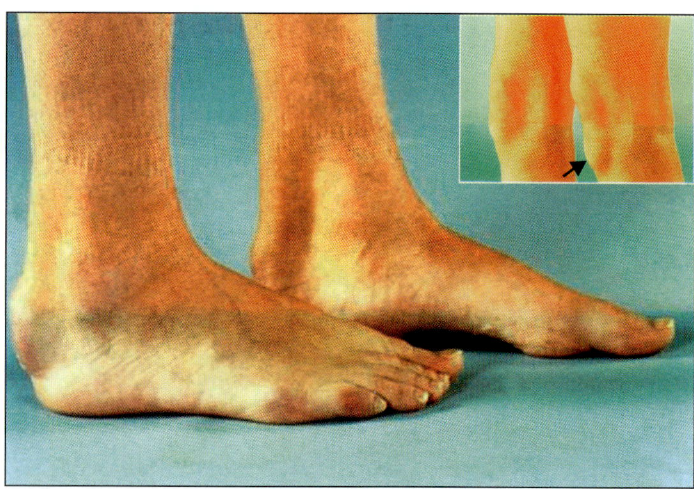

4.17 Prominent Achilles tendon xanthomas and xanthomas of the *tuberositas tibiae* in a 17-year-old girl with familial phytosterolemia. This is the same patient described in the previous figure. Given the age and the prominence of the Achilles tendon xanthomas (left) in the absence of hypercholesterolemia or hypertriglyceridemia, one could have considered cerebro-tendinous xanthomatosis in the differential diagnosis. The inset shows xanthomas of the anterior tuberosity of the tibia (arrow).

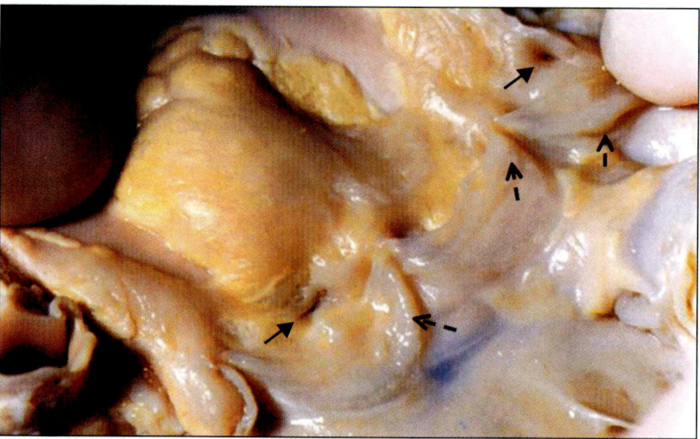

4.18 Atheroma of the aortic root in a case of familial phytosterolemia. This is an autopsy specimen of the aortic valve region taken from a girl who died suddenly at the age of 5 years. Broken arrows show the unfolded aortic leaflets of the specimen held by the pathologist. Large, confluent, protuberant atheromas which encroach upon and occlude both coronary orifices can be seen, indicated by solid arrows. Genomic DNA revealed a novel C>G mutation at the second residue of codon nucleotide 107 in exon 3 of the ABCG8 gene, resulting in a TCA to TGA stop codon and therefore a $Ser_{107} \rightarrow$ Ter mutation. The diagnosis of familial sitosterolemia was confirmed by the presence of elevated serum cholesterol and sitosterol levels in a sister, two brothers and a female cousin. These relatives have also been shown to be homozygotes for the same mutation. Courtesy of Dr David Mymin from the University of Manitoba who provided further information on this case that was also reported in *Circulation* (Mymin D *et al.* [2003]. Image in cardiovascular medicine. Aortic xanthomatosis with coronary ostial occlusion in a child homozygous for a nonsense mutation in ABCG8. *Circulation*, **107**: 791–797).

protein and is upregulated by liver X receptor (LXR) agonists. The two genes are co-ordinately upregulated by dietary cholesterol. In Caucasians, only one mutation causing familial phytosterolemia has been found in *ABCG5*, but several have been observed in the adjacent head-to-head *ABCG8* (**4.19**). In the Japanese, mutations are found in *ABCG5*. Over 25 mutations are known to cause familial phytosterolemia. A recent mutation, $Gln_{24} \rightarrow His$ (Q24H) causing a frame-shift followed by eight new codons and a premature stop codon, has been observed with a high frequency in Kosrae Islanders in Micronesia because of a founder effect (**4.22**).

Diagnosis of familial phytosterolemia is based essentially on the FH phenotype associated with a recessive mode of inheritance (parents are normolipidemic) and elevated plasma levels of plant sterols, which can be measured in lipid-research laboratories using gas liquid chromatography (**4.23**). Normal or moderately high plasma cholesterol or LDL-C levels disproportionate to xanthomatosis are a useful clue but very high levels may also be observed. In phytosterolemia, the plasma cholesterol concentration is extremely responsive to dietary cholesterol restriction and to bile acid binding resins, another diagnostic clue. It is likely that most of the cases reported in the past as having *pseudo-homozygous familial hypercholesterolemia*

may have in fact been cases of familial phytosterolemia. Typically, one of the parents had normal cholesterol, the other was hypercholesterolemic or normolipidemic and the affected person had severe xanthomatosis (**4.24–4.26**). Several of those were found to have hyperphytosterolemia *a posteriori*, and furthermore, Helen Hobbs and colleagues found *ABCG8* mutations in such cases. Familial phytosterolemia is inherited as an autosomal recessive disorder and the severe hypercholesterolemia is very sensitive to dietary cholesterol.

Paradoxically, ingestion of sitostanol (an unabsorbable sterol) results in reduced cholesterol absorption, increased fecal output of cholesterol and plant sterols, and a marked reduction in serum sterols. This observation has provided a basis for the treatment of this disease. Administration of cholestyramine and a low plant fat diet with restrictions on

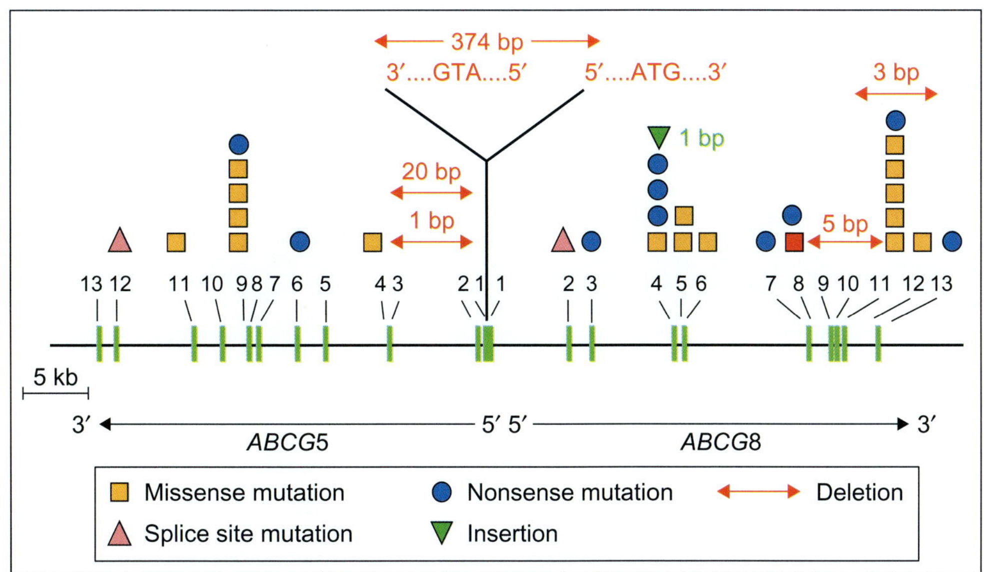

4.19 Gene structure of *ABCG5* and *ABCG8* and mutation sites. *ABCG5* and *ABCG8* are very close together on the sitosterolemia locus (*STSL*) on chromosome 2p21 that spans about 80 kb. Each contains 13 exons and they are transcribed in opposite directions in a head-to-head organization. The two transcription initiation sites are separated by 160 bp and the two translation start codons (ATG) are only separated by 374 bp. This small intergenic region serves as a bidirectional promoter. *ABCG5* and *ABCG8* have a high degree of homology between them (~28% at the protein level) and are highly conserved throughout evolution. These genes are likely to have evolved from a common ancestral gene. Mutations in either of these genes may cause familial phytosterolemia although many polymorphisms exist (not shown) that are not associated with the disease despite occurring in highly conserved regions. More mutations have been reported for *ABCG8* than for *ABCG5*. They are widely distributed on the gene and do not seem to cluster. The amino acid changes causing hyperphytosterolemia are given in the next figure. These two genes are expressed almost exclusively in the liver and intestine, and are co-regulated by the liver X receptor (LXR). Therefore, a high-cholesterol diet or LXR agonists upregulate *ABCG5* and *ABCG8*. Reproduced with permission from Berge KE (2003). Sitosterolemia: a gateway to new knowledge about cholesterol metabolism. *Ann Med*, **35**: 502–511.

nuts, chocolate and seeds constitute the first line of treatment. Recently however, ezetimibe (**4.21**) a novel sterol absorption inhibitor targeting NPC1L1, has been found to be highly effective at reducing plant sterol levels and could be a valuable adjuvant to dietary therapy.

Familial hyperalphalipoproteinemia and cholesteryl ester transfer protein deficiency

Hyperalphalipoproteinemia (HALP), abnormally high levels of plasma α-lipoprotein or HDL-C, is defined by values of HDL-C >90th percentile by age group and sex of a control population. According to the Lipid Research Clinic Prevalence Study database this corresponds to values greater than 1.81 mmol/l (70 mg/dl) before puberty for both sexes, 1.55 mmol/l (60 mg/dl) for adult men, 1.89 mmol/l (73 mg/dl) for pre-menopausal women, 1.86 mmol/l (72 mg/dl) for elderly men and 2.12 mmol/l (82 mg/dl) for

post-menopausal women). HALP may be acquired or may segregate in families where it can be associated with longevity. In most cases it is not a disease; on the contrary it may afford protection against cardiovascular diseases, given the role of HDL in reverse cholesterol transport and the anti-atherogenic properties of these lipoprotein particles. Indeed, HDL have anti-inflammatory, antioxidant, vasodilating, and antithrombotic effects. They enhance fibrinolysis, inhibit production of adhesion molecules by the endothelium and are cardioprotective. Epidemiological evidence has clearly established the inverse relationship between CAD risk and HDL-C, low HDL-C constituting an independent CAD risk factor (**4.27**). Furthermore, there is evidence that plasma levels of HDL-C are inversely related to plasma concentrations of C-reactive protein (CRP), a major atherosclerosis risk factor (**4.28**). Even in the presence of elevated atherogenic lipoproteins, high HDL-C may have some protective effects. Unfortunately, there are rare examples indicating that HALP may be associated with early CAD.

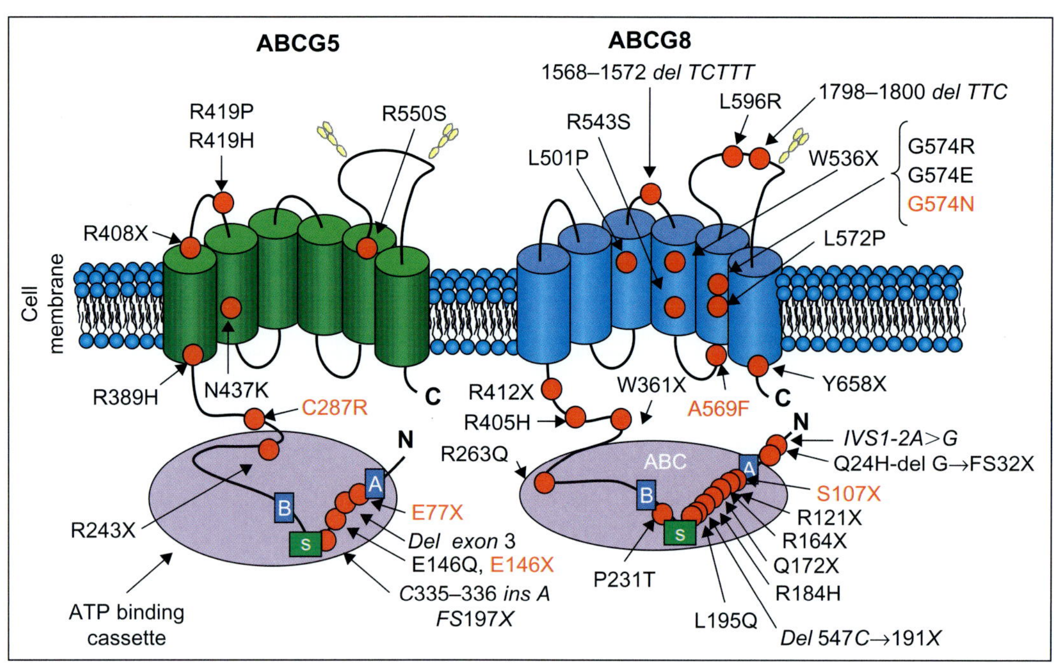

4.20 Protein structure of ABCG5 and ABCG8 and mutations causing familial phytosterolemia. *ABCG5* encodes ABCG5 or sterolin-1 protein (651 amino acids) and *ABCG8* encodes ABCG8 or sterolin-2 (673 amino acids). Sterolins are critical proteins for preventing the retention of plant sterols that are absorbed and allowing the secretion of cholesterol at the apical membrane of the hepatocytes into the biliary lumen. Putative topology of these two proteins with known mutation sites causing phytosterolemia are given in this figure. Typical of such transporters are the membrane spanning domains (six for each half transporter) represented by the cylinders and the Adenosine Triphosphate Binding Cassette (ABC) also referred to as the nucleotide binding fold (NBF) at the N terminal (N) represented by the purple ovals, from amino acid 66 to 277 in *G5* and from 88 to 295 in *G8*. They include two Walker motifs (A and B in blue rectangles) and an active transport signature (s, green rectangle). The Walker motifs are common nucleotide binding folds in the α and β subunits of ATP-requiring enzymes that can predict nucleotide binding sites. These two hemi-transporters are non-functional until they dimerize to form a protein similar to that of other full transporters such as ABCA1 (12 TMDs and 2 ABCs). The N-linked (Asn) glycosylation sites are in yellow. In a recent review, Hazard and Patel have catalogued 36 mutations (22 in *ABCG8*) associated with familial phytosterolemia and 33 polymorphisms (27 in *ABCG8*). The changes in italics are at the genomic levels (i.e. *1798–1800 del TTC*), the others are at the protein level (i.e. E77X); 'del' means deletion, 'ins' means insertion, 'FS' means frame-shift and 'X' means a stop codon (truncation of the protein). '*IVS1 -2A>G*' means a splice site mutation at base -2 in intron 1 where an A is replaced by a G resulting in the loss of exon 2. This recessive disease may be due to homozygosity for a single mutation or to compound heterozygosity.

There seem to be twice as many compound heterozygotes as there are homozygotes for *ABCG8* which is not the case for *ABCG5*. Mutations in *ABCG5* have been reported mostly in Chinese, Japanese and Indians. The $\text{Arg}_{408}\rightarrow$Ter mutation (*ABCG5* first TM domain on the left) was found in a German of Caucasian origin. The $\text{S}_{107}\rightarrow$X mutation in *ABCG8* was responsible for familial phytosterolemia in the child in **4.18** (lower right). The Q24H-*del G*→FS32X mutation is present at a high frequency in the island of Kosrae in Micronesia. Several studies have attempted to relate the sterolin polymorphisms to changes in lipid levels or disease. Carriers of the rare allele (HH or HD) of the D19H non-synonymous polymorphism in the ABCG8 gene were found to exhibit greater percentage reductions in low-density lipoprotein-cholesterol (LDL-C) on atorvastatin (39.7 vs. 36.2%, *P* = 0.036) and achieve lower levels than those with the more common DD genotype. Similarly, the T400K polymorphism of *ABCG8* influences both the baseline serum phytosterol concentrations and the lowering effect of sitostanol esters on them. They are lower and the response is smaller in carriers of the rare KK genotype. This is an update and modification of a diagram taken from Heimerl S *et al.* (2002). Mutations in the human ATP-binding cassette transporters ABCG5 and ABCG8 in sitosterolemia. *Hum Mutat*, **20**: 151–158.

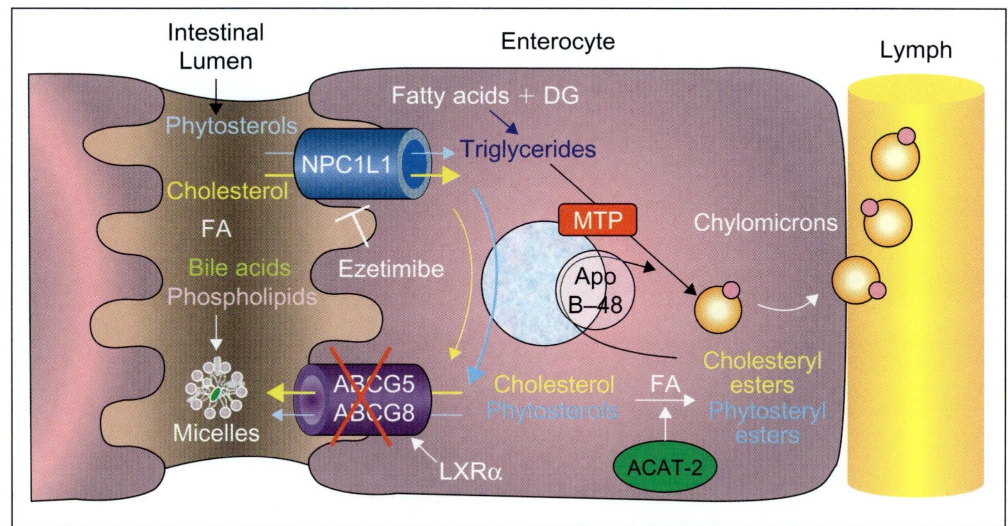

4.21 Alterations in sterol trafficking in familial phytosterolemia. The defect in familial phytosterolemia is illustrated in this diagram showing the major pathways in cholesterol and plant sterol absorption and intracellular trafficking in the intestinal mucosal cells. ABCG5 and ABCG8, also referred to as sterolin-1 and sterolin-2 are sterol efflux pumps regulating in part cholesterol absorption and hepatic sterol output. These proteins are defective in familial phytosterolemia (red X) causing an impaired exit of plant sterols and cholesterol into the intestinal lumen. In the intestinal lumen, dietary sterols are unesterified and a mixture of bile salts, fatty acids, phospholipids and cholesterol, at a critical temperature and a critical concentration, forms minute micelles, which are readily absorbed lipid carriers with hydrophilic polar groups on their surface and lipophilic molecules inside. They are taken up across the brush border membrane of the enterocytes probably in large part by the transporter Niemann–Pick C-1 like-1 protein (NPC1L1), the target of the cholesterol-lowering drug ezetimibe. In the enterocyte, cholesterol (yellow) and phytosterols (blue) that have not been returned to the intestinal lumen by ABCG5-ABCG8 are re-esterified by acyl co-enzyme A:cholesterol acyltransferase-2 (ACAT-2) and packaged into chylomicrons for release into the lymphatics along with triglycerides and apoB-48 by the enzyme complex microsomal triglyceride transfer protein (MTP) in the endoplasmic reticulum. In familial phytosterolemia, phytosterols which are, relatively speaking, more effectively exported by ABCG5-ABCG8 than cholesterol markedly accumulate and chylomicrons transport more into the circulation. Normally the activity of this transporter is regulated by the liver X receptor α (LXRα) so that LXR agonists will enhance the efflux activity of ABCG5-ABCG8. This diagram is redrawn and modified from Sehayek E (2003). Genetic regulation of cholesterol absorption and plasma plant sterol levels: commonalities and differences. *J Lipid Res*, **44**: 2030–2038.

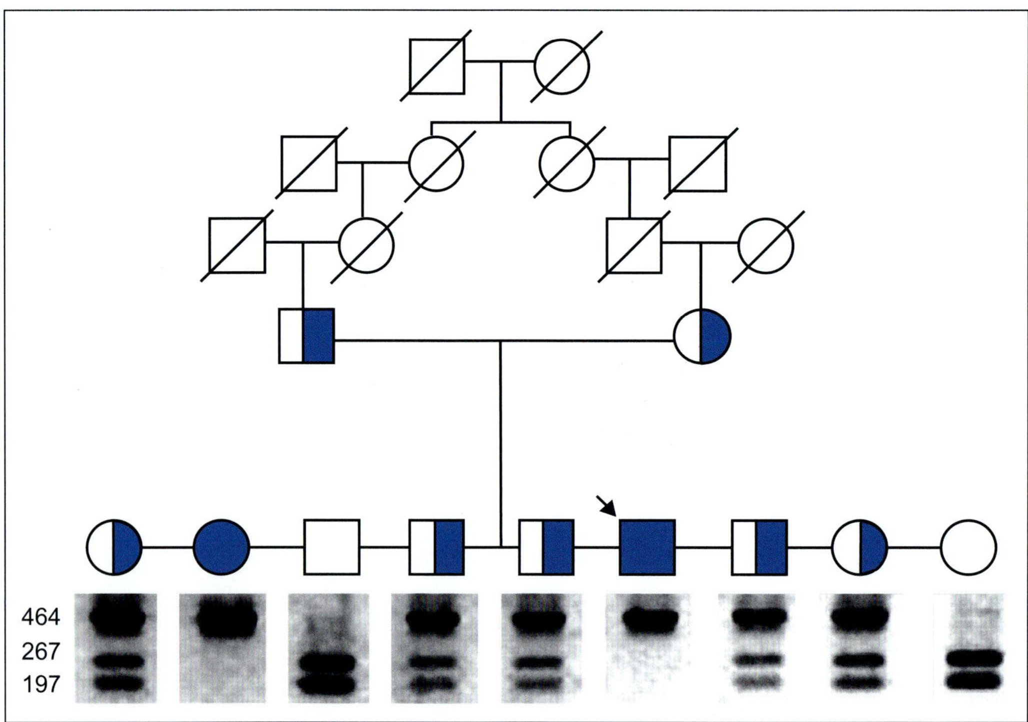

4.22 Consanguinity and familial phytosterolemia on the island of Kosrae. The Micronesian island of Kosrae in the Pacific, 4023 km northeast of Australia, was first inhabited by southeast Asians 2000–3000 years ago. Westerners, largely whalers and missionaries of Caucasian ancestry, first visited Kosrae in 1824 and in subsequent years intermarried with native Kosraeans. In the 1800s, there was a severe decline in the native population attributable to diseases brought in by visitors. This resulted in marked attrition of the native population that was most apparent in the 1880s. Modern Kosraeans are descendants of the relatively few survivors at that time. In 1945, after World War II, Kosrae became a United States Trust Territory, and most citizens carried out sedentary civil service jobs and ate high-fat, high-calorie surplus foods. This resulted in a major lifestyle change, which has caused an epidemic of obesity and diabetes. In the past 10 years, the Kosraean population has been studied for genes that cause obesity, diabetes, hypertension, and dyslipidemia. Breslow and colleagues at the Rockefeller University in New York City, while contributing to these studies, searched for mutations responsible for familial phytosterolemia. In the family illustrated here, they discovered the novel mutation Q24H-*del G*→FS32X (**4.20**) that precludes the formation of an ABCG8 protein. The phytosterolemia pedigree shows the genotyping of *ABCG8* using digestion with the PfoI restriction enzyme of the PCR-amplified 464 bp product. The enzyme fails to digest the mutated allele in the two homozygotes (filled circle and square) and digests the normal allele, producing two fragments of 267 bp and 197 bp (open circle and square, respectively). The proband (arrow) and his affected sister were 46 and 48 years of age, respectively. Their campesterol and sitosterol levels were 25-fold to 50-fold higher than normal (3.9–5.6 mg/dl and 7.5–11.6 mg/dl, respectively, compared with mean levels of 0.18 ± 0.08 mg/dl and 0.22 ± 0.13 mg/dl, respectively, in normal Kosreans). The proband had stable angina but no xanthomatosis. The half-filled circles and squares represent the heterozygotes. After genotyping 1090 subjects, Breslow *et al.* determined that the carrier rate was high (13.8%), compatible with a founder effect, and accounted for plasma campesterol and sitosterol levels in carriers that were 55% and 30% higher, respectively, than in non-carriers. The carriers also had 21% lower plasma levels of lathosterol, a surrogate marker for cholesterol biosynthesis. These results suggested that heterozygosity for a mutated *ABCG8* allele results in a modest increase in dietary cholesterol absorption and a decrease in cholesterol biosynthesis. This pedigree illustrates well the recessive mode of inheritance of familial phytosterolemia with consanguinity in a family. This diagram is reproduced with permission from Sehayek E *et al.* (2004). Phytosterolemia on the island of Kosrae: founder effect for a novel *ABCG8* mutation results in high carrier rate and increased plasma plant sterol levels. *J Lipid Res*, **45**: 1608–1613.

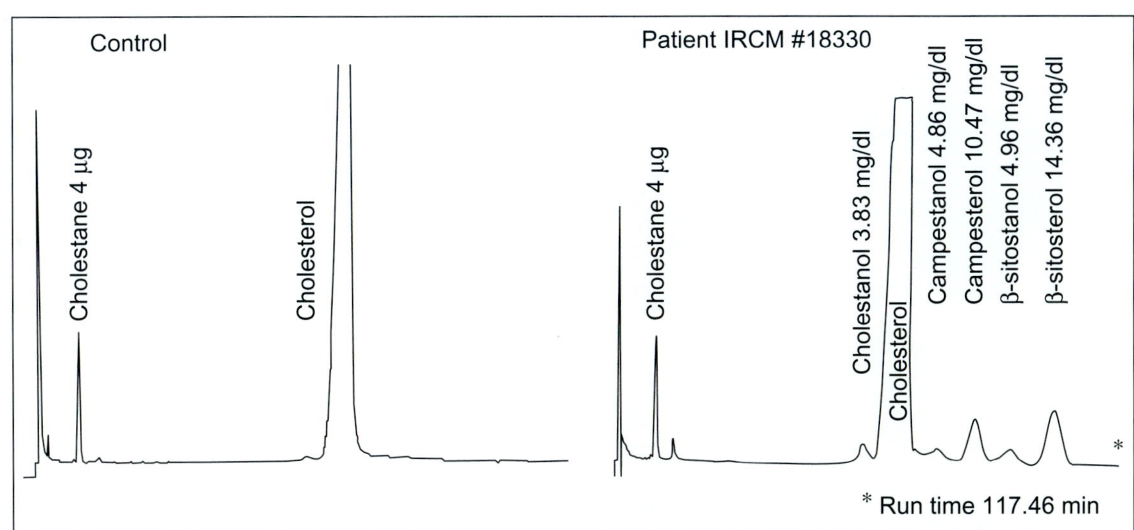

4.23 Gas liquid chromatography pattern of plasma plant sterols in a normal subject and in a patient with familial phytosterolemia. An effective way to establish the diagnosis of familial phytosterolemia is to demonstrate the excess of plant sterols in plasma. If available, gas liquid chromatography (GLC) is ideal as it allows accurate measurement of the concentrations of the various plant sterols. This separation from 100 µl of plasma, saponified and extracted with hexane was done at 220 °C on a 30 m long and 0.25 mm diameter Supelco SP-1000 capillary column of sialylated plasma sterols. It clearly shows the relatively bigger peaks of the plant sterols and stanols than those of a control subject. They are still much smaller than the cholesterol peak. 5α-cholestane was used as an internal standard. The plasma was obtained from a 13-year-old boy from the Dominican Republic referred for xanthomatosis with a relatively normal cholesterol. He presented with xanthomas of Achilles tendons and the extensor tendon of the fingers, brownish yellow tuberous xanthomas of the elbows, xanthelasma, upper corneal crescents, and planar patchy xanthomas of the popliteal space and of the cubital fossa. Total cholesterol (TC) was 7.13 mmol/l (276 mg/dl), triglycerides (TG) 0.54 mmol/l (48 mg/dl), low-density lipoprotein-cholesterol (LDL-C) 5.61 mmol/l (217 mg/dl), HDL-C 0.67 mmol/l (26 mg/dl), LDL apoB 246 mg/dl, VLDL-apoB 5 mg/dl. His apoE phenotype was E3/3. His father (not measured in mother) and one maternal aunt had a normal lipid and lipoprotein profile. He was treated with cholestyramine (he could tolerate only two measures a day) and a diet restricted in vegetable oil seeds and nuts. After nine months, the planar xanthomas had regressed completely, and the tuberous xanthomas had improved substantially without any change in tendon xanthomas. His lipid profile had also improved: TC 3.02 mmol/l (117 mg/dl), TG 0.632 mmol/l (56 mg/dl), LDL-C 1.86 mmol/l (72 mg/dl), and HDL-C 0.80 mmol/l (31 mg/dl).

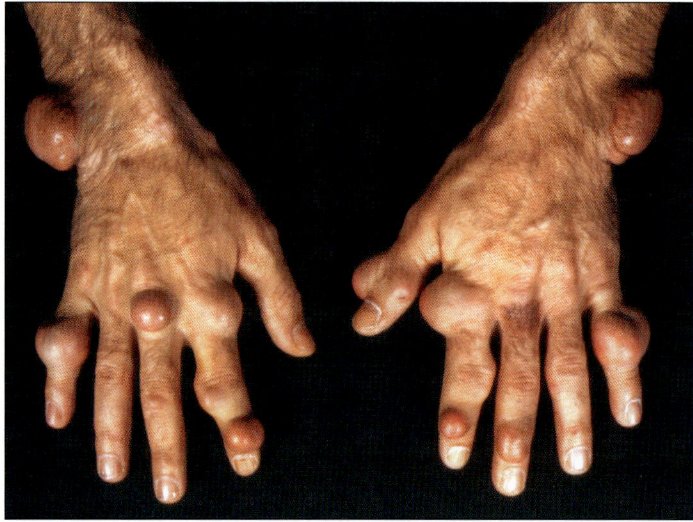

4.24 Severe xanthomatosis of hands, wrists and fingers in a subject with 'pseudo-homozygous familial hypercholesterolemia' (FH) and presumed to have familial phytosterolemia. Unusually severe xanthomatosis was present in two brothers who were referred to our lipid clinic at the ages of 30 (proband) and 27 years with severe hypercholesterolemia. They had large tuberous and tendinous xanthomas as one may observe in homozygous FH. They had first been noticed at about the age of 10. Arcus corneae were also present. Their mother had died suddenly at the age of 63, a sister also died suddenly at 43, but the father was alive, well and normolipidemic at the age of 70. Their daughters did not have hypercholesterolemia. Skin lesions had not been noticed in their parents. The proband noticed that his xanthomas were becoming softer after 6 months on a lipid-lowering diet. He died shortly afterwards of a myocardial infarction (MI). At autopsy he had generalized atherosclerosis and scars of a previous MI. In this context the tentative diagnosis of 'pseudo-homozygous hypercholesterolemia' was made. Loss to follow-up of both cases precluded further investigation. At first visit the proband lipid profile was as follows: total cholesterol 11.9 mmol/l (460 mg/dl) triglycerides 0.83 mmol/l (74 mg/dl), low-density lipoprotein-cholesterol (LDL-C) 9.23 mmol/l (357 mg/dl) and HDL-C 0.75 mmol/l (29 mg/dl). This picture was obtained from the proband. His Achilles tendon xanthomas are shown in **1.20**.

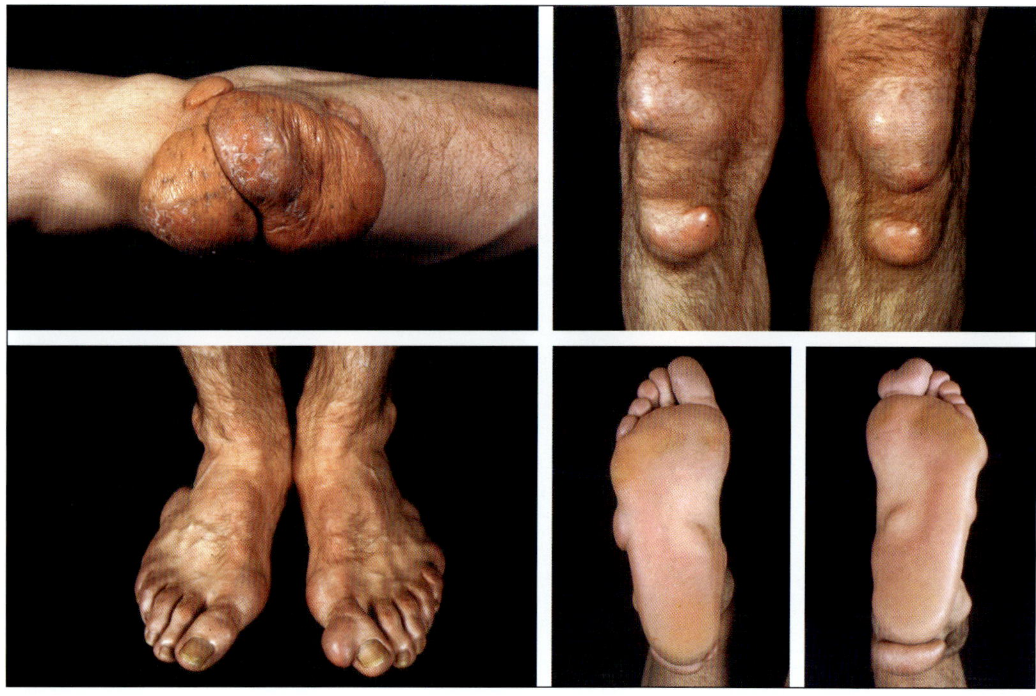

4.25 Severe xanthomatosis of elbows, knees and feet in a subject with 'pseudo-homozygous familial hypercholesterolemia' and presumed to have familial phytosterolemia. Same subject (proband) as in **4.24**. Some of the tuberous xanthomas (elbows, knees) had an orange-yellow discoloration. He had prominent subcutaneous plantar xanthomas.

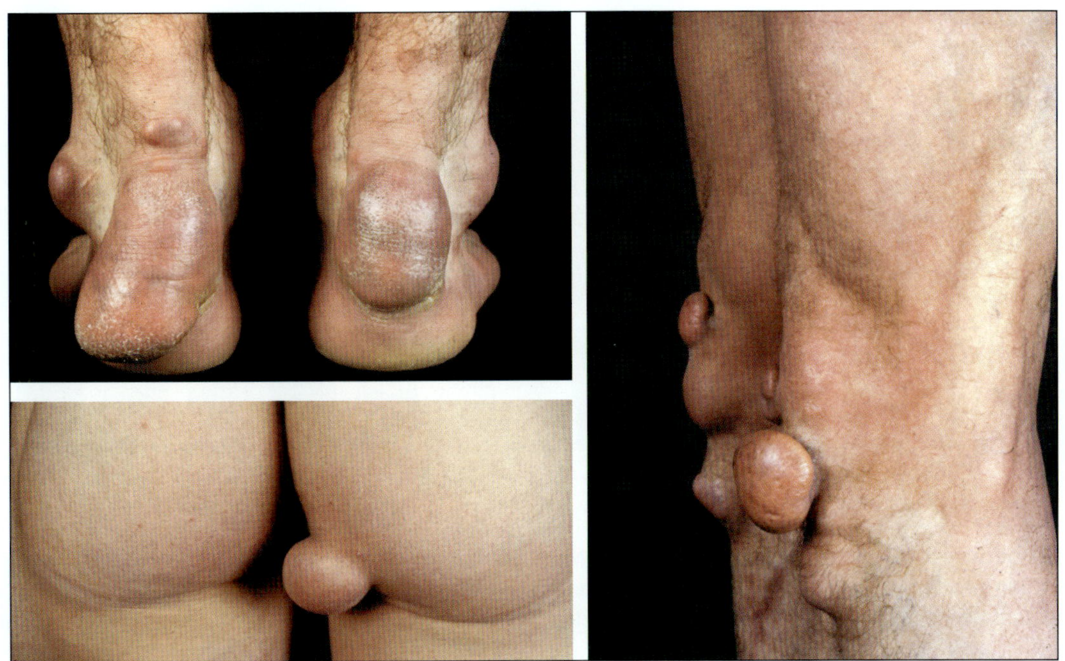

4.26 Severe xanthomas of Achilles tendons, knees and buttocks in a subject with 'pseudo-homozygous familial hypercholesterolemia' and presumed to have familial phytosterolemia. The xanthomatosis was very similar, as seen here, in the 27-year-old brother of the proband. Both were construction workers and xanthomas tended to develop at points of friction. A comparison with **1.14–1.17** demonstrates how little different from homozygous familial hypercholesterolemia these lesions are. The brother had a lipoprotein profile that was quite similar to that of the proband: total cholesterol 13.75 mmol/l (532 mg/dl), triglycerides 0.73 mmol/l (65 mg/dl), low-density lipoprotein-cholesterol (LDL-C) 12.35 mmol/l (477 mg/dl) and HDL-C 0.9 mmol/l (35 mg/dl).

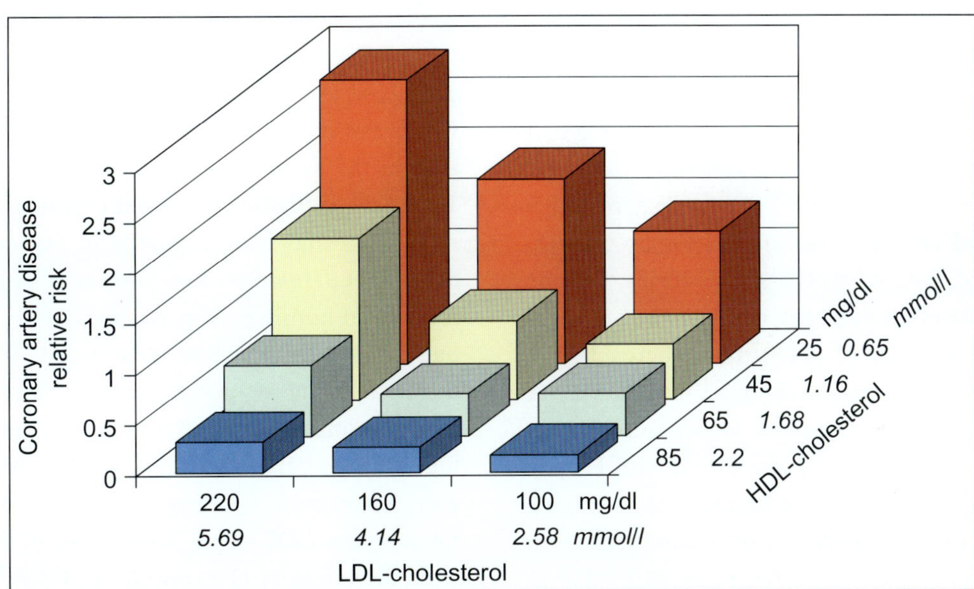

4.27 Coronary artery disease (CAD) risk as a function of low-density lipoprotein-cholesterol (LDL-C) and HDL-C in the Framingham Heart study in men (50–70 y). This is a classical epidemiological demonstration of the close association of plasma HDL-C and CAD risk in men in the town of Framingham (Massachusetts, USA). The lower the HDL-C the greater is the likelihood of developing CAD. This relationship is gradually enhanced as LDL-C levels are increased, the risk nearly reaching 30% when LDL-C is 5.7 mmol/l and HDL-C is 0.65 mmol/l. Similar findings have been obtained in many other studies including the Prospective Cardiovascular Münster Study (PROCAM) in Germany and in many clinical trials. This clearly indicates a relatively low risk in the presence of hyperalphalipoproteinemia. Redrawn and modified with permission from Castelli WP (1988). Cholesterol and lipids in the risk of coronary artery disease—the Framingham Heart Study. *Can J Cardiol*, **4**: 5A–10A.

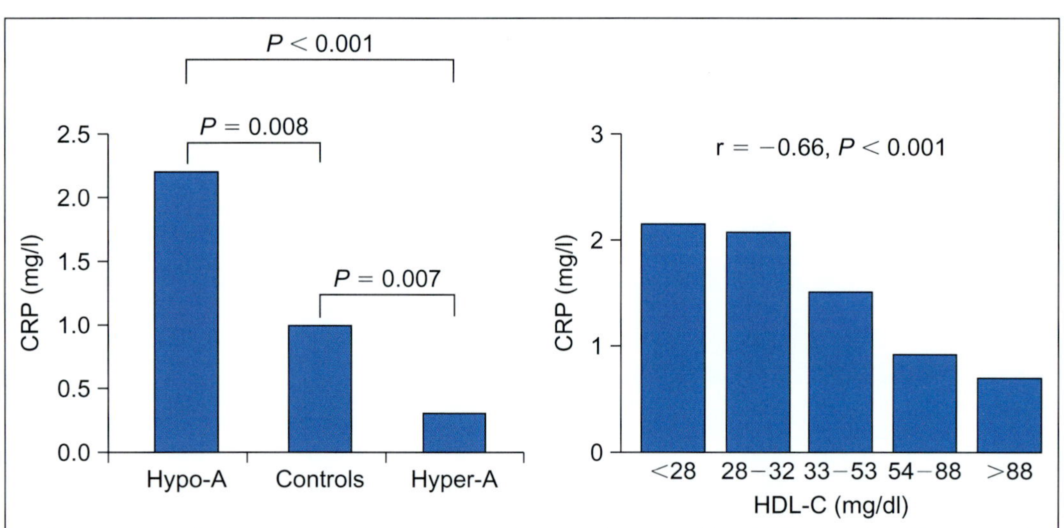

4.28 Inverse relation between C-reactive protein (CRP) and high-density lipoprotein-cholesterol (HDL-C) in hypo-, normo-, and hyperalphalipoproteinemic subjects (*n* = 52). High-density lipoproteins have several intrinsic beneficial properties besides reverse cholesterol transport that account for their cardiovascular protective effect. In addition to carrying antioxidants and exhibiting anti-inflammatory properties, their plasma levels are inversely related to the concentrations of CRP as shown here. In this study, apparently healthy subjects with hypoalphalipoproteinemia (HDL-C <5th percentile of a healthy Italian population) have plasma CRP levels more than double compared with normolipidemic healthy controls and seven times higher than subjects with hyperalphalipoproteinemia (HDL-C >95th percentile). CRP is an acute phase reactant that serves as an important marker of inflammation and its plasma levels correlate positively with atherosclerotic vascular disease risk. However, since apoAI in HDL is a negative acute phase reactant that goes down during acute inflammation, the possibility has been raised that at the onset of a systemic inflammatory state, apoAI and other constituents may be modified and HDL may become pro-inflammatory (Navab M *et al.* [2005] **15**: 158–161. The findings of this small study are in line with the recognized relationship between levels of HDL-C and coronary artery disease risk. Redrawn with permission from Pirro M *et al.* (2003). Plasma C-reactive protein in subjects with hypo/hyperalphalipoproteinemias. *Metabolism*, **52**: 432–436.

Familial hyperalphalipoproteinemia

Familial hyperalphalipoproteinemia (FHALP) (OMIM No. 143470) is an *autosomal dominant inherited lipoprotein trait* that has not been linked to any specific disease. Such families were reported in the 1970s and 1980s by Glueck, Patsch and Nestel and their co-workers in America, Europe and Australia, respectively. Longevity analysis showed prolongation of life and a rarity of premature atherosclerotic events. Lipoprotein kinetic studies revealed only a smaller pool of slowly exchangeable cholesterol. Others reported in one family overproduction of apoAI associated with HALP. The gene defect responsible for these findings has not been established but a locus was identified on chromosome 6p linked to the autosomal dominant inheritance of HALP in a Mexican kindred by Canizales-Quinteros *et al.* (2003). Haplotype analysis refined the localization to a 7.32-centi-Morgan (cM) interval (73–80 cM from pter) flanked by markers D6S1280 and D6S1275. Recently for the first time, Vergeer and colleagues in Amsterdam reported a mutation of the scavenger receptor class B type 1 (SR-B1), which has an important role in reverse cholesterol transport, in a family with HALP without other lipoprotein abnormalities (HDL-C increased 37% in carriers). This is a Pro$_{297}\rightarrow$Ser substitution in the extracellular domain of SR-B1 on chromosome 12q24.31, a highly conserved region amongst vertebrates.

FHALP has been reported in association with the *apolipoprotein CIII variant* Lys$_{58}\rightarrow$Glu in two healthy members of a German family by Von Eckardstein *et al.* (1991). The proband was detected while screening of 200 students for determination of apoE polymorphism. Two additional apoCIII bands anodal to apoCIII$_2$ were observed on isoelectric focusing (IEF) gel electrophoresis (**4.29**). Mean plasma HDL-C was 2.9 mmol/l (112 mg/dl) in the 27-year-old proband for a mean LDL-C of 3.6 mmol/l (139 mg/dl). The values were 2.66 mmol/l (103 mg/dl) and 3.83 mmol/l (148 mg/dl), respectively, in the affected mother. Triglycerides were low, 1.19 mmol/l (106 mg/dl) and 0.68 mmol/l (60 mg/dl), in the proband and the mother, respectively. This was associated with low plasma concentrations of apoCIII, considered to account for the lipoprotein profile because reduced apoCIII in VLDL would favour their clearance and enhanced lipolysis due to increased LPL activity (apoCIII is an inhibitor of

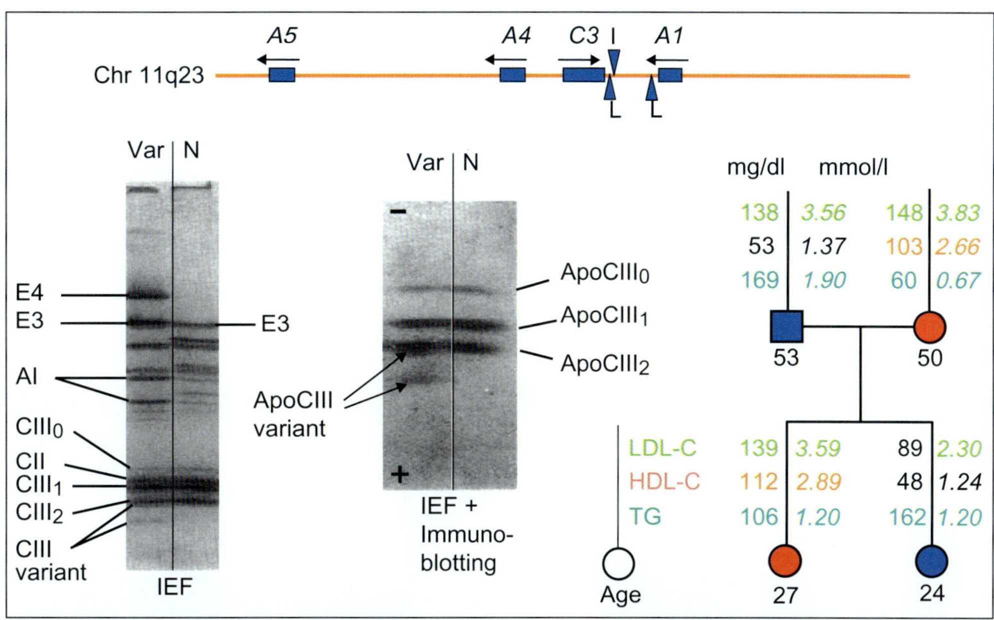

4.29 Hyperalphalipoproteinemia associated with the apoCIII Lys58→Glu variant. The genetic defect in dominant hyperalphalipoproteinemia is not yet fully established. However, Von Eckardstein and colleagues in 1991 reported two subjects from one family where heterozygous carriers of the K58E apoCIII variant had hyperalphalipoproteinemia. ApoCIII is a major protein constituent of triglyceride-rich lipoproteins (TRL) and high-density lipoproteins (HDL). It occurs in plasma in three isoforms differing in their sialic acid content hence the nomenclature ApoCIII 0–2. They are readily separated by isoelectric focusing (IEF) of delipidated very-low-density lipoproteins (VLDL) (left panel). The variant is seen as two extra bands anodal to apoCIII$_2$, one migrating very close to the apoCIII$_2$ band. Immunoblotting after IEF separation with a specific anti-apoCIII antibody (middle panel) does not reveal apoCII that migrates between CIII$_0$ and CIII$_1$ as seen in the left panel. In both panels the left part of the gel shows the separation for the variant and the right part that for a control. The apoE non-glycosylated isoform bands are indicated; the proposita had an apoE4/2 phenotype, the control an E3/3 phenotype. The mutation occurs in exon 4 of the apoCIII gene, a member of the *A1-C3-A4-A5* gene cluster (Arabic numerals are used for the gene in contrast to the protein, *APOC3* vs. *APOCIII*) on chromosome (Chr) 11 illustrated in the top drawing. The direction of transcription is different for *APOC3* in this cluster, as shown by the arrows. The triangles indicate the liver transcription element (L) and the intestinal transcription element (I). A family study revealed vertical transmission of this defect (right panel). The two variant carriers had plasma concentrations of HDL-C and apoAI above the 95th percentiles of sex-matched controls whereas the unaffected father and sister showed normal values. Because of diminished concentrations of the apoCIII variant, 15% of normal in VLDL and 25% of normal in HDL, the carriers had 30–40% lower apoCIII levels compared with unaffected family members and controls. Circulating HDL consisted mainly of HDL$_{2b}$ and contained a proportion of atypically large particles, enriched in apoE. Reproduced with permission from Von Eckardstein A *et al.* (1991). Apolipoprotein C-III(Lys$_{58}$→Glu). Identification of an apolipoprotein C-III variant in a family with hyperalphalipoproteinemia. *J Clin Invest*, **87**: 1724–1731.

lipoprotein lipase [LPL]) which would supply more surface remnants for HDL formation.

HALP has also been reported with a high prevalence in the oculocerebrorenal syndrome of Lowe (OCRL), an X-linked recessive disorder characterized by renal tubular dysfunction, congenital cataracts, and cognitive impairment (see Charnas and Gahl [1991]). Asami and coworkers (1997) reported three patients with OCRL from two families in which HALP segregated. They discovered a cholesteryl ester transfer protein (CETP) mutation, Asp$_{442}$→Gly (D442G) in exon 15, in one of three affected with OCRL, and four of seven healthy family members, but all three OCRL cases had HALP. The reason for this high incidence of HALP in OCRL remains poorly understood. HALP is also one of the features of multiple symmetric lipomatosis (MSL), a condition associated with a marked increase in adipose tissue LPL activity, and a specific defect of the adrenergic-stimulated lipolysis in lipomatous tissue with a typical clinical phenotype (**4.30A** and **B**). Finally, red blood cell macrocytosis or overt macrocytic anemia and abnormalities in liver function tests have been found in MSL patients, related to elevated alcohol intake, which is common in this condition. A 14-year follow-up of 31 MSL patients demonstrated that peripheral neuropathies and space-occupying mediastinal syndromes represent the most incapacitating, sometimes rapidly progressive, complication that may result in tracheal stenosis and superior vena cava obstructive syndrome (**4.30B**; Enzi *et al.* [2002]).

Kronenberg and colleagues in 2002 discovered a recessive (or co-dominant) form of HALP paradoxically in subjects with premature CAD and atherosclerosis by complex segregation analysis in the National Heart, Lung and Blood Institute (NHLBI) Family Heart Study (3755 subjects from 560 nuclear families, 522 with a high family risk of CAD) after adjusting for the effect of triglycerides on HDL-C. A major allele was inferred to account for this unexpected finding. The difference in HDL-C between the homozygous and the heterozygous subjects for the high HDL-C allele was 0.67 mmol/l (26 mg/dl). Specifically, the difference in

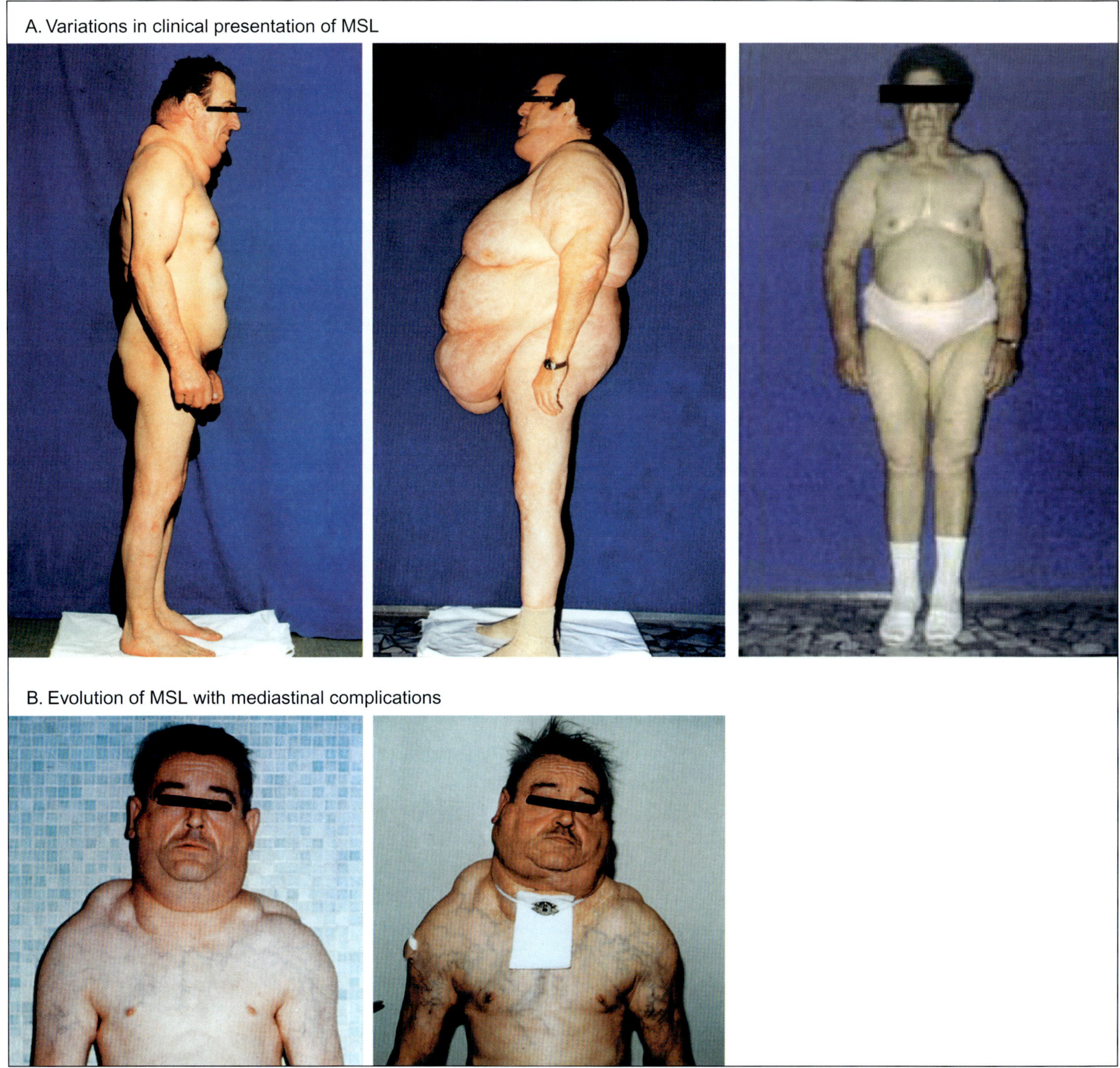

4.30 – *Figure caption opposite.*

HDL-C was 1.91 ± 0.05 mmol/l (73.9 ± 1.99 mg/dl) vs. 1.24 ± 0.01 mmol/l (48.2 ± 0.36 mg/dl). This was confirmed in a separate sample of 2013 individuals in 85 large pedigrees ascertained for early heart disease deaths, early stroke deaths, and early hypertension in Utah. This is of interest as rare cases of myocardial infarction have been reported in patients with HALP, one with a HDL-C level of 3.1 mmol/l (120 mg/dl) (Rotsztain [1978]). One could infer that this is a defence mechanism to compensate for an atherogenic environment.

As mentioned in Chapter 3, subjects with hepatic lipase deficiency have increased plasma concentrations of HDL-C that may reach the range observed in FHALP (see **3.44**).

Cholesteryl ester transfer protein deficiency

The most common form of inherited HALP in Asians is CETP deficiency due to mutations of the CETP gene on chromosome 16q21. CETP is a hydrophobic 476-amino acid glycoprotein associated with HDL particles. Its primary role is to regulate the clearance of HDL cholesteryl esters (CE) from plasma as part of the reverse cholesterol transport (RCT) process (**4.31**). HDL are lipoprotein particles that act as cholesterol acceptors in the lipid efflux process from peripheral cells, which involves the

contribution of diffusion and the activity of several lipid transporters (**4.32**) such as ABCA1, SR-B1 and ABCG1. CETP facilitates the transfer of CE from HDL to apoB-containing lipoproteins. This transfer is accompanied by a reciprocal transfer of triglycerides in the opposite direction. Thus, CETP simultaneously affects the composition and concentration of apoAI and apoB-containing lipoproteins. Absence or marked reduction of CETP will cause a decrease in the CE content of VLDL, IDL and LDL but an increase in their triglyceride content, with a reciprocal increase in HDL-CE and reduction in HDL-TG. HDL particles will become large (HDL_1 and HDL_2) and enriched in their apolipoprotein components (AI, AIV, C and E) (Asztalos *et al.* [2004]).

In a Japanese pedigree, Saito in 1984 identified two 'homozygous subjects' with 'FHAL' because of their very high levels of HDL-C (the proband and his sister having HDL-C of 4.21 mmol/l [163 mg/dl], and 4.68 mmol/l [181 mg/dl], respectively). Longevity analysis revealed that the deceased family members had a life span 9.3 years longer on average than those of an appropriate control population of the same district (Hokuriku). In 1990, however, a mutation of the CETP in this family was reported by Inazu and colleagues. They also observed that this mutation, due to a

4.30 (*Figure bottom of previous page*) **Multiple symmetric lipomatosis is associated with high levels of high-density lipoprotein-cholesterol (HDL-C).** Multiple symmetric lipomatosis (MSL) is a rare disorder discovered in the late nineteenth century and first known as the Launois–Bensaude syndrome. It is a disease of middle life characterized by large subcutaneous unencapsulated fat masses around the neck, shoulders and other parts of the trunk occurring predominantly in men. It may be associated with somatic and autonomic neuropathy, motor neurone dysfunction, increased alcohol intake (48% are heavy drinkers) and mutations in mitochondrial DNA (multiple deletions). Mediastinal growth of fat masses is a serious complication of the disease as it may lead to compression of the airways, tracheal distortion, venous stasis of the anterior chest wall from vena cava compression and palsy of the recurrent nerve. In the early 1980s, Enzi and co-workers at the University of Padova reported for the first time the association with hyperalphalipoproteinemia and elevated adipose tissue lipoprotein lipase activity. Recent studies indicate that affected patients have normal glucose, enhanced insulin sensitivity, high adiponectin and low leptin plasma levels and no excess of visceral fat. (A) The three patients demonstrate the variation in clinical expression of MSL and sex differences. On the left side is a man with type I MSL, showing circumscribed fatty masses protruding from the body surface and around the neck. The man in the middle panel has type II MSL with a widespread deposition of lipomatous tissue mimicking simple obesity. As seen in the right panel, the lipomatous deposits are distributed differently in women with MSL. In this case, there is a sparing of the submental area and prevalence of fat deposition in the proximal part of arms and legs. (B) The most important complication of MSL – mediastinal involvement. The patient on the left at the first evaluation displayed the typical symmetric lipomatous masses of the neck, supraclavicular and submental areas. On the right is the same patient 8 years later showing evidence of a progressive occupation of the thoracic inlet with a superior vena cava syndrome and a tracheal stenosis that required tracheostomy. The venous stasis is obvious on the upper thorax and arms. This patient participated in the longitudinal study of about 14.5 years that included 31 patients with MSL carried out by Enzi and colleagues. They observed that unexplained sudden death was a frequent cause of mortality. In this study, HDL-C was 1.78 ± 0.43 mmol/l (69.0 ±16.6 mg/dl) at baseline, and 1.73 ± 0.47 mmol/l (67.0 ±18.4 mg/dl) at the final visit; the hyperalphalipoproteinemia appeared to be secondary only to alcohol intake. The only measure that could improve the lipomatous deposits in MSL besides surgery was discontinuation of alcohol. These photographs are reproduced from Enzi G *et al.* (2002) Multiple symmetric lipomatosis: clinical aspects and outcome in a long-term longitudinal study. *Int J*

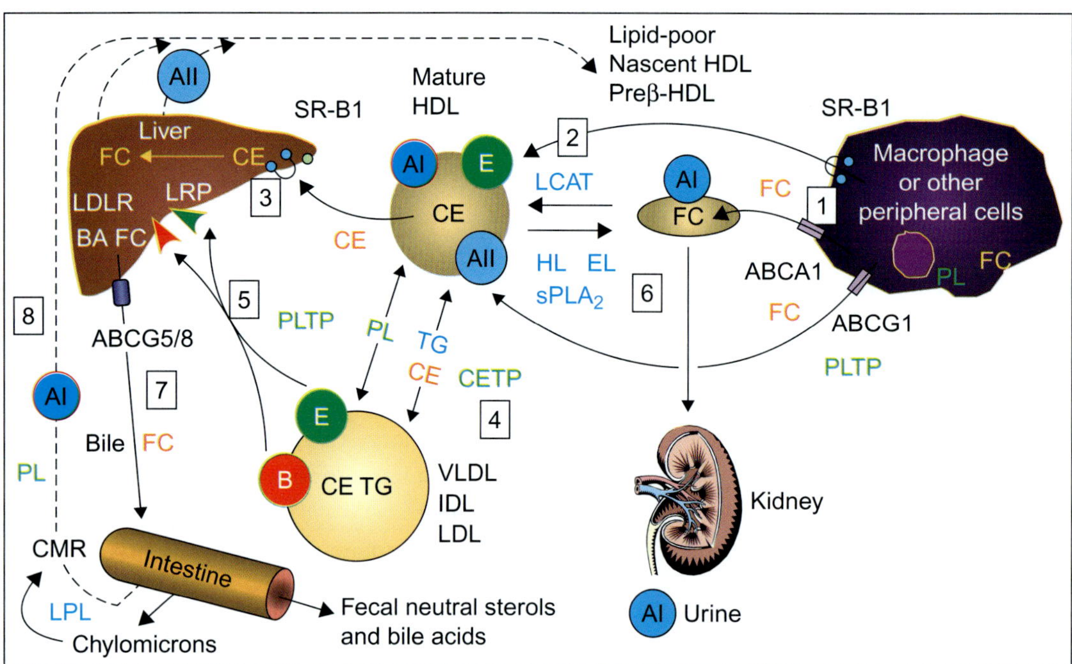

4.31 Cholesteryl ester transfer protein (CETP) is a key actor in reverse cholesterol transport. The role of CETP in reverse cholesterol transport (RCT) is depicted schematically in this diagram that should be read from the upper right hand corner. (1) Lipid-poor apoAI (AI) acquires free cholesterol (FC) and phospholipids (PL) from peripheral cells including macrophages, through an export process mediated by the cellular protein adenosine triphosphate–binding cassette A1 (ABCA1). ABCG1 and ABCG4 efflux cholesterol directly to more mature high-density lipoprotein (HDL) particles rather than to lipid-poor particles (Vaughan and Oram [2005]). Macrophages also efflux FC via the scavenger receptor class BI (SR-BI) to more mature HDL particles. (2) FC is converted to cholesteryl ester (CE) within the HDL particle through transfer of a fatty acid from phosphatidylcholine by the enzyme lecithin: cholesterol acyl transferase (LCAT). (3) HDL-CE can be targeted for and taken up selectively by the liver through the action of SR-BI and (4) HDL-CE can also be selectively transferred to apoB-containing lipoproteins (very-low-density lipoproteins [VLDL], intermediate-density lipoproteins [IDL], LDL) in exchange for triglycerides (TG) through the action of CETP and (5) returned to the liver via the low-density lipoprotein (LDL) receptor (LDLR, red arrowhead) and the LDLR related protein (LRP, green arrowhead). (6) Hepatic lipase (HL) hydrolyses HDL-TG and phospholipids, remodelling larger HDL particles to smaller HDL particles, which are then at greater risk of catabolism by the kidney. Hepatic lipase (HL) and endothelial lipase (EL) and possibly secretory phospholipase A2 (sPLA$_2$) may also participate in the remodelling of HDL from larger to smaller particles by hydrolysing lipids. (7) The liver secretes free cholesterol directly into the bile putatively via the ABCG5-ABCG8 heterodimeric transporter (see section on Familial phytosterolemia) or converts it into bile acids (BA), which are then secreted into the bile. (8) Lipoprotein lipase (LPL) contributes to HDL formation by generating redundant phospholipids and apolipoproteins on chylomicron remnants (CMR) and other remnant lipoproteins that are transferred to HDL. Phospholipid transfer protein (PLTP) interacts with ABCA1 and facilitates lipid efflux from peripheral cells, henceforth playing a role in HDL remodelling and formation of lipid-poor apoAI particles with preβ mobility (preβ-HDL). It transfers phospholipids (PL) from remnant lipoproteins to HDL and is therefore active in maintenance of HDL levels. Finally, there is recent evidence that cholesteryl ester from mature HDL may be taken up not only by SR-B1 but also via CETP itself acting as a receptor on liver cells and adipocytes (green dot). See also **2.12**, **3.3** and **3.44** for overall lipid metabolism involving CETP. Modified and expanded from Rader DJ (2003). Regulation of reverse cholesterol transport and clinical implications. *Am J Cardiol*, **92**: 42J–49J.

G→A point mutation in the splice donor site (position +1) of intron 14 of the CETP gene, yielded a null allele and was on the same haplotype in four families from three different regions in Japan (see below).

Reduced rates of CE transfer activity in plasma were first reported in Japanese patients in 1985 by two separate groups (Koizumi's and Kurasawa's). The molecular basis of this defect was reported in *Nature* in 1989 by Brown, Inazu, Tall and colleagues at Columbia University in New York. The original patients were homozygotes for the common point mutation in the 5′-splice donor site of intron 14 of the *CETP* gene (**4.33**). These *CETP* mutations are common in Japan where they are found in 5–7% of the general population and are a frequent cause of elevation of HDL-C. In homozygotes, plasma HDL-C may be increased three- to six-fold with massive elevation of apoAI and presence of

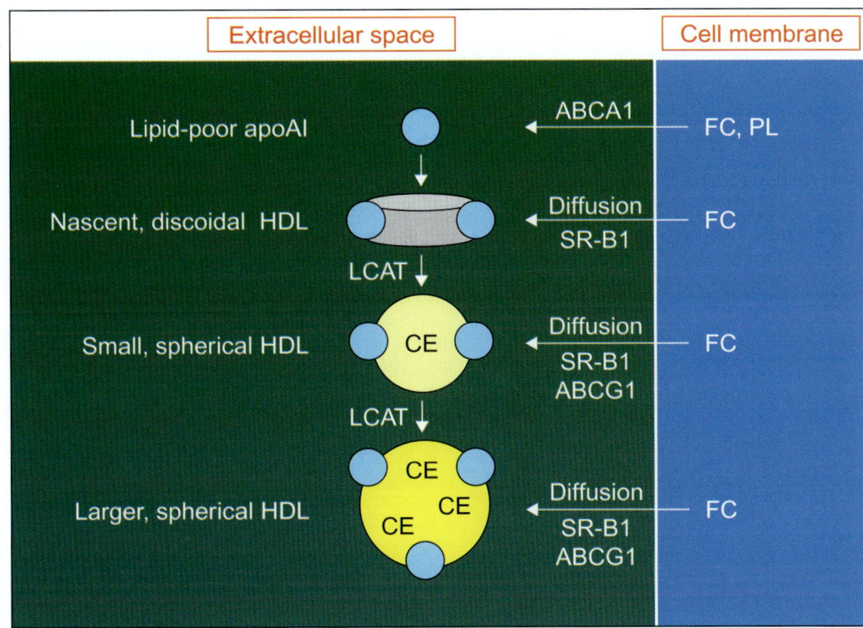

4.32 Acquisition of cholesteryl ester by high-density lipoproteins (HDL) from cellular efflux. HDL particles may accept free cholesterol (FC) from peripheral cells via several mechanisms. The ATP-binding cassette transporter A1 (ABCA1) effluxes FC to lipid-poor apoAI resulting in the formation of discoidal nascent HDL. Esterification of the FC in nascent HDL by lecithin:cholesterol acyl transferase (LCAT) generates spherical, mature HDL particles. The lipidation of lipid-poor apoAI and the conversion of discoidal HDL to spherical particles are rapid as evidenced by the very low levels of lipid-poor apoAI and discoidal HDL in normal plasma. Free cholesterol may be effluxed to mature HDL particles by passive diffusion or by a receptor-mediated pathway, including the scavenger receptor B-1 (SR-B1) or the ATP-binding cassette transporter G1 (ABCG1). Redrawn with permission from Barter PJ, Kastelein JJ (2006). Targeting cholesteryl ester transfer protein for the prevention and management of cardiovascular disease. *J Am Coll Cardiol*, **46**: 492–494.

large HDL particles rich in CE and apoE. Heterozygotes may have a normal or intermediate phenotype with moderately raised HDL-C, reduced plasma triglyceride, and low plasma glucose. CETP deficiency due to a mutation in exon 9 ($Arg_{268} \rightarrow$Stop) was the first case to be reported in a Caucasian in North America (Nova Scotia, Canada; Teh *et al.* [1998]). Occasional *CETP* mutations have also been observed in other non-Asian countries (e.g. Germany).

The diagnosis is based on the typical lipoprotein abnormalities, high HDL-C concentration, large HDL, reduced CE content of VLDL, IDL and LDL (–30%), compensated by an increased triglyceride content, normal or reduced apoB concentration (–60%) with large buoyant LDL, and a family history of HALP. Demonstration of the CETP mutation will establish the diagnosis. No specific clinical manifestation has been reported with CETP deficiency. Whether CETP deficiency is associated with reduced or increased CAD risk has been a matter of controversy for several years because reports of both have been published. Context-dependency (gene–gene and gene–environment interactions) has been a major confounder in this debate (**4.34**). Furthermore, the protection from HALP may be attenuated or lost if the circulating HDL in CETP deficiency are dysfunctional (reduced uptake capacity for effluxed cholesterol). CETP itself may be a contributor to cardiovascular risk in hypertriglyceridemic subjects (**4.35**). The *Taq*IB polymorphism of intron 1 of the *CETP* gene modulates plasma CETP and HDL-C levels, the B1 allele being associated with lower

HDL-C, increased CETP levels and increased CAD risk (**4.34**) (see also Boekholdt *et al.* [2005]). Variants and polymorphisms of *CETP* and perhaps other genes, singly or in combination, may contribute to changing a protective phenotype into an atherogenic one. This seems to be the case for a recent report of premature CAD in two hyperalphalipoproteinemic brothers free of CVD risk factors with normal triglycerides and LDL-C (**4.36**). After revisiting the Honolulu Heart Study (**4.37**) and from the bulk of evidence in humans the consensus at present is that it is generally associated with a reduced risk of CAD. However, an atherogenic potential exists and it may be more likely to occur in complete CETP deficiency than in partial CETP deficiency. The 'abnormal' lipoprotein profile in CETP deficiency can be corrected by giving probucol, a cholesterol-lowering agent with antioxidant properties that increases CETP mass in plasma and reduces HDL-C (**4.36**). Probucol may be indicated in complete CETP deficiency with a family history of atherosclerotic cardiovascular disease. Several CETP inhibitors such as torcetrapib, and a vaccine against CETP have been developed to raise HDL-C as a protective measure against CAD.

In practice, hyperalphalipoproteinemia is important to recognize because it has many causes (*Table 4.1*) and also may mislead physicians into thinking that the patient has hypercholesterolemia secondary to high LDL, when in fact it is due to increased HDL levels in the presence of normal LDL-C. Fortunately, this is rare now that HDL-C

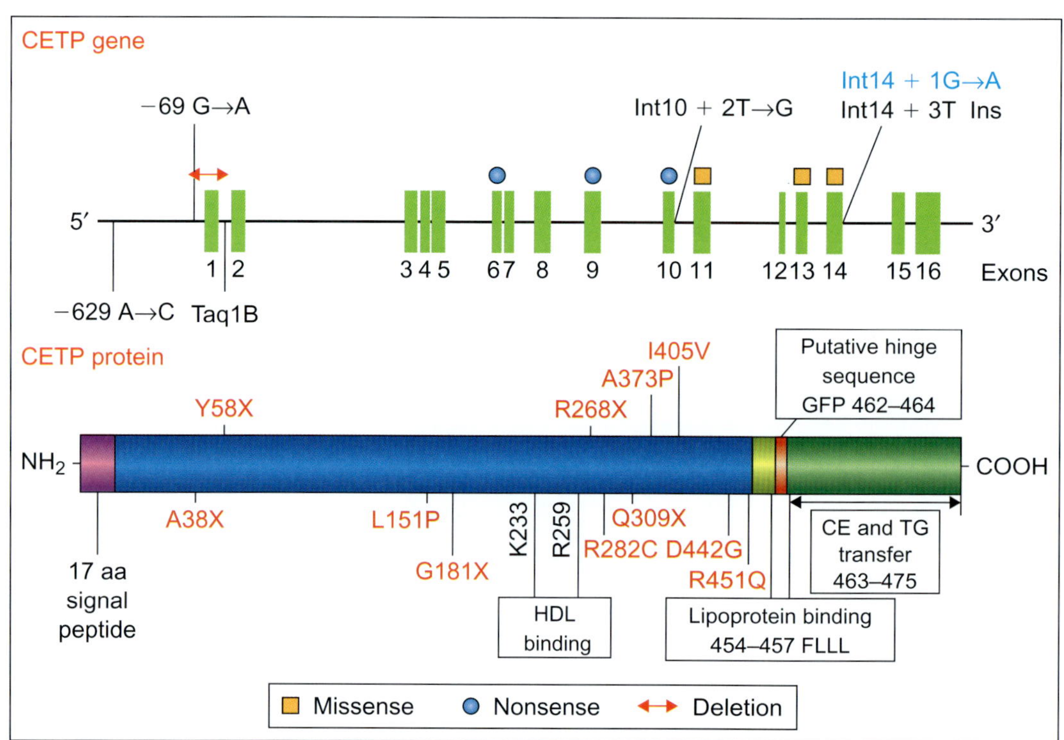

4.33 Cholesteryl ester transfer protein (CETP) gene and protein structure, mutations and polymorphisms. The CETP gene structure is given in the top part of this figure. Above the gene, the types of mutations in the various exons as well as the intronic mutations are indicated. Two polymorphisms are depicted under the gene. The -629 A→C substitution polymorphism influences cardiovascular (CV) mortality. The −629A allele (*AA* and *CA* genotypes) confers a strong protective effect against future CV death; the mortality is reduced from 10.8% in *CC* homozygotes to 4.6% in *CA* heterozygotes, and 4.0% in *AA* homozygotes. The *Taq*1B polymorphism of intron 1 has been shown to influence plasma high-density lipoprotein-cholesterol (HDL-C) levels and the risk of coronary artery disease. The G→A point mutation in the splice donor site (position +1) of intron 14 (Int14 + 1G→A) of *CETP* (blue), that yields a null allele, is the most common mutation in the Japanese population. In the homozygotes, there is complete absence of CETP. The bottom part of the figure illustrates the major domains of the 493-amino acid (aa) (including a signal peptide of 17 aa) CETP precursor protein. The mature protein has 476 aa since the signal peptide residues are discounted. Putative functional domains are indicated in boxes: the HDL binding site, the helical hydrophobic stretch (FLLL: Phe-Leu-Leu-Leu) for lipoprotein binding, and the C terminal domain responsible for CE and triglyceride (TG) exchange (amphipatic helix flexible tail). Amino acid changes leading to CETP deficiency are given. The D442G mutation is the second most frequent mutation in Japan and has been reported in China, Korea and Vietnam. It is associated with partial CETP deficiency. It has also been reported in the oculo-cerebrorenal syndrome of Lowe. The G181X of exon 6, another mutation found in Japan, is also associated with complete CETP deficiency. The R268X has been observed in Canada. The I405V variant is a polymorphism, and its relationship to healthy ageing is still controversial. It is in linkage disequilibrium with the CETP -629 A→C polymorphism and shares some of its effects on CV risk. Diagrams redrawn and expanded from Teh EM *et al.* (1998). Human plasma CETP deficiency: identification of a novel mutation in exon 9 of the CETP gene in a Caucasian subject from North America. *J Lipid Res*, **39**: 442–456, and Yamashita S *et al.* (2000). Molecular mechanisms, lipoprotein abnormalities and atherogenicity of hyperalphalipoproteinemia. *Atherosclerosis*, **152**: 271–285.

measurement is more widely available and requested. In the LRC collaborative study, among adults aged 20–79 years, 3% of white men, 10% of white women, 17% of black men, and 25% of black women had predominant hyperalphalipoproteinemia (HDL-C ≥95th percentile, but LDL-C <95th percentile) which accounted for their hypercholesterolemia (Morrison *et al.* [1980]). The proportion was even greater in children. Furthermore, hyperalphalipoproteinemia may reduce the risk of CAD related to an atherogenic dyslipidemia. This has been reported in a Mexican family with FH-3 (PCSK9-related) (Canizales-Quinteros *et al.* [2003]). Importantly, on occasion, the opposite is true: hyperalphalipoproteinemia in the presence of an otherwise normal lipoprotein profile may be associated with premature CAD in a family as shown by Sirtori and colleagues in their case report (**4.36**). Hyperalphalipoproteinemia may also be the first clue to the diagnosis of hepatic lipase deficiency which has been associated with severe atherosclerosis when combined with

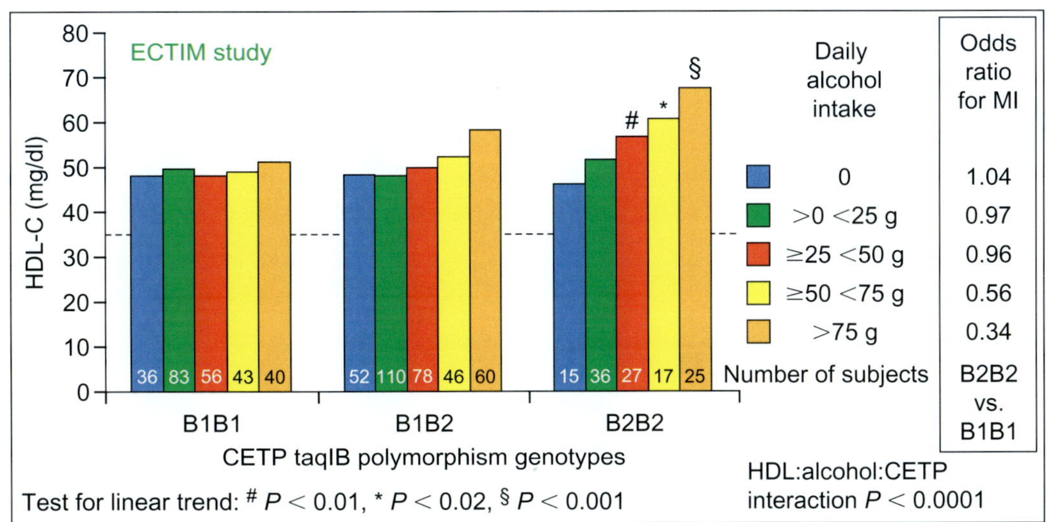

4.34 Alcohol consumption influences the effect of the CETP *Taq*IB B2 allele on plasma high-density lipoprotein-cholesterol (HDL-C) and risk of myocardial infarction. The common cholesteryl ester transfer protein (CETP) gene *Taq*IB (or *Taq*1B) polymorphism with two alleles B1 (60%) and B2 (40%) has been widely studied since its discovery in 1989. There is absence of a cutting site for the restriction enzyme *Taq*I in the B2 allele. Its relation to lipid variables and risk of myocardial infarction (MI) was studied by Frédéric Fumeron and co-workers in the large case–control study called 'ECTIM' (*Étude Cas-Témoin de l'Infarctus du Myocarde*) of men aged 25–64 from Strasbourg, Toulouse, Lille and Belfast. There were 608 cases and 724 controls. The B2 carriers had reduced levels of plasma CETP ($P < 0.0001$) and increased levels of HDL-C, apoAI, and apoAII ($P < 0.0001$) as well as LpAI ($P < 0.0002$) and LpAI:AII ($P < 0.02$) lipoprotein particles. The effect of alcohol on plasma HDL-C and CETP was studied as a function of the B1B2 genotype. The B2 allele had no effect in subjects drinking <25 g/day of alcohol but HDL-C increased commensurably, with higher values of alcohol consumption (interaction: $P < 0.0001$). A similar interaction was not observed for plasma CETP, stressing the independent role of CETP and HDL-C on the alcohol effect. The odds ratios were computed from the regression coefficients estimated in the logistic regression analysis of case–control status for MI of B2 homozygotes. It decreased from 1.0 in non-drinkers to 0.34 in those drinking 75 g/day or more (right panel). These results provided the first demonstration of a gene–environment interaction affecting HDL-C levels and coronary artery disease risk. It confirmed the protective role of increased HDL-C levels with alcohol consumption but indicated that the desirable effect was limited to the carriers of the 'good' B2 allele. A recent meta-analysis of data from seven population-based studies and three randomized, controlled trials has since demonstrated that *Taq*IB polymorphism is firmly associated both with HDL-C plasma levels and with risk of CAD. Figure drawn from data reported in Fumeron F *et al.* (1995). Alcohol intake modulates the effect of a polymorphism of the cholesteryl ester transfer protein gene on plasma high density lipoprotein and the risk of myocardial infarction. *J Clin Invest*, **96**: 1664–1671.

CETP mutations (Hirano *et al.* [1995]). MSL should be suspected if lipomatosis is present (**4.30**). In children, OCRL will be identified before the hyperalphalipoproteinemia is detected. CETP deficiency should be suspected in an Asian patient with high HDL-C, and identified as well in Caucasians, even if rare, because of its relationship to atherosclerosis. The authors routinely ask hyperalphalipoproteinemia patients questions about longevity and family history of heart disease to determine whether the lipoprotein trait is anti- or pro-atherogenic. High levels of abnormal HDL not alpha-migrating on lipoprotein electrophoresis have been reported in biliary obstruction. Hyperalphalipoproteinemia of unknown etiology has been observed in a patient with elevated levels of lipoprotein lipase, elevated immunoglobulin M (IgM) levels, a high erythrocyte sedimentation rate and a circulating HDL-albumin complex (Demacker *et al.* [1994]). The differential diagnosis must also be made with secondary causes of hyperalphalipoproteinemia. In the Heart and Estrogen/progestin Replacement Study (HERS), 20% of post-menopausal women on HRT who developed CAD had hyperalphalipoproteinemia without a concomitantly higher prevalence of other CAD risk factors. Some patients with primary biliary cirrhosis may have high levels of HDL-C; this has been ascribed to decreased hepatic lipase activity. Several agents may raise HDL-C (i.e. estrogens, fibrates, niacin, statins, long-term administration of amiodarone), but only a few, such as the anti-epileptic drugs phenytoin and carbamazepine will induce hyperalphalipoproteinemia ≥90th percentile (*Table 1.4*). Similarly, several conditions – alcohol intake, exercise, weight loss and smoking cessation –

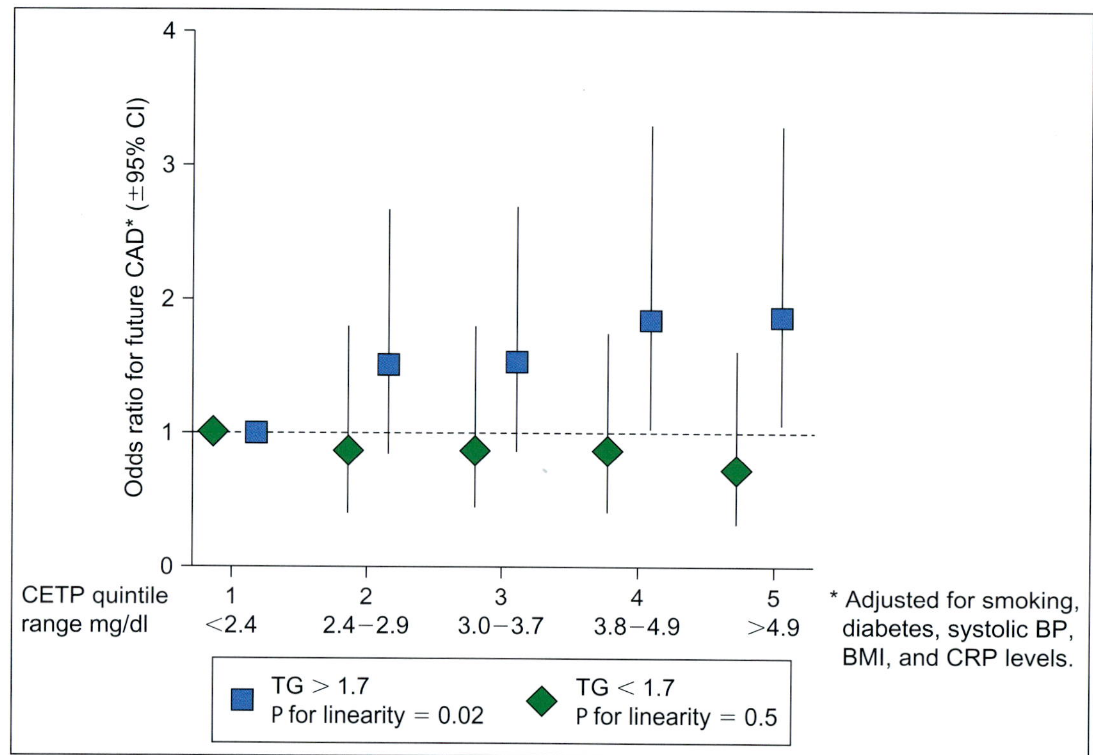

4.35 Elevated CETP levels are predictive of future coronary artery disease (CAD) in subjects with high plasma triglycerides only. This figure shows the results of a nested case–control study conducted among 25 663 apparently healthy men and women aged between 45 and 79 years who participated in the European Prospective Investigation into Cancer and Nutrition (EPIC)-Norfolk Population study. The 755 individuals who went on to develop fatal or non-fatal CAD during an average follow-up of 6 years were compared with age-, sex- and time- or enrolment-matched control subjects who remained free of CAD during follow-up. At baseline plasma C-reactive protein (CRP) concentrations were not significantly different between cases and controls (4.0 ± 2.2 vs. 3.8 ± 2.1 mg/l, $P = 0.07$). The risk of CAD increased with increasing cholesteryl ester transfer protein (CETP) quintiles, although this relationship was present in subjects with triglycerides above the median level (blue squares) but not in those with triglycerides below the median 1.7 mmol/l (150 mg/dl). The relationship between CETP levels and CAD risk was strong among those with high triglyceride levels such that those in the highest CETP quintile had an odds ratio (OR) of 1.87 (95% CI 1.06–3.30, $P < 0.02$). Redrawn from Boekholdt *et al.* (2004). Plasma levels of cholesteryl ester transfer protein and the risk of future coronary artery disease in apparently healthy men and women – The prospective EPIC (European Prospective Investigation into Cancer and Nutrition) – Norfolk population study. *Circulation*, **110**: 1418–1423.

raise HDL-C, but only a few, such as severe alcoholism or regular intense exercise, will cause hyperalphalipoprotein-emia. The most notorious environmental cause of hyperal-phalipoproteinemia is exposure to chlorinated hydrocarbon pesticides (lindane, DDT and others) where HDL may reach levels greater than 3.8 mmol/l (146 mg/dl) (Carlson and Kolomodin-Hedman [1972]).

Alagille's syndrome and progressive familial intrahepatic cholestasis

Obstructive liver disease may be associated with hyper-lipoproteinemia. Indeed, conditions leading to cholesta-sis, such as primary biliary cirrhosis, are associated with hypercholesterolemia and an increase in an unusual form of plasma lipoprotein, lipoprotein X (LpX). Two conditions with cholestasis and hyperlipoproteinemia are genetically transmitted, Alagille's syndrome (AGS, also called arterio-hepatic dysplasia, syndromatic ductopenia and hepatic ductular hypoplasia) and progressive familial intrahepatic cholestasis (PFIC). They are rare primarily pediatric dis-eases that could be confused with other causes of inherited lipid transport disorders.

Alagille's syndrome (OMIM No. 118450) was first reported in 1969 by Daniel Alagille and co-workers in Paris. It is a heritable developmental disorder that was formerly classified among the contiguous gene syndromes (CGS)

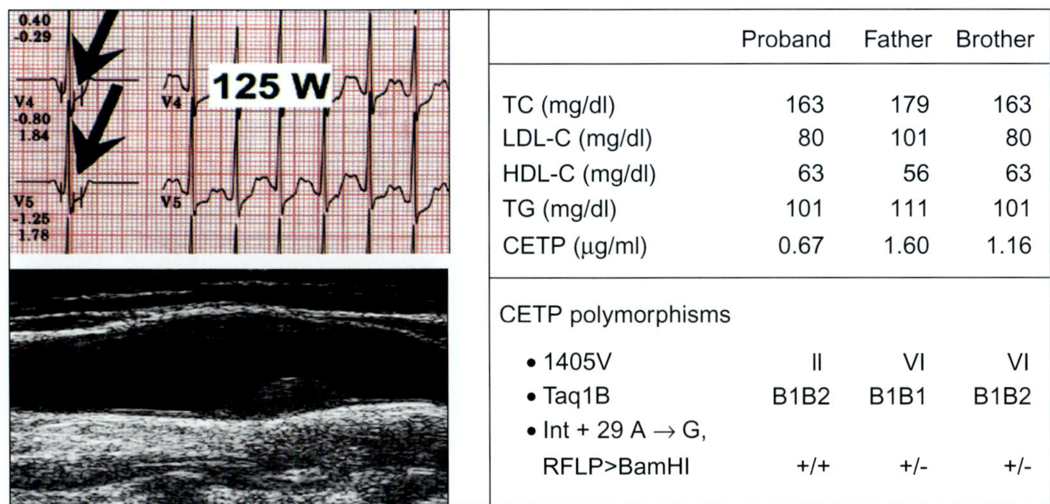

	Proband	Father	Brother
TC (mg/dl)	163	179	163
LDL-C (mg/dl)	80	101	80
HDL-C (mg/dl)	63	56	63
TG (mg/dl)	101	111	101
CETP (µg/ml)	0.67	1.60	1.16
CETP polymorphisms			
• 1405V	II	VI	VI
• Taq1B	B1B2	B1B1	B1B2
• Int + 29 A → G,			
RFLP>BamHI	+/+	+/-	+/-

4.36 Early coronary artery disease (CAD) in two brothers with high high-density lipoprotein-cholesterol (HDL-C) and low cholesteryl ester transfer protein (CETP) levels. Sirtori and colleagues reported early coronary artery disease in a 34-year-old male athlete (star quarter-miler and competitive participant in marathons) who complained of chest pain after a ski marathon. A stenotic lesion was detected in the left anterior descending coronary, treated by balloon angioplasty and stenting. The patient was thin, normotensive, non-smoker, with a total cholesterol of 160 mg/dl (4.13 mmol/l), low-density lipoprotein-cholesterol (LDL-C) 88 mg/dl (2.27 mmol/l), HDL-C 74 mg/dl (1.91 mmol/l) and triglycerides 62 mg/dl (0.7 mmol/l). He was prescribed aspirin and reduction of competitive exercise. Seven years later he again complained of exertional chest pain compatible with ischemia (confirmed by stress electrocardiogram, upper left panel), he had bilateral carotid bruits associated with markedly increased intima-media thickness (IMT) (bottom left panel). Low LDL, normal triglycerides and high HDL-C was confirmed as seen in the table on the right. Both father and brother of the patient had suffered early coronary events and had high HDL-C levels. Plasma CETP concentrations were low in the proband, 0.67 µg/ml (normal 0.8–2.2 µg/ml), with low normal findings in father and brother. The CETP gene was sequenced. The proband had a homozygous substitution of isoleucine for valine at codon 405 (I405V), was homozygous for a common polymorphism (Int + 29 A>G, RFLP > *Bam*HI; *Bam*HI digestion in intron 9 generates either a 390 bp or a 460 bp fragment, RFLP> *Bam*HI refers to generation of the larger one) and had one B1 allele of the *Taq*IB polymorphism. This familial occurrence of premature CAD in the absence of major CVD risk factors associated with a combination of CETP gene abnormalities and low CETP in subjects with normal plasma LDL and triglycerides but with high plasma HDL-C levels is consistent with other reports that CAD may develop in some cases of isolated hyperalphalipoproteinemia. After treatment with probucol 500 mg twice daily, an antioxidant that increases CETP levels, there was a reduction in HDL (to 32 mg/dl or 0.83 mmol/l), an increase of CETP into the normal range and a reduction of the anginal symptoms and exertional ischemia on electrocardiogram over 3 years. Reproduced from Sirtori CR *et al.* (2006). CETP levels rather than polymorphisms as markers of coronary risk: healthy athlete with high HDL-C and coronary disease – effectiveness of probucol. *Atherosclerosis*, **186**: 225–227.

because a few patients had cytogenetic deletions in chromosome 20p11.23–12.2. Later cases, however, were ascribed to mutations at this locus (20p12) in a gene called *JAG1* (OMIM No. 601920). It encodes a ligand (JAG1 or Jagged-1) in the Notch signalling pathway that interacts with the Notch transmembrane receptor and releases an intracellular form of Notch. This stimulates transcription from downstream promoters of several target genes, such as HES-related repressor proteins (HERP-1, -2 and -3) (HES stands for Hairy and Enhancer of Split from the *Drosophila* nomenclature). *JAG1* is crucial for arterial development and cell fate and differentiation in embryogenesis. It is expressed in the cardiovascular system and is associated with blood vessels in the liver. The frequency is estimated to be 1 in 100 000 to 1 in 70 000 births; it is the second most common cause of infantile intrahepatic cholestasis. Although some mutations are sporadic or perhaps explained by the phenomenon of skipped generation due to incomplete penetrance (15%), it is mostly inherited as an autosomal dominant trait with variable expressivity. It has been surmised that non-genetic factors may account for the wide variability in clinical expression because the same *JAG1* genotype in monozygotic twins has been associated with a discordant phenotype. There are over 230 mutations of *JAG1*, which spans 36 kb and has 26 exons on chromosome 20p12. Nonsense and missense mutations, mutations affecting splicing or resulting in frameshift and premature truncation, as well as large deletions (some encompassing the whole gene), have been identified. The

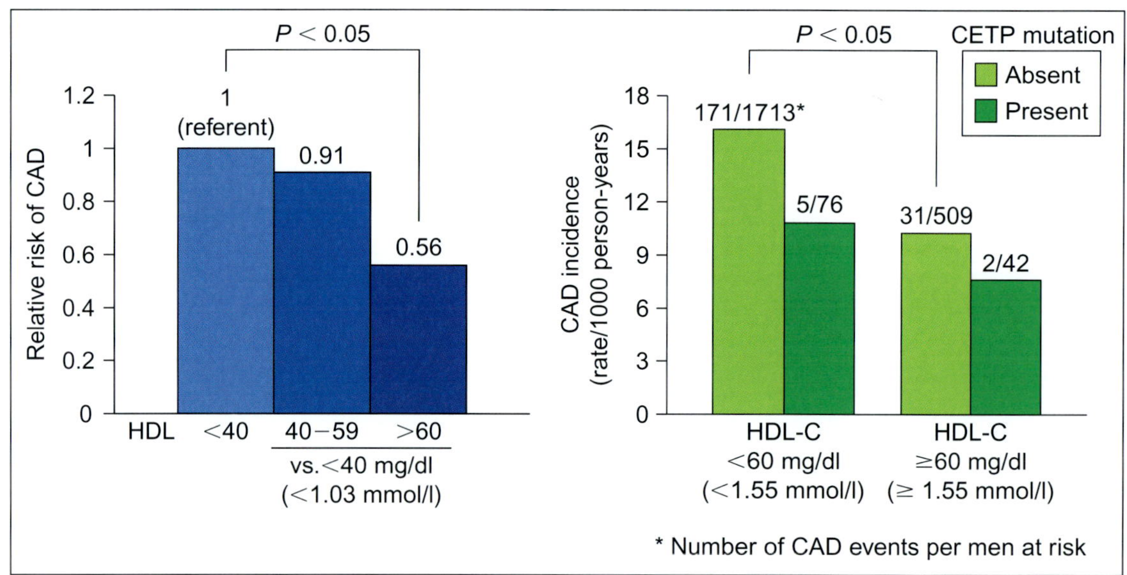

4.37 Cholesteryl ester transfer protein (CETP) mutations may be associated with higher high-density lipoprotein cholesterol (HDL-C) and lower coronary artery disease (CAD) risk. There is an ongoing controversy about whether CETP deficiency and the resultant rise in HDL-C are anti-atherogenic, or whether impaired CETP activity has the opposite effect due to CETP's role in reverse cholesterol transport. This question was investigated in the elderly (71–93 years) participating in a 7-year follow-up of 2340 men in the Honolulu Heart Program. The age-adjusted CAD incidence rates were significantly lower in men with high versus low HDL-C levels. After adjustment for age, hypertension, smoking, and total cholesterol the relative risk of CAD for those with HDL-C levels ≥60 mg/dl, compared with those with HDL-C levels <40 mg/dl, was 0.56 (left panel). Men with a CETP mutation had the lowest rates of CAD, although this was not statistically significant (right panel, age-adjusted incidence). These data indicate that low HDL-C remains an important risk factor for CAD in the elderly. Whether a CETP mutation offers additional protection against CAD warrants further investigation, but there is no indication that it worsens the risk. Redrawn from Curb JD *et al.* (2004). A prospective study of HDL-C and cholesteryl ester transfer protein gene mutations and the risk of coronary heart disease in the elderly. *J Lipid Res*, **45**: 948–954.

Table 4.1 Major presumed and established causes of hyperalphalipoproteinemia

- Dominant familial hyperalphalipoproteinemia (FHAL)
- Recessive or co-dominant FHAL with premature coronary artery disease
- ApoCIII Lys$_{58}$→Glu variant
- Oculocerebrorenal syndrome of Lowe
- Multiple symmetric lipomatosis
- Cholesteryl ester transfer protein (CETP) deficiency
- Hepatic lipase deficiency ± CETP deficiency
- High plasma levels of IgM, high-density lipoprotein (HDL)-albumin complex and high lipoprotein lipase
- Primary biliary cirrhosis, cholestasis
- Chlorinated hydrocarbon pesticide exposure
- Alcohol intoxication – chronic misuse
- Hormone replacement therapy in post-menopausal women
- Drugs: phenytoin, carbamazepine, valproic acid, phenobarbital, CETP inhibitors

majority of mutations, many clustering in exons 2 and 6, lead to complete inactivation of Jagged-1 causing the phenotype. Haplo-insufficiency has been suggested for *JAG1* because a single copy of the normal gene is incapable of providing sufficient protein production to assure normal function (Iso *et al.* [2003]. Not all patients with typical Alagille's syndrome have *JAG1* mutations. Recently, mutations in the receptor for Jagged-1, the NOTCH-2 receptor coded by *NOTCH2* on chromosome 1p12–13, were found to cause Alagille's syndrome; all affected individuals with *NOTCH2* mutations had renal involvement (McDaniell *et al.* [2006]).

AGS is a multi-organ disorder characterized by chronic cholestasis (91%) secondary to paucity of small intrahepatic bile ducts, dysmorphic facies (95%) with a broad forehead, widely spaced deep-set eyes, bulbous nose tip and pointed chin (**4.38**), pulmonary artery hypoplasia or stenosis (systolic murmur) (85%), vertebral anomalies (87%) ('butterfly' vertebrae, synostosis) (**4.39**), congenital heart defect (85%) (tetralogy of Fallot, septal defects, coarctation of the aorta) and eye abnormalities (88%) (posterior embryotoxon – an asymptomatic congenital opacity of the margin of the cornea in the anterior chamber revealed by slit lamp examination – microcornea, optic disc anomalies and others) (**4.40**). Jaundice, pruritus, hypogonadism, failure to thrive and learning disability accompany these manifestations in the typical presentation of infancy (before six months of age). Xanthomatosis may develop because of the presence of marked hypercholesterolemia that appears after the age of 2 (**4.39**). There may be diverse types of xanthomas and they may be widespread (**4.41** and **4.42**). Xanthelasma, eruptive, tuberous, tubero-eruptive, planar and even tendon xanthomas have been reported. When present, xanthomas may be discrete, but massive eruptive and tuberous xanthomas of the palms and soles rarely seen in other lipid disorders, except perhaps in familial dysbetalipoproteinemia, have been reported (**4.43**). They may also be disfiguring and the pruritus may be intractable, leading to auto-mutilation, loss of sleep and even suicide (**4.42**). Emerick and colleagues in 1999 also reported renal disease and strokes in a large series of patients. Associated conditions include mechanical obstruction of the small intestine, tubulo-interstitial nephropathy, exocrine pancreatic insufficiency, pancreas atrophy with diabetes, hepatomas or hepatocarcinomas and coproporphyrin abnormalities with photosensitivity. The

20-year life expectancy is 75%. Therefore, affected patients may be referred to adult lipid clinics. The hypercholesterolemia is in large part explained by the high levels of LpX, an albumin-containing lipoprotein with a unique lipid composition associated with some but not all forms of intrahepatic cholestasis and present in familial lecithin:cholesterol acyl transferase (LCAT) deficiency. LpX is a lamellar lipoprotein composed of phospholipids (66% by weight), free cholesterol (22%), small amounts of proteins (6%), mostly albumin (present in the core) with some apoAI, apoE and apoCs (located on the surface). It is poor in triglycerides (3%) and cholesteryl esters (3%). The commonest factors affecting mortality are congenital heart disease, hepatic cirrhosis, intracranial bleeding and renal disease. The wide range of expression, from normal to a severe lethal phenotype, renders diagnosis difficult especially when the affected subjects reach adulthood. A history of neonatal jaundice, presence of the quasi pathognomonic butterfly vertebrae and typical facies should lead to the diagnosis when coupled with evidence of cholestasis, very high plasma LDL-C (may reach 20 mmol/l or more [>800 mg/dl]) paradoxically associated with relatively low apoB, moderately elevated triglycerides and high HDL-C (HDL-C may be low if bilirubin levels are very high), and the presence of LpX. PFIC should be

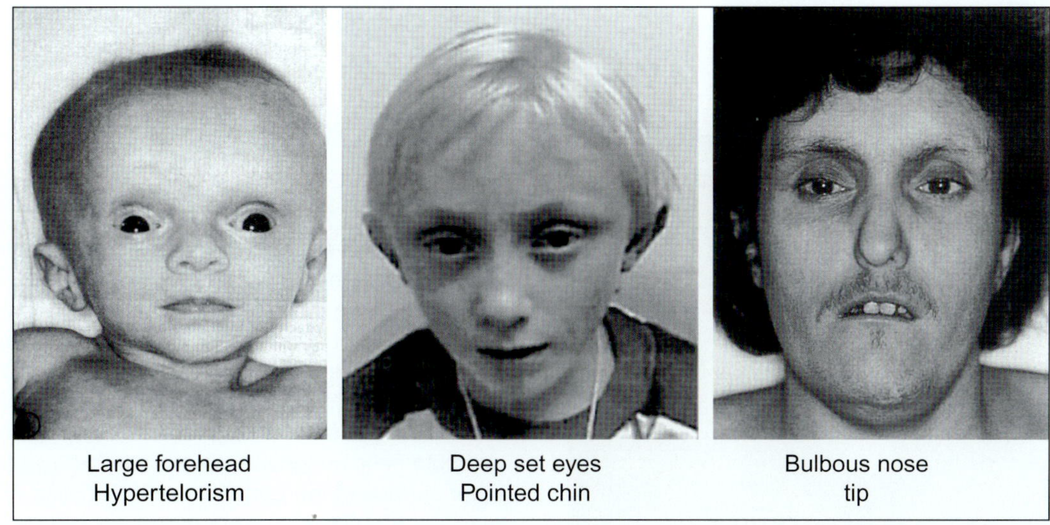

4.38 Facial features in Alagille's syndrome (AGS). Three patients affected with Alagille's syndrome demonstrating the typical facial characteristics of broad forehead, widely spaced deep-set eyes, bulbous nose tip and sharply pointed chin. The left picture is that of an infant among a series of 80 cases of AGS reported in one of the early articles published by Alagille (Alagille D *et al.* [1987]. *J Pediatr*, **110**: 195–200). The central photograph of an 8-year old boy comes from Kamath *et al.* who reviewed the facial dysmorphism of individuals with or without Alagille's syndrome showing that the typical facies could be readily recognized from photographs (79% accuracy) and did not appear to be shared by other disease entities. The identification is more difficult in adult cases; the picture on the right is that of an adult with the features of the syndrome. Reproduced with permission from Braverman IM (1998). Disease of the gastrointestinal tract. In: *Skin Signs of Systemic Disease*, 3rd edn. WB Saunders, Philadelphia, Chapter 12, pp. 405–437.

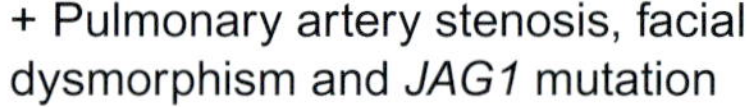

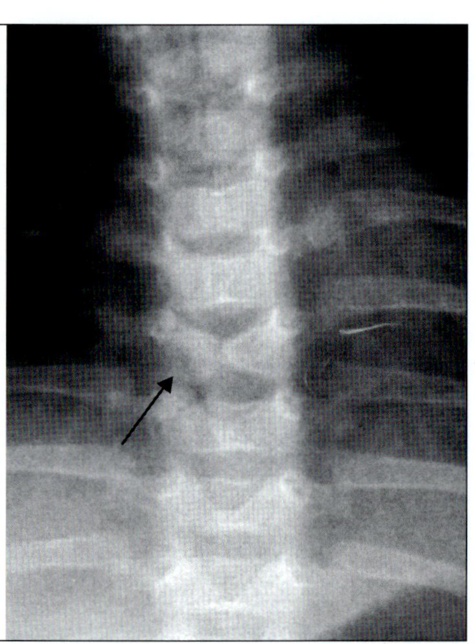

Laboratory results		Normal range	
Total bilirubin	36	3–18	µmol/l
Direct bilirubin	27	0–7	µmol/l
ALT	283	4–30	U/l
γGT	833	4–26	U/l
Alk. phosphatase	770	70–258	U/l
Total cholesterol	13.4	3.6–5.2	mmol/l
Triglycerides	0.7	0.6–1.7	mmol/l
HDL-C	2.2	0.9–2.6	mmol/l
LDL-C	10.9	0.5–3.4	mmol/l
ApoAI	185	107–199	mg/dl
ApoB	64	50–100	mg/dl

+ Pulmonary artery stenosis, facial dysmorphism and *JAG1* mutation

4.39 Biochemistry profile and 'butterfly vertebra' in a 40-month-old child with Alagille's syndrome (AGS). This is the case of a 40-month-old girl with neonatal jaundice and the classical features of AGS including facial dysmorphism, pulmonary artery stenosis, and butterfly vertebrae (right panel). Embryotoxon was not present. In this multi-organ disease, the 'butterfly vertebrae' are observed in 63% of cases. This is secondary to a fusion defect of the central portion of the vertebral body giving a butterfly-looking image on X-ray of the vertebral column (arrow). The X-ray image here is typical of the anterior fusion defect in the seventh thoracic (dorsal) vertebra. The patient was referred to Dr David Mymin's lipid clinic at the University of Manitoba in Winnipeg, Canada. The laboratory profile on the left demonstrates the cholestasis with elevated total and direct bilirubin and alkaline phosphatase, and liver dysfunction with increased levels of alanine aminotransferase and γ-glutamyl transferase. Note the very high level of low-density lipoprotein-cholesterol (LDL-C) at 10.9 mmol/l (421 mg/dl), the relatively high HDL-C at 2.2 mmol/l (85 mg/dl) and apoAI (185 mg/dl) and the low normal triglycerides. Characteristically, in spite of the very high LDL-C, the total plasma apoB is low at 64 mg/dl. This difference is due to the presence of LpX associated with intrahepatic cholestasis (not measured in this case). In 168 of 233 patients reported by Spinner MB *et al.* in 2001 the mutations led to frame-shifts that caused a premature termination codon as in this case. The causal mutation here was $Trp_{876} \rightarrow Ter$. This case report is reproduced courtesy of Dr David Mymin.

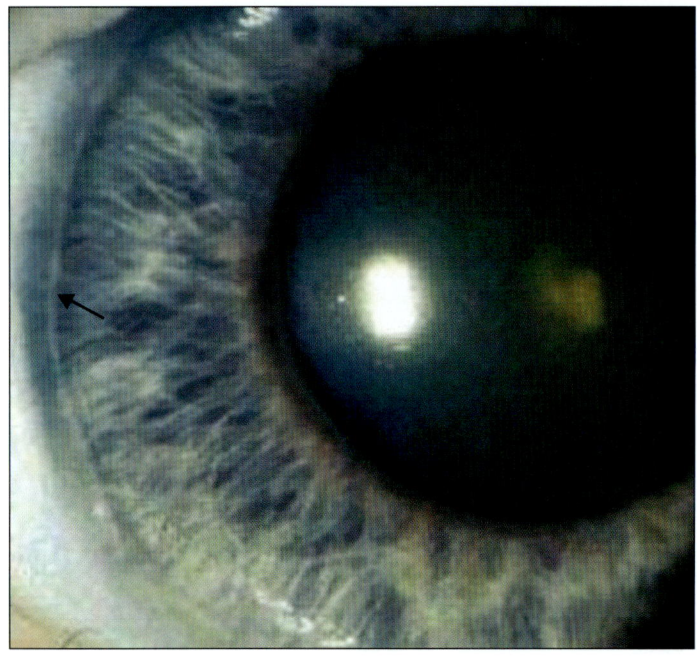

4.40 Posterior embryotoxon in Alagille's syndrome. This close-up view made with a slit lamp illustrates the thickened Schwalbe's ring displaced anteriorly in the back of the cornea and visible through the clear cornea as a sharply defined concentric white line anterior to the limbus at the edge of the sclera constituting the embryotoxon (black arrow). Details of the normal iris are seen through the anterior chamber. These are asymptomatic congenital membrane-like opacifications of the inner surface of the periphery of the cornea. They occur in 95% of cases of AGS along with other eye defects including optic disk anomalies (79%), diffuse fundus hypopigmentation (57%), iris anomalies (45%) and microcornea without apparent serious functional significance. Posterior embryotoxon may be present in approximately 15% of normal eyes. They may be seen with the naked eye on close inspection. This image was downloaded from and reproduced with permission from Welcome to success in MRCOpth (www.mrcophth.com/corneacommoncases/anteriorcleavagesyndrome.html).

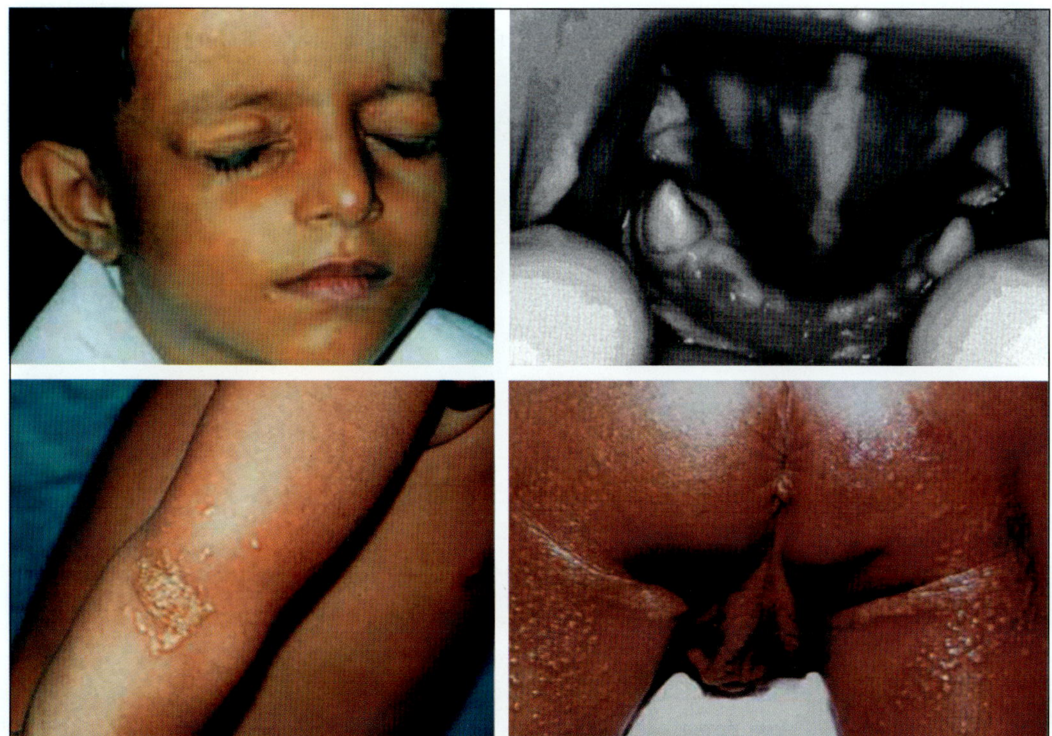

4.41 Xanthomas in Alagille's syndrome (AGS). The top left picture is of a 6-year-old boy from Kolkata, India, presenting a typical case of AGS featuring many of the manifestations of this disease. The case was studied by Sengupta and colleagues ([2005]. *Indian J Dermatol Venereol Leprol,* **71**: 119–121). The boy presented for evaluation of non-itchy lesions over the face, hands and body folds present from the age of 18 months. Examination showed well-defined painless, indurated papules and plaques on the skin over the metacarpophalangeal and interphalangeal joints of the hands, eyelids, and the axillary, antecubital, inguinal and popliteal folds bilaterally. Newer lesions were softer and yellowish in colour but older ones were mostly fibrotic and skin-coloured. His growth was stunted and he had the typical facies of AGS. Progressive jaundice had developed after one month of life. Pruritus was generalized and moderate but resistant to treatment. His serum cholesterol was 413 mg/dl (10.6 mmol/l) and triglycerides 257 mg/dl (2.9 mmol/l). He had anemia, conjugated (direct) hyperbilirubinemia, raised alkaline phosphatase, alanine aminotransferase (ALT) and γ-glutamyl transferase. He had a sub-aortic ventricular septal defect and severe pulmonary stenosis. The liver biopsy showed a paucity of interlobular bile ducts with a ratio of bile duct to portal triad of 0.66 (normal = 0.8). There were no vertebral or ophthalmologic defects.

The top right intraoral photograph from a 3-year-old Asian boy shows a rare form of xanthomas on the palate and the gums associated with hypodontia (only two molars and canines were present), an unusual dysmorphism for AGS. This patient was referred by an oral pathologist in Singapore, Dr Victor Ho, studied at the Medical Genetics Branch of the National Human Genome Research Institute (NHGRI) at the NIH in Bethesda and reported by Ho *et al.* ([2000]. *Am J Med Genet*, **93**: 250–252). The typical facial features including a flat nasal bridge and low-set ears were present. He had multiple bruises, hepatomegaly, widespread eruptive tendon and oral xanthomas as well as xanthelasmas and florid tubero-eruptive xanthomas of the plantar aspect of the feet. Total cholesterol, triglycerides, low-density lipoprotein-cholesterol (LDL-C) and HDL-C were 41.5 mmol/l, 2.86 mmol/l, 39.5 mmol/l, and 0.74 mmol/l, respectively (1604 mg/dl, 253 mg/dl, 1527 mg/dl and 28 mg/dl, respectively). HDL-C may be very low when serum bilirubin is very high, conversely bilirubin levels <100 μmol/l are associated with high HDL-C (Davit-Spraul A *et al.* [1996] *Gastroenterol,* **111**: 1023–1032). Total apoB was 181 mg/dl, a relatively small increase in concentration compared with the marked elevation of LDL-C. In contrast with the previous patient, this one presented butterfly vertebrae and bilateral embryotoxon. In 38 patients between 2 months and 15 years of age studied by Garcia and co-workers in Buenos-Aires, 11 (28%) had xanthomas associated with plasma cholesterol ranging from 220 mg/dl to 1600 mg/dl (5.7–41.4 mmol/l) (Garcia MA *et al.* [2005]. *Pediatr Dermatol,* **22**: 11–14). The xanthomas were present in the nape of the neck, extensor surfaces of the fingers, palmar creases, popliteal fossae, elbows, palms, ear helixes, inguinal area, gluteus, and knees. The confluence of the eruptive xanthomas of the elbow is depicted on the left lower panel. Xanthomas located in the folds had a 'stony' aspect and appeared in crops (right lower panel). Excoriations were often present because of the intense pruritus. Not all patients with hypercholesterolemia had xanthomas. Neonatal cholestasis was present in 92%, 82% developed the typical facies, 76% had growth retardation, 63% displayed the butterfly or hemi-vertebrae in the spine, 58% had heart or vascular anomalies, and 58% had embryotoxon. These cases and that of the previous figure illustrate not only the worldwide distribution of the disease but also the wide variation in clinical expression. The images are reproduced with permission from the respective journals and authors.

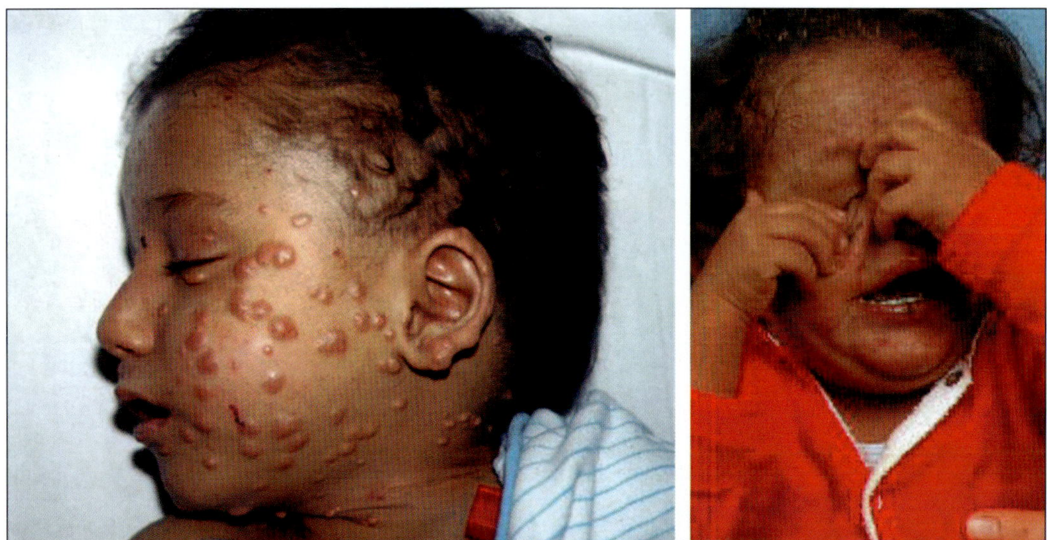

4.42 Disfiguring xanthomas in Alagille's syndrome and severe pruritus (AGS) in progressive familial intrahepatic cholestasis (PFIC). Two story-telling pictures of disease severity in Alagille's syndrome are shown, the presence of disfiguring xanthomas and the severe, sometimes intractable, generalized pruritus associated with the hyperbilirubinemia. Note the lesions on the ear lobe and helix in the left panel. The patient illustrated on the right has progressive familial intrahepatic cholestasis which is also associated with severe pruritus but not with xanthomas. These images were obtained on the web from the *Atlas of Pediatrics*, Catholic University of Louvain (Service de pédiatrie générale, Université Catholique de Louvain, cliniques St Luc. 10 ave. Hippocrate, B-1200 Bruxelles, Belgium).

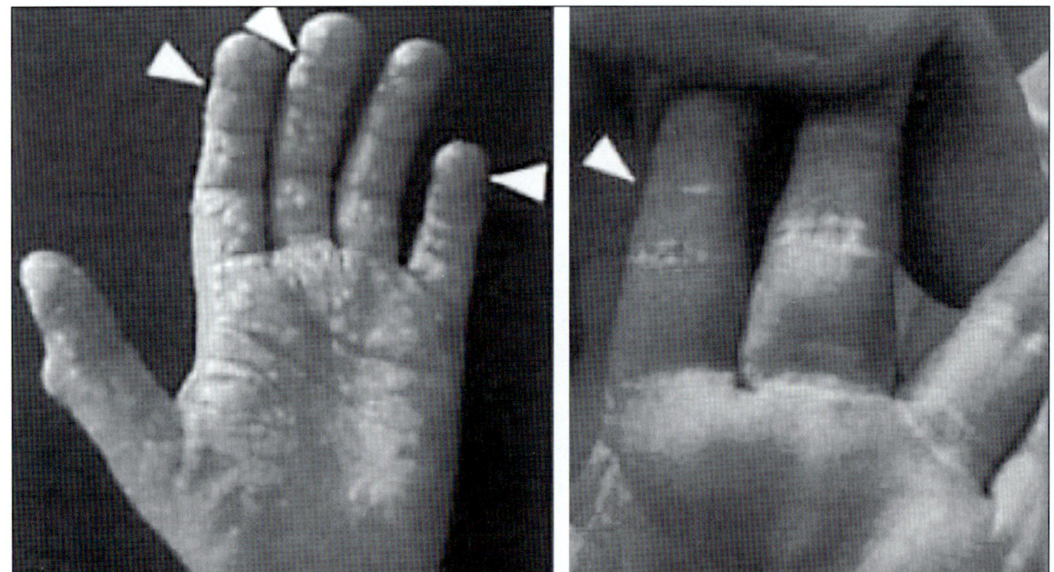

4.43 Palmar and digital xanthomas and supernumerary digital flexion creases in Alagille's syndrome. Extensive xanthomatous involvement of the palms and soles has been reported in AGS but as shown here the presentation is quite unusual (left panel). In addition, as illustrated in the right panel, xanthomas may involve the digital and palmar creases as in familial dysbetalipoproteinemia and primary biliary cirrhosis. Both patients presented supernumerary digital flexion creases (white arrowheads). This is another rare and peculiar sign of the disease that is rare in the general population (frequency varies widely among populations) but has been reported in sickle cell anemia (24–90%) and some rare chromosomal aberrations. In this series of 46 patients, Kamath and colleagues ([2002]. *Am J Med Genet* **112**: 171–175) report this dysmorphism in 35% of cases including a mother and daughter, both affected with AGS. This picture is reproduced with permission.

excluded in the differential diagnosis of intrahepatic cholestasis in childhood but the lipoprotein abnormalities are quite different (**4.44**). Study of the first-degree relatives and a search for a *JAG1* mutation should be undertaken if any doubt subsists to establish a definitive diagnosis. Aggressive screening procedures to detect mutations in *JAG1* or *NOTCH2* have been developed recently by Spinner and colleagues at the University of Pennsylvania to facilitate the molecular diagnosis.

The pruritus and high plasma bilirubin may respond partly to bile acid-binding resins and fat-soluble vitamin supplementation, but the hypercholesterolemia is resistant to medical therapy. Choleretics such as ursodeoxycholic acid and phenobarbital, hydroxyzine, antihistamines, rifampin and ultraviolet light exposure have also been used. Refractory cases may respond to cholecystojejunostomy or partial external biliary diversion. Liver transplantation has been done with success for patients with liver failure and/or severe hypercholesterolemia and xanthomatosis. This has resulted in xanthoma regression, control of pruritus and gradual recovery from growth retardation.

PFIC is a heterogeneous autosomal recessive disorder characterized by a reduced biliary excretion due to defective transport proteins (Nagasaka *et al.* [2005]) that have a role in the regulation of the enterohepatic bile salt pool and in the elimination of hydrophobic substances from the enterohepatic circulation (**4.45**). There are three types of PFIC caused by different gene defects. PFIC-1 or Byler disease was first reported in an Amish kinship in 1969. It is due to complete or near complete absence of the P-type adenosine triphosphatase (ATP8B1) encoded by the *FIC1* gene (also called *ATP8B1*) on chromosome 18q21.

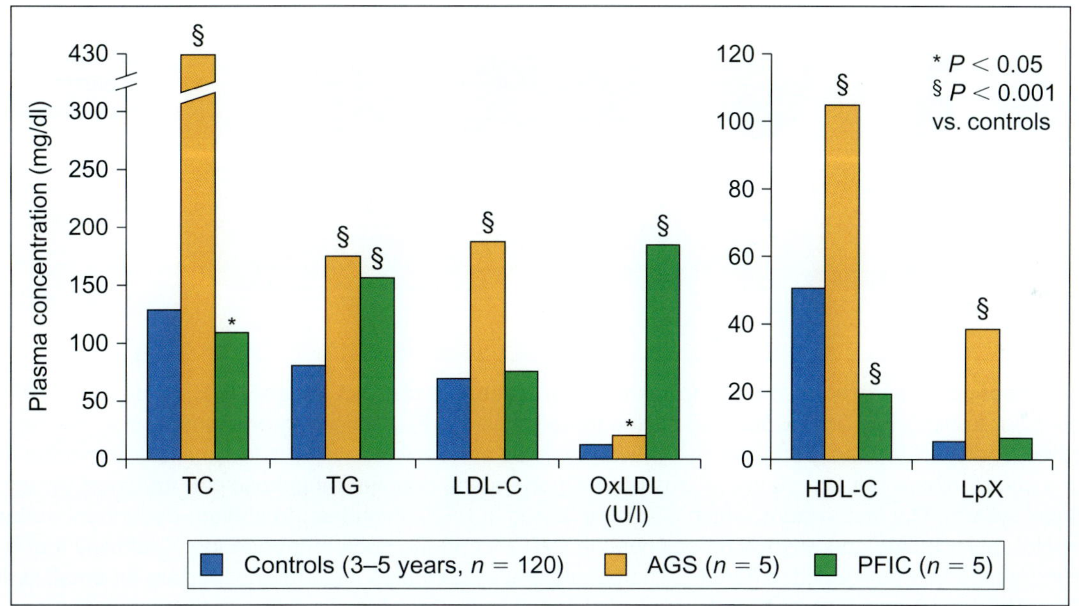

4.44 Lipoprotein abnormalities in Alagille's syndrome (AGS) and in progressive familial intrahepatic cholestasis (PFIC). Five patients with AGS and five with PFIC, 3–4 years of age, were compared with 120 age-matched controls by Nagasaka *et al.* The aim was to determine whether they were at risk of developing atherosclerosis on the basis of their lipoprotein profile, intima-media thickness and wall stiffness of the common carotid artery. Lipoprotein composition and uptake of low-density lipoproteins (LDL) by peripheral mononuclear cells harvested from a single normal volunteer and foam cell formation *ex vivo* were also determined. As shown in this figure, the lipid and lipoprotein profiles are strikingly different between AGS and PFIC. Values are expressed in mg/dl except for oxidized LDL (OxLDL) for which they are given in U/l. In AGS, plasma levels of low-density lipoprotein-cholesterol (LDL-C), HDL-C and lipoprotein X (LpX) were high, and a modest increase in oxidized LDL was observed. In PFIC, LDL-C, and HDL-C were low and LpX was normal but the distinguishing feature was a marked elevation of oxidized LDL, which are notoriously atherogenic. LDL separated by a combination of ultracentrifugation and Sepharose gel filtration from AGS patients induced foam cell formation (5 ± 2%) to the same extent as control native LDL (6 ± 2%). In contrast the foam cell formation ability of PFIC LDL was six times that of normal (36 ± 4%). This effect was not far from that induced by $CuSO_4$-oxidized LDL (52 ± 3%, n = 10). LDL from patients with PFIC were strikingly enriched in triglycerides, whereas the content of cholesteryl ester was strikingly low. Bar graph made from data in Nagasaka H *et al.* (2005). Evaluation of risk for atherosclerosis in Alagille's syndrome and progressive familial intrahepatic cholestasis: Two congenital cholestatic diseases with different lipoprotein metabolisms. *J Pediatr*, **146**: 329–335. The carotid IMT and wall stiffness results are presented in **4.46**.

FIC1 is present in several tissues and has been identified in human liver and small intestine. It is located on the canalicular membrane of the hepatocyte and is responsible for phospholipid translocation (a membrane 'flippase'). FIC1 activates the transcription of the farsenoid X receptor (FXR), an important modifier of bile acid homeostasis genes. Patients have cholestasis, severe pruritus, steatorrhoea, and reduced growth. They have normal γ-glutamyl transferase, high alkaline phosphatase, normal cholesterol, high TG, and also a high concentration of primary bile acids in serum and very low or absent levels of primary bile acids in the bile. The differential diagnosis includes inborn defects of primary bile acid synthesis; these are also associated with low γ-glutamyl transferase and raised primary bile acids but no pruritus. **PFCI-2** with a similar clinical and biochemical picture is caused by mutations of the ATP-binding cassette family B type 11 gene (*ABCB11, or FIC2*) on chromosome 2q24 that encodes the hepatocyte ATP-dependent bile salt

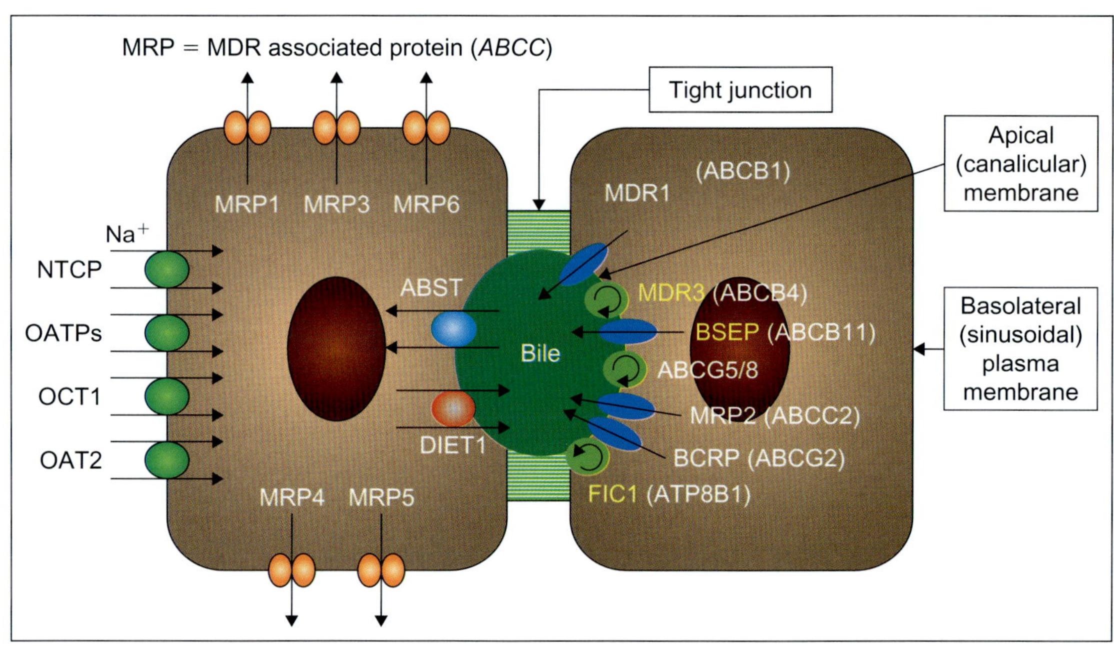

4.45 Hepatocellular transporters, three of them implicated in progressive familial intrahepatic cholestasis (PFIC). Defects in different hepatocellular transporters are responsible for the three forms of PFIC. This diagram summarizes the major transporters responsible for active hepatocellular transport processes. Two liver cells are depicted with a bile canaliculus and the tight junction between them in the centre. There are two main systems of transporters: the basolateral (sinusoidal) transport system and the apical (canalicular) transport system. The first system, which is not implicated in PFIC, includes the sodium-dependent pathway. This is represented by the Na⁺-taurocholate co-transporting polypeptide (NTCP) and the sodium-independent pathway that is represented by the organic anion transporting polypeptides (OATP). The basolateral system also include transporters for small hydrophilic organic compounds (OCT or OAT family) and several ATP-dependent efflux pumps, part of the family of multi-drug resistance associated proteins (MRPs ABCC), which are multi-specific transporters for different organic anions. These are involved in transporting a large variety of albumin-bound amphipathic organic compounds such as conjugated and unconjugated bile salts, neutral steroids, glucuronides as well as thyroid hormones and numerous drugs (antihistamine, opioid peptides, digoxin, pravastatin, etc.). The apical (canalicular) transport system mediates the secretion of bile salts and other bile constituents across the canalicular membrane of hepatocytes by various ATP-binding cassette (ABC) transporters. It is among those that the three defective transporters causing PFIC are included (in yellow letters). These transporters comprise members of the family of multi-drug resistance P-glycoproteins such as MDR1 (ABCB1) and MDR3 (ABCB4) defective in PFIC-3 and the bile salt export pump BSEP (ABCB11) defective in PFIC-2. In addition, the canalicular membrane includes MRP2 (ABCC2) and the ABC half transporters 'breast cancer resistance protein' (BCRP, ABCG2) and the 'cholesterol flippase' ABCG5/G8 (ABCG5, ABCG8) and FIC1 (ATP8B1) defective in PFIC1 or Byler's disease. ABST (SLC10A2) the apical bile salt transporter, works in the other direction and is responsible for bile salt reabsorption; it is suppressed during cholestasis preventing the hepatocyte from further accumulating toxic bile acids when the hepatocellular bile acid concentrations are already too high. It mediates sodium-dependent reabsorption of conjugated bile salts at the apical membranes of intestinal, bile ductular, and renal proximal tubular cells, whereas the sodium taurocholate co-transporting polypeptide NTCP (SLC10A1) is exclusively expressed at the basolateral membrane of hepatocytes. DIET1, a recently described apical transporter, moves bile salt in a direction opposite to that of ABST. Modified with permission from Pauli-Magnus C, Meier PJ (2005). Hepatocellular transporters and cholestasis. *J Clin Gastroenterol*, **39**: S103–S110.

export pump (BSEP). Reduced bile acid secretion and deposition of bile acids leads to hepatocellular damage and progressive liver disease. **PFIC-3** presents later in life and is caused by mutations of the ATP-binding cassette family B type 4 (*ABCB4*) gene on chromosome 7q21.1 coding for hepatocyte MDR3 (multidrug resistance-3 P-glycoprotein) that is responsible for phosphatidylcholine translocation. The MDR3 makes phospholipids available for elution into canalicular bile. Low or absent phospholipids prevents bile micelle formation causing bile duct injury. It is associated with high risk of cirrhosis with portal hypertension, gastro-intestinal bleeding and eventually liver failure. Pruritus is usually mild or may be variable in nature. Serum bile acid levels are elevated but biliary bile acid levels are normal. Portal fibrosis, inflammatory infiltrates and extensive bile ductular proliferation are seen early on liver biopsy. In con-trast with PFIC-1 and PFIC-2, γ-glutamyl transferase levels are elevated in PFIC-3 as is the case in AGS. For all three, mutations include nucleotide deletions, insertions and mis-sense mutations in highly conserved regions of the amino acid sequences. Death may often occur before adulthood at ages ranging between infancy and adolescence, especially in

PFIC-1 and PFIC-2. Affected individuals develop very high serum bile acid levels. All PFIC forms are characterized by paucity of interlobular bile ducts and may be associated with hepatocellular carcinoma. Defects in the causal genes may also cause a milder form called benign recurrent intrahe-patic cholestasis (BRIC). This is characterized by episodic bouts of cholestasis and may lead to intrahepatic cholestasis of pregnancy. PFIC-1 and PFIC-2, but not PFIC-3, are associated with normal levels of γ-glutamyl transferase. In contrast with AGS, PFIC is not associated with any typical facial features.

Nagasaka and co-workers in Chiba, Japan, compared the lipoprotein profiles of children with AGS with those of children with PFIC and determined susceptibility to ath-erosclerosis by measuring the intima-media thickness and wall stiffness of the common carotid artery in 3- and 4-year-old children (**4.46**). The lipid and lipoprotein profiles are strikingly different. In AGS, plasma levels of LDL-C, HDL-C and LpX are high, and there is a modest increase in oxidized LDL. In PFIC, LDL-C and HDL-C levels are low and LpX is normal, but the distinguishing feature is a marked elevation of oxidized LDL, an until recently

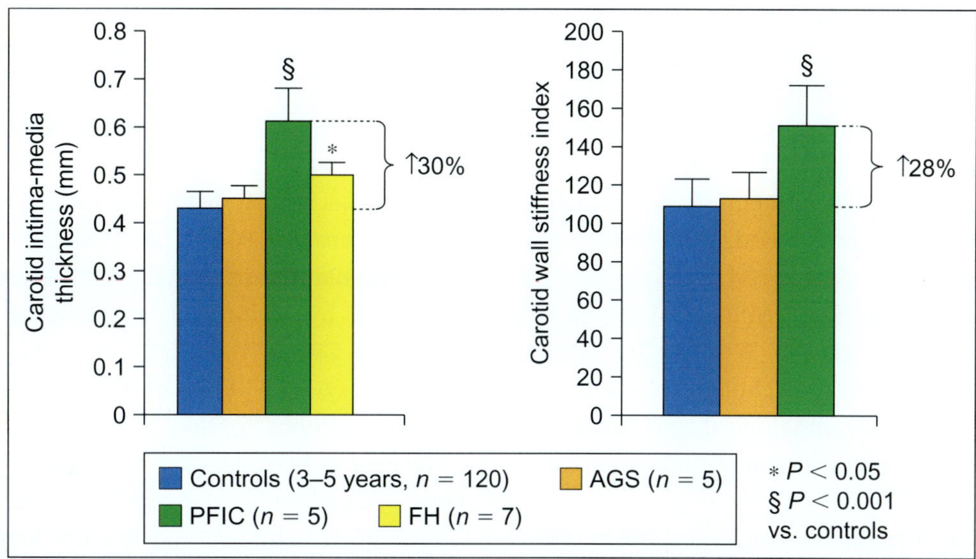

4.46 Surrogate measurements of atherosclerosis in Alagille's syndrome (AGS), progressive familial intrahepatic cholestasis (PFIC) and heterozygous familial hypercholesterolemia (FH). This figure demonstrates that both intima-media thickness (IMT) and wall stiffness of the common carotid artery measured by ultrasonography are significantly increased relative to controls in PFIC but not in AGS. Carotid wall stiffness was calculated by measuring change in lumen diameter during the cardiac cycle. IMT was increased 30% in PFIC and 3% in AGS. This unexpected difference could be accounted for by the differences in lipoprotein profile and composition as well as the propensity of PFIC lipoproteins to promote foam cell formation between the two diseases (see text and **4.44**). Patients affected with heterozygous familial hypercholesterolemia (n = 7, same age group) served as a positive control group with high low-density lipoprotein (LDL) levels and absence of lipoprotein X and hyperbilirubinemia; they had only a modest increase in IMT. Bar graph derived from data in Nagasaka H *et al.* (2005). Evaluation of risk for atherosclerosis in Alagille syndrome and progressive familial intrahepatic cholestasis: Two congenital cholestatic diseases with different lipoprotein metabolisms. *J Pediatr*, **146**: 329–335.

unrecognized manifestation. In this study, intima-media thickness and wall stiffness were increased in patients with PFIC but not in patients with AGS. Increased propensity to atherosclerosis may be ascribed to the high levels of oxidized LDL, low HDL and the fact that triglyceride-enriched LDL from PFIC readily induced foam cell formation *ex vivo*. In contrast, high LpX levels (LpX has antioxidant properties) and relatively low apoB are deemed responsible for the reduced atherosclerosis risk in AGS. The current therapeutic approach for PFIC, as for AGS, is both medical and surgical. Hepatocyte transplantation in two cases was unsuccessful because fibrosis was already present (Dhawan *et al.* [2006]).

Further reading

Familial lipoprotein(a) hyperlipoproteinemia

Berglund L, Ramakrishnan R (2004). Lipoprotein(a). An elusive cardiovascular risk factor. *Arterioscler Thromb Vasc Biol*, **24**: 2219–2226.

Boffa MB, Marcovina SM, Koschinsky ML (2004). Lipoprotein(a) as a risk factor for atherosclerosis and thrombosis: mechanistic insights from animal models. *Clin Biochem*, **37**: 333–343.

Danesh J, Collins R, Peto R (2000). Lipoprotein(a) and coronary heart disease. Meta-analysis of prospective studies. *Circulation*, **102**: 1082–1085.

Deb A, Caplice NM (2004). Lipoprotein(a): new insights into mechanisms of atherogenesis and thrombosis. *Clin Cardiol*, **27**: 258–264.

Edelstein C, Pfaffinger D, Hinman J, Miller E, Lipkind G, Tsimikas S, Bergmark C, Getz GS, Witztum JL, Scanu AM (2003). Lysine-phosphatidylcholine adducts in kringle V impart unique immunological and potential pro-inflammatory properties to human apolipoprotein(a). *J Biol Chem*, **278**: 52841–52847.

Jenner LJ, Seman LJ, Millar JS, Lamon-Fava S, Welty FK, Dolnikowski GG, Marcovina SM, Lichtenstein AH, Barrett PHR, DeLuca C, Schaefer EJ (2005). The metabolism of apolipoproteins (a) and B-100 within plasma lipoprotein (a) in human beings. *Metabolism*, **54**: 361–369.

Koschinsky ML (2005). Lipoprotein(a) and atherosclerosis: new perspectives on the mechanism of action of an enigmatic lipoprotein. *Curr Atheroscler Rep*, **7**: 389–395.

Lackner C, Boerwinkle E, Leffert CC, Rahmig T, Hobbs HH (1991). Molecular basis of apolipoprotein (a) isoform size heterogeneity as revealed by pulsed-field gel electrophoresis. *J Clin Invest*, **87**: 2153–2161.

Luc G, Bard JM, Arveiler D, Ferrieres J, Evans A, Amouyel P, Fruchart JC, Ducimetiere P, Study Group PRIME (2002). Lipoprotein(a) as a predictor of coronary heart disease: the PRIME Study. *Atherosclerosis*, **163**: 377–384.

McLean JW, Tomlinson JE, Kuang WJ, Eaton DL, Chen EY, Fless GM, Scanu AM, Lawn RM (1987). cDNA sequence of human apolipoprotein(a) is homologous to plasminogen. *Nature*, **330**: 132–137.

Naruszewicz M, Selinger E, Davignon J (1992). Oxidative modification of lipoprotein(a) and the effect of β-carotene. *Metabolism*, **41**: 1215–1224.

Seed M, Boerwinkle E, Thompson GR, Utermann G (1990). Lipoprotein(a) and coronary heart disease in patients with familial hypercholesterolemia. Reply. *N Engl J Med*, **323**: 1774.

Sun HJ, Unoki H, Wang XF, Liang JY, Ichikawa T, Arai Y, Shiomi M, Marcovina SM, Watanabe T, Fan JL (2002). Lipoprotein(a) enhances advanced atherosclerosis and vascular calcification in WHHL transgenic rabbits expressing human apolipoprotein(a). *J Biol Chem*, **277**: 47486–47492.

Utermann G (1999). Genetic architecture and evolution of the lipoprotein(a) trait. *Curr Opin Lipidol*, **10**: 133–141.

Familial phytosterolemia (ABCG5-ABCG8 defects)

Berge KE, Tian H, Graf GA, Yu LQ, Grishin NV, Schultz J, Kwiterovich P, Shan B, Barnes R, Hobbs HH (2000). Accumulation of dietary cholesterol in sitosterolemia caused by mutations in adjacent ABC transporters. *Science*, **290**: 1771–1775.

Bhattacharyya AK, Connor WE (1974). Beta-sitosterolemia and xanthomatosis. A newly described lipid storage disease in two sisters. *J Clin Invest*, **53**: 1033–1043.

Graf GA, Cohen JC, Hobbs HH (2004). Missense mutations in ABCG5 and ABCG8 disrupt heterodimerization and trafficking. *J Biol Chem*, **279**: 24881–24888.

Hazard SE, Patel SB (2007). Sterolins ABCG5 and ABCG8: regulators of whole body dietary sterols. *Pflugers Arch*, **453**: 745–752.

Heimerl S, Langmann T, Moehle C, Mauerer R, Dean M, Beil FU, Von Bergmann K, Schmitz G (2002). Mutations in the human ATP-binding cassette transporters ABCG5 and ABCG8 in sitosterolemia. *Hum Mutat*, **20**: 151.

Kwiterovich PO Jr, Bachorik PS, Smith HH, McKusick VA, Connor WE, Teng B, Sniderman AD (1981). Hyperapobetalipoproteinemia in two families with xanthomas and phytosterolemia. *Lancet*, **317**: 466–469.

Sehayek E, Yu HJ, Von Bergmann K, Lujohann D, Stoffel M, Duncan EM, Garcia-Naveda L, Salit J, Blundell ML, Friedman JM, Breslow JL (2004). Phytosterolemia on the island of Kosrae: founder effect for a novel *ABCG8* mutation results in high carrier rate and increased plasma plant sterol levels. *J Lipid Res*, **45**: 1608–1613.

Sudhop T, Lütjohann D, Von Bergmann K (2005). Sterol transporters: targets of natural sterols and new lipid lowering drugs. *Pharmacol Ther*, **105**: 333–341.

Familial hyperalphalipoproteinemia and cholesteryl ester transfer protein deficiency

Asztalos BF, Horvath KV, Kajinami K, Nartsupha C, Cox CE, Batista M, Schaefer EJ, Inazu A, Mabuchi H (2004). Apolipoprotein composition of HDL in cholesteryl ester transfer protein deficiency. *J Lipid Res*, **45**: 448–455.

Barter PJ, Kastelein JJP (2006). Targeting cholesteryl ester transfer protein for the prevention and management of cardiovascular disease. *J Am Coll Cardiol*, **47**: 492–499.

Boekholdt SM, Kuivenhoven JA, Wareham NJ, Peters RJG, Jukema JW, Luben R, Bingham SA, Day NE, Kastelein JJP, Khaw KT (2004). Plasma levels of cholesteryl ester transfer protein and the risk of future coronary artery disease in apparently healthy men and women – The prospective EPIC (European Prospective Investigation into Cancer and Nutrition) – Norfolk population study. *Circulation*, **110**: 1418–1423.

Boekholdt SM, Sacks FM, Jukema JW, Shepherd J, Freeman DJ, McMahon AD, Cambien F, Nicaud V, De Grooth GJ, Talmud PJ, Humphries SE, Miller GJ, Eiriksdottir G, Gudnason V, Kauma H, Kakko S, Savolainen MJ, Arca M, Montali A, Liu S, Lanz HJ, Zwinderman AH, Kuivenhoven JA, Kastelein JJP (2005). Cholesteryl ester transfer protein TaqIB variant, high-density lipoprotein cholesterol levels, cardiovascular risk, and efficacy of pravastatin treatment – Individual patient meta-analysis of 13,677 subjects. *Circulation*, **111**: 278–287.

Busetto L, Strater D, Enzi G, Coin A, Sergi G, Inelmen EM, Pigozzo S (2003). Differential clinical expression of multiple symmetric lipomatosis in men and women. *Int J Obes Relat Metab Disord*, **27**: 1419–1422.

Canizales-Quinteros S, Aguilar-Salinas CA, Reyes-Rodríguez E, Riba L, Rodríguez-Torres M, Ramírez-Jiménez S, Huertas-Vázquez A, Fragoso-Ontiveros V, Zentella-Dehesa A, Ventura-Gallegos JL, Vega-Hernández G, López-Estrada A, Aurón-Gómez M, Gomez-Perez F, Rull J, Cox NJ, Bell GI, Tusié-Luna MT (2003). Locus on chromosome 6p linked to elevated HDL choesterol serum levels and to protection against premature atherosclerosis in a kindred with familial hypercholesterolemia. *Circ Res*, **92**: 569–576.

Carlson LA, Kolomodin-Hedman B (1972). Hyperalphalipoproteinemia in men exposed to chlorinated hydrocarbon pesticides. *Acta Med Scand*, **192**: 29.

Charnas LR, Gahl WA (1991). The oculocerebrorenal syndrome of Lowe. *Adv Pediatr*, **38**: 75–107.

De Grooth GJ, Klerkx AHEM, Stroes ESG, Stalenhoef AFH, Kastelein JJP, Kuivenhoven JA (2004). A review of CETP and its relation to atherosclerosis. *J Lipid Res*, **45**: 1967–1974.

Demacker PNM, Jansen RTP, Hijmans AGM, Van Gorp HPWM (1994). A case of hyperalphalipoproteinemia associated with albumin complexing. *Atherosclerosis*, **111**: 13–23.

Fumeron F, Betoulle D, Luc G, Behague I, Ricard B, Poirier O, Jemaa R, Evans A, Arveiler D, Marques-Vidal P, Bard JM, Fruchart JC, Ducimetiere P, Apfelbaum M, Cambien F (1995). Alcohol intake modulates the effect of a polymorphism of the cholesteryl ester transfer protein gene on plasma high density lipoprotein and the risk of myocardial infarction. *J Clin Invest*, **96**: 1664–1671.

Glueck CJ, Fallat RW, Millett F, Steiner PM (1975). Familial hyperalphalipoproteinemia. *Arch Intern Med*, **135**: 1025–1028.

Hirano K, Yamashita S, Kuga Y, Sakai N, Nozaki S, Kihara S, Arai T, Yanagi K, Takami S, Menju M, Ishigami M, Yoshida Y, Kameda-Takemura K, Hayashi K, Matsuzawa Y (1995). Atherosclerotic disease in marked hyperalphalipoproteinemia – Combined reduction of cholesteryl ester transfer protein and hepatic triglyceride lipase. *Arterioscler Thromb Vasc Biol*, **15**: 1849–1856.

Morrison JA, Khoury P Laskarzewski P, Gartside P, Moore M, Heiss G, Glueck CJ (1980). Hyperalphalipoproteinemia in hypercholesterolemic adults and children. *Trans Assoc Am Physicians*, **93**: 230–243.

Kronenberg F, Coon H, Ellison RC, Borecki I, Arnett DK, Province MA, Eckfeldt JH, Hopkins PN, Hunt SC (2002). Segregation analysis of HDL cholesterol in the

NHLBI Family Heart Study and in Utah pedigrees. *Eur J Hum Genet*, **10**: 367–374.

Pirro M, Siepi D, Lupattelli G, Roscini AR, Schillaci G, Gemelli F, Vaudo G, Marchesi S, Pasqualini L, Mannarino E (2003). Plasma C-reactive protein in subjects with hypo/hyperalphalipoproteinemias. *Metabolism*, **52**: 432–436.

Rotsztain A (1978). Risk factors and HDL. *Circulation*, **57**: 1032.

Teh EM, Dolphin PJ, Breckenridge WC, Tan MH (1998). Human plasma CETP deficiency: identification of a novel mutation in exon 9 of the CETP gene in a Caucasian subject from North America. *J Lipid Res*, **39**: 442–456.

Vaughan AM, Oram JF (2005). ABCG1 redistributes cell cholesterol to domains removable by high density lipoprotein but not by lipid-depleted apolipoproteins. *J Biol Chem*, **280**: 30150–30157.

Von Eckardstein A, Holz H, Sandkamp M, Weng W, Funke H, Assmann G (1991). Apolipoprotein C-III(Lys$_{58}$→Glu). Identification of an apolipoprotein C-III variant in a family with hyperalphalipoproteinemia. *J Clin Invest*, **87**: 1724–1731.

Yamashita S, Maruyama T, Hirano K, Sakai N, Nakajima N, Matsuzawa Y (2000). Molecular mechanisms, lipoprotein abnormalities and atherogenicity of hyperalphalipoproteinemia. *Atherosclerosis*, **152**: 271–285.

Alagille's syndrome and progressive familial intrahepatic cholestasis

Alagille D, Estrada A, Hadchouel M, Gautier M, Odievre M, Dommergues JP (1987). Syndromic paucity of interlobular bile ducts (Alagille syndrome or arteriohepatic dysplasia): review of 80 cases. *J Pediatr*, **110**: 195–200.

Dhawan A, Mitry RR, Hughes RD (2006). Hepatocyte transplantation for liver-based metabolic disorders, *J Inherit Metab Dis*, **29**: 431–435.

Harris MJ, Le Couteur DG, Arias IM (2005). Progressive familial intrahepatic cholestasis: genetic disorders of biliary transporters. *J Gastroenterol Hepatol*, **20**: 807–817.

Iso T, Hamamori Y, Kedes L (2003). Notch signaling in vascular development. *Arterioscler Thromb Vasc Biol*, **23**: 543–553.

McDaniell R, Warthen DM, Sanchez-Lara PA, Pai A, Krantz ID, Piccoli DA, Spinner NB (2006). NOTCH2 mutations cause Alagille syndrome, a heterogeneous disorder of the notch signaling pathway. *Am J Hum Genet*, **79**: 169–173.

Nagasaka H, Yorifuji T, Egawa H, Yanai H, Fujisawa T, Kosugiyama K, Matsui A, Hasegawa M, Okada T, Takayanagi M, Chiba H, Kobayashi K (2005). Evaluation of risk for atherosclerosis in Alagille syndrome and progressive familial intrahepatic cholestasis: two congenital cholestatic diseases with different lipoprotein metabolisms. *J Pediatr*, **146**: 329–335.

Pauli-Magnus C, Meier PJ (2005). Hepatocellular transporters and cholestasis. *J Clin Gastroenterol*, **39**: S103–S110.

Sengupta S, Das JK, Gangopadhyay A (2005). Alagille syndrome with prominent skin manifestations. *Indian J Dermatol Venereol Leprol*, **71**: 119–121.

van Mil SWC, Houwen RH, Klomp LW (2005). Genetics of familial intrahepatic cholestasis syndromes. *J Med Genet*, **42**: 449–463.

Warthen DM, Moore EC, Kamath BM, Morrissette JJ, Sanchez P, Piccoli DA, Krantz ID, Spinner NB (2006). Jagged1 (JAG1) mutations in Alagille syndrome: increasing the mutation detection rate. *Hum Mutat*, **27**: 436–443.

Conclusion

The authors hope that this *Atlas* has pointed out the importance of recognizing clues, even the most discrete ones, which may reveal the presence of dyslipoproteinemias. One may make a presumptive diagnosis of familial hypercholesterolemia (FH) on spotting extensor tendon xanthomas in the bus or when shaking hands. Some of these clues may be pathognomonic, such as the orange palmar creases of familial dysbetalipoproteinemia, a faint discoloration often missed by the inattentive physician. Hopefully, it has become obvious from reading this text that the family history is essential to establish the hereditary nature and the mode of transmission of the disease. Examination of first-degree relatives can be very helpful, especially when trying to sort out the difference between familial combined hyperlipidemia and familial endogenous hypertriglyceridemia or when assessing the impact on cardiovascular risk. It should be clear that a phenotype is not synonymous with a disease, as several diseases may share the same or a very similar phenotype as is the case for the FH phenotype (LDLR, apoB-100, PCSK9, ARH gene defects).

The practitioner who can identify a rare disease from among the many common entities encountered in daily practice has an edge. Using key images, this *Atlas* endeavours to alert physicians to the existence of such rarities and to provide a rapid means of securing the diagnosis and understanding the underlying metabolic defect. Alagille's syndrome, homozygous familial hypercholesterolemia, familial dysbetalipoproteinemia, multiple symmetric lipomatosis and Wolman's disease are all cases in point; a picture is worth a thousand words. It is hoped that the book has also helped the reader to understand some discordance in the literature attributable to variations in nomenclature, for instance, the different numbering of amino acids for hepatic lipase used in the sequence of Cai *et al.* (1989) and that of Ameis *et al.* (1990). A ready reference to websites has been provided for those looking for more information, such as the OMIM number or a website address for those not familiar with the letters used for amino acid nomenclature (http://www.chem.qmul.ac.uk/iupac/AminoAcid/AA1n2.html #AA1).

This is a tool that the authors hope will be useful in daily practice and will serve as a reference text for interested physicians and scientists.

Index